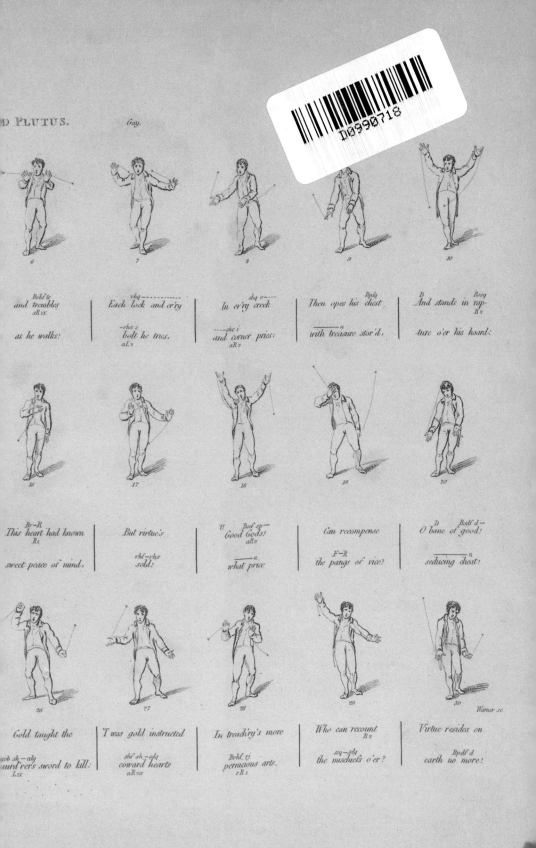

D PLUTUS.   Gay.

6   7   8   9   10

Beh'd te
and trembles
sR ix
as he walks!

vhq - - - - - - - - - - -
Each lock and cv'ry
-vhx c
bolt he tries,
aR 2

chq o - - -
In ev'ry creek
- - - - she i
and corner pries:
aR 2

Bpdq
Then opes his chest,
- - - - - - n
with treasure stor'd,

D   Bseq
And stands in rap-
R 2
ture o'er his hoard:

16   17   18   19   20

By - R
This heart had known
R i
sweet peace of mind,

But virtue's
vhf - vhx
sold!

U   Bcef sp -
Good Gods!
ait e
- - - - a
what price

Can recompense
F - R
the pangs of vice?

D   Bsdf d -
O bane of good!
- - - - - - n
seducing cheat!

26   27   28   29   50   Warner sc.

Gold taught the
cb ch - aq
urd'rer's sword to kill:
Lix

T was gold instructed
shf sh - aq
coward hearts
aR 2x

In treach'ry's more
Bvhf, rj
pernicious arts.
r R i

Who can recount
R 2
the muschet's o'er?

Virtue resides on
Bpdf d
earth no more!

I SEE A VOICE

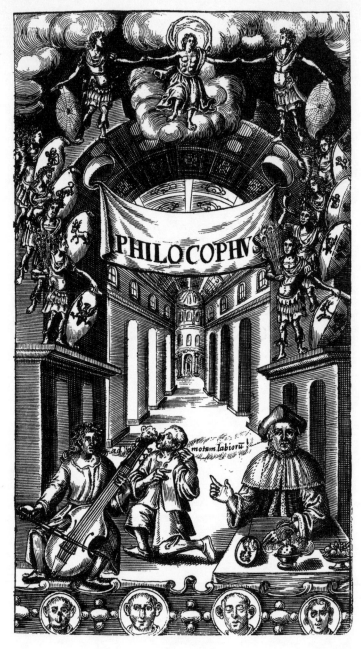

FRONTISPIECE: The correspondence of the five senses as seen by
John Bulwer (1648)

I SEE A VOICE

*A Philosophical History
of Language, Deafness
and the Senses*

JONATHAN RÉE

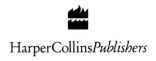

HarperCollins*Publishers*

Endpapers: 'The Miser and Plutus' on
chironomical principles
(cf. pp. 294–6), from Gilbert Austin,
Chironomia; or a Treatise on Rhetorical Delivery,
London 1806, by permission of the Bodleian Library,
University of Oxford.

HarperCollins*Publishers*
77–85 Fulham Palace Road,
Hammersmith, London W6 8JB

Published by HarperCollins*Publishers* 1999
1 3 5 7 9 8 6 4 2

A catalogue record for this book is
available from the British Library

ISBN 0 00 255793 2

Set in Postscript Linotype Galliard by
Rowland Phototypesetting Ltd,
Bury St Edmunds, Suffolk

Printed and bound in Great Britain by
Caledonian International Book Manufacturing Ltd, Glasgow

I see a voice; now will I to the chink,
To spy an I can hear my Thisbe's face.

SHAKESPEARE,
A Midsummer Night's Dream
V.i.190–1

CONTENTS

ILLUSTRATIONS

FRONTISPIECE: The correspondence of the five senses (cf. p. 123), from John Bulwer, *Philocophus: or the Deafe and Dumbe Man's Tutor*, London, 1648, (Art. 8° B 11, frontispiece), by permission of the Bodleian Library, University of Oxford.

CHAPTER EMBLEMS: Chapters 1–24, Artificial manual signs in John Bulwer's chirograms, as Figure 6; Chapters 25–30, Natural manual signs in John Bulwer's chirograms, as Figure 7, by permission of the Bodleian Library, University of Oxford.

A history of metaphysics (p. 13): from 'The Miser and Plutus' by Gilbert Austin (as Endpapers), by permission of the Bodleian Library, University of Oxford.

FIGURE 1 (p. 77): The letter ALEPH, from Franciscus Mercurius van Helmont, *Een zeer Korte Afbeedling van het Ware Natuurlyke Hebreuwse A.B.C.*, Amsterdam 1697, (Opp Adds 8° I 424, plate 1), by permission of the British Library.

FIGURE 2 (p. 79): Helmont in prison, from Franciscus Mercurius van Helmont, *Alphabeti vere Naturalis Hebraici brevissima delineatio*, Saltzbach 1667, (621 A 15, frontispiece), by permission of the British Library.

A history of science (p. 83): from 'The Miser and Plutus' by Gilbert Austin (see endpapers), by permission of the Bodleian Library, University of Oxford.

FIGURE 3 (p. 102): The letter A, from Juan Pablo Bonet, *Reducción de las Letras, y arte para enseñar à ablar los mudos*, Madrid, 1620, (71 A 18, frontispiece), by permission of the British Library.

FIGURE 4 (p. 103): R, S and T, from Juan Pablo Bonet, *Reducción de las Letras, y arte para enseñar à ablar los mudos*, Madrid, 1620, (71 A 18, frontispiece), by permission of the British Library.

FIGURE 5 (p. 106): Dalgarno's Dactylological Glove, from George

London, 1668, (A 9 310, p. 378), by permission of the Bodleian Library, University of Oxford.

Introduction

There is nothing more personal than a voice. Shyness about using your voice in public – speaking out, screaming, singing, even just saying your own name – is probably the most elementary form of self-consciousness. If we need to attract a stranger's attention, most of us prefer ringing a bell or sounding a horn, or coughing, knocking, or clapping, rather than piping up with our own voices: it may not be so convenient, but it is certainly less embarrassing.

It is as if your voice were as private and vulnerable as your defenceless naked body. In fact the voice can be so reticent that it will seem to hide itself even from its owner, and discovering a voice of your own is sometimes said to be the task of a lifetime. Singers and actors are constantly trying to find their voice; and silent solitary writers, anxious to hit their stride in poetry or prose, also like to picture themselves as seeking for a voice. Given all this self-concealing intimacy, it may seem quite surprising that we are ever willing to speak openly at all – that we feel so little shame about letting off sounds from a hole in the middle of our faces, and doing it in public too: displaying the inner secrets of our vocal parts to the prurient curiosity of all who have ears to hear.

But voices are also destined for other people: you speak, primarily, in order to be heard. And the idea of being heard, of possessing a voice or having it neglected or denied, of seeking, vindicating, giving or offering a voice – the voice of the people, the voice of God – nearly coincides with that of human and civil rights. Having a voice is much the same as having a vote, it seems (some languages use the same word for both).[1] Voices could almost be seen as part of the constitution of

---

1 The fortuitous similarity between *vox* and *votum* no doubt helped naturalize the connection in Latin; but even without such encourgagement the German *Stimme* covers both meanings.

1

representative government, or even the meaning of politics itself.

On the other hand, a voice is never a voice in general: it is always a voice of a particular kind. According to Jaques's disquisition in *As You Like It*, each of the stages of a man's life has its vocal peculiarity: to begin with, there is the infant, mewling and puking in its nurse's arms, and soon to turn into a whining schoolboy; then a lover, sighing like furnace; a soldier, full of strange oaths; a justice, dispensing wise saws; and lastly, before the onset of oblivion, his voice will whistle and pipe again, reverting to its childish treble.[2] It would be a different story, of course, if Jaques were describing the career of a female voice; and apart from gender and age, voices also vary with region, class, and sexual and cultural allegiance, not to mention fluctuations in your situation, your temperament and the tone of your feelings.[3]

Distinctive vocal styles can identify people as sharply as their bodies or their faces. A voice, with its own particular texture, pitch and volume, its tunes, rhythms and dynamics, can be the most immediate and poignant object of tenderness, recognition or regret – as in *King Lear*, for instance, when Gloucester suddenly catches the 'trick' of his poor king's voice.[4] Or the moment when Proust's Marcel realized, thinking back, how the girls in the little gang put whole 'philosophies of life' into their artless intonations; how their voices had more sounds in them than the finest musical instruments; and how they left him with the impression of unfathomable depths of hopeless, giddying kisses.[5] The 'loved, idealized voices of those who have died, or of those lost for us like the dead', as Cavafy has it, are surely the most sensitive trigger and the most natural material for sentiment, grief, and nostalgia.[6]

It may even be that where grey-faced philosophers have talked pallidly about 'spirituality', 'identity', 'conscience', 'mentality', 'interiority' or

---

2 William Shakespeare, *As You Like It*, II. vii. 143–63.
3 Cf. the connection between *Stimme* (voice) and *Stimmung* (mood) in German.
4 'The trick of that voice I do well remember:/Is't not the King?' See Shakespeare, *King Lear*, IV. vi. 109–10.
5 Marcel Proust, *A l'ombre des jeunes filles en fleurs* (1918), *A la recherche du temps perdu*, Paris, Pléiade, 1954, Vol. 1, pp. 909, 918; *Within a Budding Grove, Remembrance of Things Past*, translated by C. K. Scott Moncrieff and Terence Kilmartin, London, Chatto and Windus, 1981, Vol. I, pp. 969–70, 980.
6 C. P. Cavafy, *Collected Poems*, translated by Edmund Keeley and Philip Sherrard, London, Chatto and Windus, 1990, p. 15.

'subjectivity', they have really been referring, in their evasive and Latinate way, to the vibrant principle of the living voice itself. Perhaps the idea of the soul is just a furtive and inhibited metaphor for normal healthy vocality. The theme of the voice has certainly proved irresistible for thinkers who are not too particular about correctness and logical propriety: metaphysicians, occultists, and other bold practitioners of intellectual exoticism and self-indulgence. The seventeenth-century genius Francis Mercury van Helmont, for instance, was convinced that the voice is an expression of male sexual strength: if a man's reproductive potency was not squandered elsewhere, it could be sublimely recycled and transferred to his voice, so that he would be able to populate the world with articulate sounds – spoken words, his own 'off-spring and children, viz., his outflown spirits and Angels'.[7] For, as one of Helmont's disciples expressed it, 'nothing emanates from us which bears a more vivid character of life than the Voice . . . the *breath or Spirit of life* resides in the voice, transmitting its light through it.'[8]

Such notions are amongst the most robust commonplaces of popular belief and common sense, or what might be called folk metaphysics. The idea of magic is inseparable from invocations, mantras and prayers, after all; and disciplined critical knowledge defines itself, in contrast, by its imperviousness to vocal fetishism. It is a point of scientific honour to be unimpressed by fine-sounding words: science prides itself on knowing how to abstract from them, how to sift facts and concepts from the vocal noises by which they happen to be conveyed. It sees itself as essentially the opposite of the chanting of spells, the singing of charms, the swearing of oaths, and all kinds of abracadabra, mumbo-jumbo and verbal hocus-pocus. The attribution of special powers to words, Freud thought, is the defining mark of all kinds of pre-scientific superstition, from primitive animism, through religion and theology, all the way up to the tedious meanderings of (he said) modern philosophy.[9]

In the twentieth century, meditations on the voice were hitched to another popular theme: the fate of 'modernity' or 'the Western world',

7 Francis Mercury van Helmont, *The Paradoxical Discourses Concerning the Macrocosm and Microcosm, set down in writing by J. B.*, London, 1685, Part Two, p. 63.
8 Johann Conrad Amman, *Dissertatio de Loquela*, Amsterdam 1700, p. 8; translated by Charles Baker, *Dissertation on Speech*, London, 1873, p. 8.
9 Sigmund Freud, 'The Question of a Weltanschauung', *New Introductory Lectures* (1933), translated by James Strachey, *Standard Edition of the Complete Psychological Works of Sigmund Freud*, Vol. XXII, London, Hogarth Press, 1964, pp. 165–6.

and its relation to art, science and bodily experience. Oswald Spengler spent the period following the First World War announcing a cata-strophic 'decline of the West', and tracing the tragedy to the historic triumph, thousands of years before, of vision and the eye over hearing and the ear. Old-style auditory creatures were essentially gentle and complacent herbivores, Spengler argued: responsive, obedient, and sweetly at one with their existence. We ocular moderns, by contrast, are aggressive predators: through vision we distance ourselves from our environment, and treat it as an intrinsically meaningless collection of hostile objects, targets and victims – in short, a battlefield.

> The act of fixation by two eyes . . . is equivalent to the birth of the *world*, in the sense that Man possesses a world – that is, as a picture, as a world before the eyes, as a world . . . of perspective distance, of space and motions in space . . . This way of seeing . . . implies in itself the notion of *domination*. The world-picture is the environment insofar as it is *dominated* by the eyes . . . The *world* is the prey, and in the last analysis human culture itself has arisen from this fact.[10]

The 'thought of the eye', as Spengler called it, gave birth to a proud, solitary and resolute subjectivity, cynically surveying the abstract light-world that surrounds it. The optical soul was the master of mechanical invention, but too fascinated by 'static, optical details' to have any sense of the tragedy and mystery of 'life'. Vision had cut us off from the ancient wisdom of ordinary pre-theoretical mutuality, annihilating the 'inward kinship of I and Thou'. Now that modern civilization was confronting its ultimate crisis – a crisis of its own making, a crisis of technology – it was stumbling uncomprehendingly towards catas-trophe: twentieth-century humanity, Spengler thought, having lost its voice and its sense of hearing, was destined to 'go downhill *seeing*'.[11]

After Spengler, theoretical anxieties about the voice grew to a point where one might talk of a stand-off between its friends and its enemies. The friends of the voice understood it as a token and symbol of the warm human togetherness which optical modernity was threatening

---

10 Oswald Spengler, *Der Mensch und die Technik: Beitrag zu einer Philosophie des Lebens*, Munich, Beck, 1931, pp. 19–20; translated by C. F. Atkinson as *Man and Technics*, London, George Allen and Unwin, 1932, pp. 24–5 (translation modified).
11 *Der Mensch und die Technik*, pp. 30, 15, 12; *Man and Technics*, pp. 39, 20, 14.

to repress and destroy,[12] whilst the enemies saw it as embodying the lures of a deluded and suffocating humanism. The friends perhaps took their cue from Heidegger, with his doleful ruminations about the destiny of western thought, and how, at the time of Socrates, it had pinned all its hopes on 'theories' and 'ideas', thus tacitly promoting the cold unfeeling procedures of vision at the expense of the more personal and kindly practices of hearing, listening and speech.[13] Or, pursuing another theme in Heidegger, they might identify visualism with the mathematical style of reasoning with which Descartes had inaugurated modern philosophy nearly two thousand years later. Through Descartes's efforts, experience had supposedly been uprooted from the real world: apprehensions got flattened into representations, human existence was reduced to private subjectivity, and time became trivialized into mere novelty: 'the fact that the world becomes picture,' as Heidegger put it, 'is what distinguishes the essence of the modern age.'[14]

The enemies of the voice – notably the French structuralists of the 1960s – were sickened by these nostalgic pieties about life, inwardness and pre-modern communality, and therefore called for a revolt against what Julia Kristeva called 'the phonetic consciousness'. Literature, or written language in general, was not the companion of speech, but its opponent, because it belonged to the open world of light, space and the eye, not the closed world of sound, time and the ear. We needed to break out of the ancient prison-house of speech and one-dimensional temporality, and disport ourselves in the multi-dimensional spaces of writing or 'textual productivity' instead.[15] As Roland Barthes put it in

12 See Walter J. Ong, *Orality and Literacy: The Technologising of the Word*, London, Methuen, 1982, and Gemma Corradi Fiumara, *The Other Side of Language: a Philosophy of Listening and Hearing* (1985), translated by Charles Lambert, London, Routledge, 1990.
13 Martin Heidegger, *Being and Time* (1927), translated by John Macquarrie and Edward Robinson, Oxford, Blackwell, 1962. The 'remarkable priority of "seeing"' is discussed at §36, p. 215, and §31, p. 187; and the value of 'hearing the voice' at §34, p. 206.
14 Martin Heidegger, 'Die Zeit des Weltbildes' (1939), in *Holzwege*, Frankfurt, Klostermann, 1950, pp. 69–104, p. 83; translated by William Lovitt as 'The Age of the World Picture', in *The Question concerning Technology and other Essays*, New York, Harper and Row, 1977, pp. 115–54, p. 130.
15 See Julia Kristeva, 'The bounded text' (1966–7), first published in *Semiotiké*, Paris, 1969, and translated in *Desire in Language: A Semiotic Approach to Literature and Art*, edited by Leon S. Roudiez, New York, Columbia University Press, 1980, pp. 58–9. Derrida's investigations of the same themes (in *La Voix et le Phénomène*, Paris, Presses Universitaires de France, 1967, and *De la grammatologie*, Paris, Minuit, 1967) are far more circumspect, as are Kristeva's of a later date.

1968, 'modern society . . . believes itself to be ushering in a civilization of the image, but what it actually establishes is a civilization of speech.' The crisis of modern times, he concluded, was a crisis of the voice: 'the voice', according to Barthes, 'is what is really at stake in modernity.'[16]

By the end of this book it will have become clear, I hope, that these quarrels between the friends and enemies of the voice are actually rather inane: that they have been generated not by a definite set of solid problems, but by a congeries of shadowy metaphysical prejudices. There are, as we shall discover, four such delusions in particular, implicitly shared by both parties to the dispute: first, that the voice is intrinsically connected with the existence of a self-identical soul, spirit, or inward subjectivity; second, that experience must ultimately be analysed into the contributions made by the various bodily senses; third, that hearing is specifically concerned with time, and vision with space; and fourth, that language has two fundamentally different forms: audible speech which occupies time but not space, and visible writing which occupies space but not time.

But even if all these notions can be shown to be misconceived, that would not mean they can be corrected and then shrugged off and forgotten, like miscalculations in a column of figures. For if the trustworthy edifices of scientific knowledge arise from our experience, so too do the treacherous mirages of metaphysics. We may keep dismissing them from our minds, but that will not stop them crowding back in when we next pause to consider the nature of our perceptions and their connections with the rest of the world. An inability to be seduced by such notions would be like an inability to love or die or mourn: quite enviable from an abstract point of view perhaps, but chillingly remote from the ordinary conditions of human existence.

16 Roland Barthes, 'Leçon d'écriture', *Tel Quel* 34, Summer 1968, translated as 'Lesson in Writing', in *Image, Music, Text*, edited by Stephen Heath, London, Fontana, 1977, pp. 170–8, p. 175. Martin Jay's *Downcast Eyes: the Denigration of Vision in Twentieth-Century French Thought* (Berkeley, University of California Press, 1993) offers a broad and solemn survey of 'ocularcentrism': Jay begins with the Greek 'privileging of vision' (p. 33), and exposes Descartes as 'a quintessentially visual philosopher' (p. 69), whilst arguing that the counter-Enlightenment Germans tended to 'privilege the ear over the eye' (p. 106). See also David Michael Levin, ed., *Modernity and the Hegemony of Vision*, Berkeley, University of California Press, 1993. For some weary scepticism, see Jonathan Rée, 'Writing and the Ring of Words', in *Culture & History* 12, 1992, pp. 23–54.

The metaphysical misinterpretations that experience suggests to us can be as elusive as they are pervasive; in the last logical analysis, they may even be strictly nonsensical. Like a half-remembered dream that haunts our waking hours, their content will be impossible to pin down with unambiguous exactitude. They will never be detected by an investigation that considers the world and all that is in it as an objective and unhistorical thing-in-itself, rather than as a *phenomenon*. For to treat something as a phenomenon means approaching it not as an object, but as a topic or theme: a great onion, as you might picture it, made of nothing but layer upon layer of more or less intelligent experiences – a topic of human perceptions, weighed down by history, saturated with memories, fears and desires; a theme of love, hatred, obsession and fascination; in short a hubbub of conflicting interpretations, accessible only through the multiple obliquities of a philosophical history.

In order to keep the structure of the narrative as uncluttered as possible, I shall be making three distinct cross-sections through the phenomenon of the voice: the first a kind of history of the metaphysics of the senses; the second a kind of history of scientific theories of language; and the third a kind of history of philosophy.

Part One describes certain notions about sensory experience that suggest themselves pretty naturally to anyone who has ever taken an interest in their body and how it responds to the world: in particular, the idea that perception is based on 'the five senses', and the idea of the voice as 'the breath of life' and the perfect means for 'expressing' inner feelings. These notions of experience and subjectivity are ones which practically all of us must, as children, have formed or rediscovered for ourselves; they belong to no specific historical period and no particular place, and provide the subject-matter for an emphatically non-chronological kind of history.

Part Two, in contrast, recounts a series of episodes in the history of European and American linguistic theory from the middle of the seventeenth century to the end of the twentieth, all connected in some way with the difficult predicaments of those born deaf. It is a complicated story, in which good will is repeatedly subverted by bad science, especially by botched or uncomprehending attempts to 'make language visible', whether by writing it in some kind of phonetic notation, or by such exotic means as picture-writing, manual spelling, lip-alphabets, gestural signing or vocal photography. In the end the theoretical problems of deaf communication have been satisfactorily solved, thanks both to the activities of the deaf and to Saussure's revolution in linguistics, making for a gratifying tale of progress in the history of science.

Part Three is about the accounts of perception propounded in the high tradition of Western philosophy, both through its theories of knowledge, and through its theories of art. The story is punctuated by the three great revolutions of modern philosophy: the creation of a general doctrine of ideas by Descartes in the first half of the seventeenth century, the construction of a concept of mind-dependent natural objectivity by Kant at the end of the eighteenth, and the formulation of the phenomenological method by Husserl at the beginning of the twentieth. Descartes, Kant and Husserl can be seen as accomplishing successive stages in the demolition of traditional metaphysical notions of subjectivity and the senses, which thus prove to have been an obstacle to progress in philosophy no less than in linguistics.

But the great philosophers were not just conducting a private conversation amongst themselves. Their doctrines were responses to intellectual discomforts that are either too broad or too specific to be comprehended by a history of philosophy, as distinct from a history of popular metaphysics or a history of scientific theories and technical and educational practices. To get a fairer philosophical understanding of ourselves we need to superimpose several different histories in our imaginations; and that is why, in place of a conclusion, I will appeal to the kind of self-knowledge we can construct with the help of the arts, including the arts of philosophy.

As far as its content is concerned, this three-tiered philosophical history will begin at the beginning, in the platitudes of everyday experience. Part One will explore the obvious assumption (shared by philosophers and children, poets, scientists and inventors) that all our perceptions can be traced back to several parallel supply-routes, namely the five senses, each conceived as a separate conduit giving access to different qualities of the real world. But this idea will be seen encountering difficulties when the differences between the various senses begin to be taken into account. For instance vision is likely to appear better attuned to the realities of the natural world than hearing; and again, the sense of hearing will distinguish itself from the other senses because it alone is partnered by an active faculty, namely the voice. We not only hear, but also vocalize, and we hear ourselves vocalizing, too. We cannot make ourselves seen or smelt, or tasted or felt in the way we can make ourselves heard: a minuscule contingency in a way, but a metaphysical anomaly as well, and not unconnected with the special values and anxieties that have woven themselves into the phenomenon of the human voice.

And vocality has had to bear some very heavy symbolic freight indeed. The fact that our voice is carried by our breath means that it is easily taken as a kind of messenger despatched from our soul, a metaphorical or even literal exhalation of some original inwardness hidden away in our head or breast. But on the other hand our voice can also speak: it can articulate words, that is to say, or rather be articulated by them, through repeating the conventional signs of a public language. ('If words be made of breath, And breath of life . . .' as Gertrude says in *Hamlet*.)[17] The voice is thus a double phenomenon, located at a kind of metaphysical cusp where the inward subjectivity of individual spirits intersects with the social realities of linguistic history.

Part Two will examine this phenomenological tapestry from the reverse side. Just as Foucault once analysed the phenomenon of philosophical reason by investigating the history of madness or unreason,[18] so the phenomenon of the voice can be approached by way of voicelessness – the experience of the mute or dumb, that is to say, or more accurately the deaf, together with the troops of doctors and teachers who have struggled to release them from their silent world (or perhaps expel them from it against their will) by devising ways of making them participate in spoken language, despite their inability to hear it.[19]

The historical experience of the deaf is like a vast philosophical

17 Shakespeare, *Hamlet*, III.iv.199–200.
18 See Michel Foucault, *Folie et déraison: Histoire de la folie à l'âge classique*, Paris, Plon, 1961; translated and severely abridged by Richard Howard, *Madness and Civilization*, New York, Pantheon, 1965.
19 For the history of the deaf, my first guide has been Harlan Lane's brilliant *When the Mind Hears: A History of the Deaf*, New York, Random House, 1984. I now disagree with much of Lane's analysis (it is distorted by partisan hindsight on behalf of deaf nationalism, and too impatient with metaphysical, scientific and philosophical complexities), but I would never have known how to criticize it without its initial help and inspiration.

experiment concerning the relations between language and the senses. The fundamental assumption has always been that the key to imparting linguistic knowledge to the deaf must be to substitute another sense for the missing sense of hearing. Attention was therefore concentrated on the task of making speech visible – visible on a permanent surface in the form of writing, visible on the hands through finger-spelling, visible on the body through non-linguistic gestural signs, or directly visible in the features of a speaker's face. And a huge metaphysical quarrel then broke out amongst the educators of the deaf, between supporters of the 'method of speech' and partisans of the 'method of signs', with the generally conservative 'oralists' appealing to a link between spoken language and human spirituality, and the more radical 'gesturalists' or 'manualists' arguing for the expressive and intellectual superiority of a visual 'language of signs'. Both approaches were to bring joy and enlightenment to some deaf people; but they also, on occasion, deprived them of their childhoods, their friendships, their families and their cultures, perhaps even of any life worth living. By the end of the twentieth century, however – thanks to developments both in scientific linguistics and in the social and political organization of the deaf community – the assumptions that had presided over centuries of controversy in deaf education were exposed as fundamentally flawed. The differences between sight and hearing had, it turned out, no essential bearing on the nature of language, and sign languages proved to be neither better nor worse than spoken ones: they were structurally much the same, and given the chance they would develop into flourishing natural languages just like any others.

The vindication of sign languages was a philosophical revolution, one might say; but although philosophers had been constantly commenting on the problems of deaf education, and occasionally intervening in them, they did not contribute much to their resolution. So it is only in Part Three that this history touches down where it might have been expected to begin: on philosophical concepts of intellect, sensation and knowledge as they appear through the lens of the History of Philosophy. First, there is the story of Locke and his followers with their solemn but often bizarre attempts to break up human experience into the separate contributions of the five senses. Then there is the even stranger story of how philosophers before and after Kant tried to account for the phenomena of 'fine art' in terms of the theory of the senses, dividing the field into 'visual' arts (supposedly concerned with space) and 'auditory' arts (supposedly concerned with time): a theory which was valiantly maintained despite being constantly contradicted both by ordinary visual and auditory experience and by artistic activity itself.

These confusions in the philosophy of experience were not to be sorted out till the twentieth century, when Husserl demonstrated that the notion of the world could never be attained by piecing together the separate deliverances of the various senses. There is no experience that is not experience of the world: the world precedes everything else in our experience, and must be present to us before we can perceive anything at all. And we do not really perceive the world through our five separate senses, but with our bodies as a whole. It is only with the world and our bodies as background that we have been able to construct the metaphysical notions of sensation, vocality and subjectivity with which we have distracted and bemused ourselves so long.

In the end the narrative will return to the history of the voice, and it should become possible to look back and see how both philosophy and linguistic theory have been impaled for centuries on a misleading contrast between vision and writing on the one hand, and hearing and speech on the other – a contrast which is continuously belied, however, not only by the practice of the vocal arts (including the arts of storytelling), but also, if we care to listen out for it, by the oceanic indeterminacy of the human voice itself.

ONE

SOUND, VOICE AND THE SOUL

A history of metaphysics

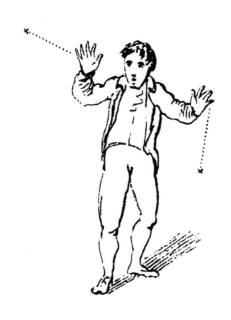

It is rather obvious that our experience of the world begins with our senses; and equally clear, after a moment's thought, that we have several of them: touch, smell, taste, hearing and vision, according to the usual reckoning. So it is natural, when we come to reflect on our experience, that we should start by trying to make sense of this five-fold sensory world.

We may begin by worrying about mirages, hallucinations, dreams, and illusions: if our senses sometimes delude us, how can we ever rely on them to acquaint us with real physical objects, as opposed to the state of our own subjective perceptions? But soon we will feel the need to make some distinctions between the different senses. Touch will probably be reckoned the most robustly realistic of them, followed by taste and smell: they make real physical contact with their objects. Vision and hearing, by comparison, are indirect and abstract, since they connect us not with physical things, but only with the light and sound they emit or reflect.

Vision may perhaps have an advantage over hearing in that it imparts distinct information about the shapes of things and their spatial relations, whereas hearing informs us only about sounds, not about real objects in space. On the other hand, hearing has an advantage over vision in terms of our ability to affect it at will. Simply by making sounds with our voices, we can enter into our auditory world in a way that has no analogue amongst the other senses: our voices are like an extra antenna, even an honorary sixth sense.

Metaphysicians and mystics have always liked to associate the voice with an immortal soul or divine spirit; and although we may be impatient with such unmodern notions, we will still have to admit that individual voices have a rather special significance in human life. We respond to them as we do to faces: as immediate embodiments of personal character and sensitive indicators of fluctuating mood. At the same time, they are marked by an enigmatic inner divide: the elusive fault-line between the voice that simply makes sounds, and the voice that speaks and utters the words of a language.

When a little baby whimpers or cries or yells, its voice gives uncontrived expression to its emotions; but when a child begins to speak, it is using its voice to participate in social communication in accordance with artificial linguistic conventions. Voices thus encode an intriguing human tension, even a contradiction: they are both expression and communication, both feeling and intellect, both body and mind, both nature and culture. The whole of us, it would seem, is included in the compass of the human voice.

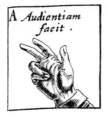

1

Sound and Substance

Which would be the greater calamity: losing your sight or losing your hearing? That, as I remember, was the most absorbing question in the whole of my ramshackle childhood metaphysics. I would keep screwing up my eyes or sticking my fingers in my ears, and comparing the results. But my preference in those days was always the same: given the choice, I would far rather be deaf than blind. Blindness would mean never knowing where I was or what was going on around me. It would be like stumbling and fumbling through a pitch-dark dungeon – and my mind was stocked with enough stories and images and dreams to make that prospect terrifying: rats and spiders and ganglions of fleshy roots; putrefying bodies, gaping chasms, quicksands, and pits of slurping slime. The thought of blindness made me shudder.

Someone told me I could ruin my eyes by straining or tiring them, and the idea of going blind terrified me so much that I tried to remember to keep them shut whenever possible. If I lost my eyesight, I thought, I would never be able to tell what was brushing up against me, or what I was about to tread on or sit in. I would not even know what I was picking up and putting in my mouth.

Compared with that, what would it really matter if I lost my hearing, as long as I still had the use of my eyes? The world of sound had little to offer me except interruptions and interferences, or the drone of grown-up conversations, so in some ways I could imagine deafness more as a liberation than a deprivation. Of course I would not be able to hear what was going on downstairs or out in the street. But I could always go and have a look, so it seemed that deafness would not be much more than a mild inconvenience.

What is more, sounds seemed peculiarly thin and unimportant: flimsy, wispy nonentities, almost entirely disconnected from the real world. They lacked palpable solidity; and solidity – as I learned when reading John Locke many years later – is not only the most constant of our sensations, but also 'the Idea most intimately connected with, and essential to Body'.[1] Blithe little materialist that I was, I presumed that nothing really existed except pieces of solid matter: as far as I was concerned, body and being meant more or less the same. I might hear something, or taste it or smell it or see it, but unless I could hit it or kick it or lean up against it, or feel its weight or its impact, I would not be convinced that it was really and truly there.

And touch seemed to me the most central kind of sensation, as well as the most reliable and realistic. If your eyes left you uncertain how far away something was, or what it was made of, you could always reach out and feel it, at least if you were close enough and had the nerve. In general you can expect the things you see to correspond one for one to those you can touch. Taste was much the same: you could touch your food before tasting it, and you could also feel it, crisp or soft or chewy in the mouth. Once again, the evidence of one sense appeared to interlock with that of the others in mutual support. To some extent, the same kind of reassuring correspondences are available with smells: they might waft around unpredictably in the wind, but they were clearly composed of physical matter, even if they were not exactly tangible. You could watch the smoke drifting towards you before you caught its smell, and you could feel your bowl of soup and see the steam rising from it towards your nostrils. Sight, taste and smell therefore made an integrated team, under the reliable leadership of touch: they huddled snugly together round the same solid palpable objects.

With sounds it appeared rather different. Compared to other deni-

---

1 John Locke, *An Essay concerning Human Understanding* (1690), edited by Peter H. Nidditch, Oxford, Clarendon Press, 1975, Book II, Chapter IV, 'Of Solidity', §1, p. 123.

zens of our sensory worlds, they were out on a limb. Of course I could hear a car go past, as well as seeing it; or I could pick up a watch and put it to my ear to find out if it was working. I could drop a stone down a well and listen for it splashing into the water. But in and of themselves, what exactly were the things that I could hear? Often, lying in bed in the dark, I could not place or even recognize the sounds that crowded in on me – the dripping of a tap or the ticking of a clock – until I turned on the light to have a look. And even when my ordinary curiosity was satisfied and I could see where the noises came from, I was still baffled when I tried to pin them down to a particular bodily existence at a definite point in space. I could quickly get myself lost in metaphysical mazes by asking: what exactly are all these tickings and drippings, and what precisely are they made of? I knew where they originated; but how did they spread out from their place of origin, and where were they at any given point in time? That I could not understand.

Sounds seemed to me to be nature's waifs and strays: they did not fit into the familiar world of physical things, and they could not be tracked down by my other senses either. After hatching in the dripping tap or ticking clock, they plunged into empty space, fanning out through the room, passing my ears on the way, and then spreading through the rest of the house, growing weaker and weaker all the time, and then the garden, the sky, the moon, becoming more diluted, mile after mile, year after year; but never, I supposed, reaching any absolutely definitive end. They were colourless, tasteless, odourless, and intangible. They were not part of the material world, and they had no weight to them, no substance. Is it surprising that I thought I could happily do without them?

It probably did not occur to me at the time, but I wonder what it would be like if we had only one sense instead of five. Our lives would be impoverished of course, even though we could have no idea what we were missing; but would they not also be profoundly and structurally *altered*?

Just how different they would be might depend which sense we were left with. Touch on its own should enable us to understand our world in much the same way as with a full set of five senses: we would be able to feel our way towards the idea of a spatial world filled with plants and trees and animals and stones and water and earth, not to mention our own bodies and those of other people. We could still frame an idea of ourselves as individuals, each making a unique journey through space and time; and we would still be able to conceive of objects and other people coming into our lives, leaving it, and being recognized again if they turned up on another occasion. Even if we had nothing to go on but our sense of touch, we could still imagine ourselves as a locus of feelings, a continuous subject of experiences, and we would still be able to distinguish between our subjective sensations and the objectivity of the real world outside us.

Perhaps we would not be quite so well off if we had no sense organs except our eyes, so that we could see things but not feel them. At the best of times it is unsettling to come across things that can be seen but not touched: rainbows, mirages, the sky, or the fruit in a *trompe l'œil* painting. The idea of untouchable apparitions is positively uncanny. Ghosts, of course, are supposed to look like ordinary solid people: the chilling truth is revealed when you try to hit them, or grasp them by the hand, and find you meet with no resistance. Perhaps we should agree with the celebrated blind man from Puiseaux, who was sought out by Diderot in the 1740s as a source of first-hand testimony in the philosophy of the senses. Diderot commiserated with him for having been plunged since birth into impenetrable darkness: Would he not be overjoyed to be granted the use of his eyes at last? Not particularly, the old man replied, unimpressed. 'I would just as soon have long arms: it seems to me that my hands would tell me more about what happens on the moon than you can find out with your eyes and your telescopes.'[2]

The blind man of Puiseaux had a good point: eyesight on its own does not always enable you to distinguish appearances from realities, and when in doubt it is wise to call on the sense of touch to settle the matter. All the same, we could probably develop some notion of our position in the world on the basis of sight alone, if not quite so securely as we would by means of touch. If we were left relying on one of the other senses, however, our predicament would be far more desperate.

2 Denis Diderot, *Lettre sur les aveugles, à l'usage de ceux qui voient* (1749), in Paul Vernière, ed., *Œuvres Philosophiques*, Paris, Garnier, 1964, p. 89.

The problem is not that life might get boring, but that the whole structure of our experience would be indescribably impoverished. It would be impoverished *ontologically*, one might say: our whole idea of what it means to experience the world would be degraded beyond recognition. Strictly speaking, in fact, we might have no use at all for the idea of a world of real objects distinct from our experience and set over against it. Scents or tastes might appear and disappear, but we would be in no position to wonder whether they existed in reality or only in our imagination; we could not even raise the question whether they ceased to exist when we stopped experiencing them, or just went away from us for a while, perhaps to come back later. When the same sensation recurred, we could not ask ourselves if it was the very same flavour or perfume which had returned, or only another one that we could not tell apart from it. If our sensations faded or intensified, we could not ask if this was because of some real change in the world, or merely some alteration in the vividness of our perceptions. The problem is not so much that we would be uncertain which experiences came from within us and which from outside: we would not even be able to make sense of the alternatives. Without visual or tactile clues, it seems, we could not begin to frame an idea of space, so it would not occur to us that there might be a difference between our own bodies and a world of objects independent of it. We would not distinguish between perceiving two similar objects in immediate succession, and perceiving the same one continuously. An experience of tastes and smells would not give a hint of anything but sensations of taste and smell: we would not live our lives as spatial beings at all, and we would have no sense of our own individuality or our own separate lives, let alone of other people.

The same would seem to apply, most starkly of all, to the world of sound. A purely auditory creature might enjoy a rich and various experience, taking delight in the most subtle patterns of loudness, pitch and timbre, but it would never have an inkling of a distinction between the private symphony of its sensations and a real world outside. It would have no conception that its experience might be limited to a small portion of reality, no notion of permanent objects existing out of reach of its hearing, or of itself as a creature that moves amongst them, acting and responding. In short it would not have *experiences* in any meaningful sense of the word; indeed it would not really have a world either: it would be nothing but the sum of its sensations.[3]

Abstract considerations like these may have been latent in my childish sense of the flimsy insubstantiality of sounds; but probably not. What really impressed me at the time was the simple observable fact that sounds do not perpetuate themselves on their own. The piano may sustain a note, and the church bell may be tolled over and over again; but the sound will linger only a fleeting instant before sinking back into silence. A sound can barely survive the moment of its creation. As Hegel noted – and Hegel, like Locke, was a marvellously attentive chronicler of the stirrings of ordinary metaphysical fantasy – the peculiarity of a sound it that 'the ear has scarcely grasped it before it is mute'.[4]

In Baldassare Castiglione's *Book of the Courtier*, there is a story about an Italian merchant who was in Poland one winter, and wanted to trade with some Muscovites on the opposite bank of the Dnieper. The river was iced over, hard as marble, but the hostility between the King of Poland and the Duke of Muscovy meant that neither party would cross over to the other side. Accordingly the Muscovites resorted to shouting their terms across the frozen river. But the cold was so bitter that their very words froze before reaching the ears of the Italian merchant, and the messages were left suspended in mid-air, congealed and unable to move. After a while the Italian merchant appealed to some Polish accomplices for help. They knew all about cold weather, and lit a great fire in the middle of the rock-solid river. At length the words began to thaw, and trickle down from the sky like snow melting from the mountains in May. (The Muscovites had left by then, but when the Italian merchant heard the prices they were asking he came away without regrets.)[5]

Castiglione's story may be beguiling, but the more you think about

3 The point has been persuasively argued by P. F. Strawson in Chapter 2 ('Sounds') of his *Individuals: an Essay in Descriptive Metaphysics*, London, Methuen, 1959. See especially pp. 73–4: 'the crucial idea . . . of a spatial system of objects through which oneself, another object, moves, but which extends beyond the limits of one's observation at any moment' cannot be translated into 'purely auditory terms'.
4 G. W. F. Hegel, *Aesthetics: Lectures on Fine Art*, translated by T. M. Knox, Oxford, Clarendon Press, 1975, p. 892.
5 Baldassare Castiglione, *The Book of the Courtier* (1528), translated by Charles S. Singleton, New York, Doubleday, 1959, Book Two, §55, p. 155.

it, the less sense it makes. How could sounds be captured and preserved and then released later? How would they have lasted all that time, and how could they have perpetuated themselves in silence? And when they were eventually unfrozen, could they actually be the same sounds, after all? Surely it is like listening for the breaking waves in an old sea shell: you may be entranced at first, and hear them quite clearly; but the magic will be silenced once you ask yourself which particular waves you are hearing, or where they broke, and when.

The basic truth about sounds, it would seem, is that they never last. You cannot collect and keep a beloved sound, as you can a letter or a flower or a lock of hair. You may have a recording of it of course – a recording on a wax cylinder or magnetic tape, or, if you lack these technical facilities, directly in your heart (the word *recording* literally means learning by heart, after all). But recording is not the same as preservation: it is a technique for generating copies of an original, rather than maintaining it in existence. Recording is a technique of mimicry, imitation, or reproduction – like making a mould of a carving, so that replicas can be cast from it even if the original does not survive. It is a peculiarity of sounds, it seems, that they cannot be conserved, but only recorded and reproduced.

It would seem impossible, therefore, to hear exactly the same sound twice – but for one very striking exception: echoes. Thomas Hobbes was deeply intrigued by the way we can '*hear double* or *treble*, by multiplication of *echoes*', and regarded the phenomenon of echoing as positive proof that sounds are purely subjective, existing not 'in the thing we hear, but in ourselves'. Echoes, as he put it, 'are sounds as well as the original; and *not* being in one and the *same place*, cannot be *inherent* in the body that maketh them'. It followed, Hobbes thought, that sounds do not exist, at least not '*really*'.[6] In any case, even echoes quickly fade, and you will be lucky to catch them a third time, let alone a fourth or a fifth. After that, as Hegel said, they can 'reecho only in the depths of the soul'.[7]

If there are such things as natural symbols, then sounds are surely the natural symbol of transience and the lostness of past time. They are essentially evanescent, an exact correlative of wistfulness and poignant

6 Thomas Hobbes, *First Discourse, of Human Nature* (1640), in *English Works*, Vol. IV, edited by William Molesworth, London 1840, pp. 7–8.
7 Hegel, *Aesthetics*, p. 892.

regret, not to mention sentimentality. They seem to be nature's way of mourning, and in the inevitable metaphor, they are born only to die away. Perhaps that is why, as some would have it, beautiful music is always sad. But I was still only a cheerful child. I had not yet reached the age of nostalgia, and did not care for the world of sound.

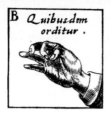

2

Physics and colour-music

From an objective and scientific point of view, of course, all this musing about which of my senses gave me the best contact with the world of solid physical realities must seem a complete waste of time. My child-hood doctrine of the five senses and my partiality towards what I could see with my eyes and touch with my hands was based on images and fables, wishes and compulsions, not dispassionate, self-critical, con-trolled inquiries. Science tells us, after all, that seeing is simply what happens when light enters our eyes, and hearing when sound enters our ears. Sound and light are nothing but different kinds of physical turbulence, which propagate themselves through space and spark off sensations or perceptions in us if our ears or eyes happen to be in their path. My idea that ears give on to a more fleeting and inconsequential world than that revealed to the eyes must therefore have been mere childish fantasy. Sound is just as solid and substantial as light; in some ways, in fact, physical science suggests that they are much the same sort of thing.

Sonus lucis simia: sound is light's ape or monkey. That was the motto of the ingenious German Jesuit Athanasius Kircher, author of a bulky treatise on music published in 1650.[1] Sound was the earthly counterpart to heavenly light, a ponderous and imperfect translation

---

1 Athanasius Kircher, *Musurgiae Universalis*, 2 Vols, Rome, 1650, Vol. 2, p. 240.

of it, a fleshly analogue for its spiritual purity – a point which Kircher illustrated in a practical way by developing a 'hearing lens' or 'speaking trumpet' which made distant sounds seem close, just as a telescope does with distant sights.[2] And if sound corresponded to light, it was reasonable to suppose that different tones corresponded to different colours. Furthermore, since musical harmony was already the topic of a well-established branch of mathematics, it should not be difficult to work out the mathematical basis for the higher harmonies of light, and even to base a new, visual music on them.

That was Kircher's dream, though the task of defining the exact form of the parallel between colours and tones proved too hard for him. But in 1669 the young Isaac Newton was lecturing on the 'harmonies of colours', and proceeding on the assumption that they were 'perhaps analogous to the concordances of sounds'.[3] Many years later, he was still worrying at 'the harmony and discord of Colours', suggesting rather desperately that the phenomenon might arise from 'the proportions of the Vibrations propagated through the Fibres of the optick Nerves'.[4]

Newton's main argument was that just as all the different tones can be located on a single scale running from the highest to the lowest pitch of audible sound, so all the different colours must have their place on a single scale of visible light. The natural and intrinsic order of colours, he thought, was revealed when sunlight is refracted to produce the array seen in rainbows. He regarded this latent structure as the phantom or ghost of sunlight – its spectre or *spectrum* – and observed, at an early stage in his researches, that it ran from Red to Violet, passing through Yellow, Green and Blue in an unalterable five-colour sequence. But there is nothing necessary about seeing five colours in the rainbow. The naming and counting of colours is an arbitrary matter: it depends where you choose to say that one colour ends and another one begins. And Newton eventually revised his perceptions, adding the jargon words 'Orange' and 'Indigo' to his vocabulary so as to bring the number of colours in the spectrum up to seven:

2 See Louis Bertrand Castel, 'Clavessin pour les yeux', in *Esprit, Saillies et Singularités du P. Castel*, Amsterdam, 1753, pp. 279–86.
3 Quoted in John Gage, *Colour and Culture: Practice and Meaning from Antiquity to Abstraction*, London, Thames and Hudson, 1993, p. 232.
4 Isaac Newton, *Opticks* (1704), Book Three, Query 14, New York, Dover, 1952, p. 346.

Red, Orange, Yellow, Green, Blue, Indigo and Violet – the seven colours which schoolchildren are still instructed to look for whenever they see a rainbow.

Newton's reason for preferring to find seven colours in the spectrum of sunlight was that it helped clinch his analogy between light and sound.[5] For if there were seven colours, ascending from Red to Violet, then they could be aligned with the seven tones of the ancient Greek musical scale – that is to say, the octave, which later became the basis of early Christian church music as well.

But there was a complication, though Newton chose to ignore it. In the late Middle Ages, when attempts were made to standardize the pitches and harmonies of the octaves used in different parts of Christendom, it became necessary to produce finer gradations of tone by inserting extra steps into the scale. 'Half-tones' were therefore inserted between the old tones, except in two cases (B-C and E-F) where they sounded close enough already; and so it was that the octave acquired five new tones. The resulting twelve-tone scale is, like any other, somewhat arbitrary and imperfect; but it is exceptionally rich in near-perfect consonances, and therefore has a plausible claim to natural authority.[6] In any case it has entered deep into musical performance and memory; and in addition, no less immovably, it has been built into the physical fabric of keyboards, which, from the fifteenth century on, were reconstructed with five black keys amongst the traditional seven whites.

Keyboards were to play a central part in subsequent experiments with the analogies between sound and light – projects which were dominated by an eighteenth-century Parisian Jesuit named Louis Bertrand Castel. As a young man, Castel was inspired by the writings of Kircher, and began to dream of building sound-machines which would enable the blind to 'hear the beauty of colours', and light-machines which would transform sounds and make them 'present to the eyes, as they are to the ears, so that the deaf could relish and appreciate the joys of music just like anyone else'. All that was needed was a device for making sounds visible, so that whenever we listened to music we

5 See John Gage, *Colour and Culture*, esp. pp. 168, 232.
6 Particularly the most simple consonances after octaves, namely fifths and major thirds, which correspond to frequency ratios of 3:2, and 5:4 respectively. See James Jeans, *Science and Music*, Cambridge, Cambridge University Press, 1937, pp. 152–190.

would also 'find the air blooming with brilliant and harmonious colours'. Here, Castel said, Kircher had hit on 'one of those ideas that I call seeds of discovery'.[7]

Castel devoted a lifetime to cultivating Kircher's seed of discovery. His approach was based on Newton's spectrum and the twelve-tone musical scale. Following Newton, Castel conceived the colours of the spectrum as joining up at their two extremes, with Red and Violet merging into each other to form a kind of circle or wheel which could then be mapped onto the cycle of tones in the scale. (Castel did, however, believe that Newton's spectrum was inverted: he held that the sequence from Red through Yellow to Green, Blue and Violet corresponded to a falling scale, not a rising one.) And just as the octave was supposed to start at C, so, he argued, the colour scale originated in Blue. (It might have been more natural to run from Violet to Red, as in the rainbow; but Père Castel was a practical man of science, and observation taught him that the basic colour at the root of all others was in fact Blue.) Starting with this 'fundamental tonic colour', Castel noted other colours developing out of it 'by a kind of substantial or even transcendent generation'. Castel's primary colours corresponded to the white notes: after the Blue of C, D was Green, E Yellow, F Apricot, G Red, A Violet and B Indigo. The black notes were intermediate colours: C sharp Celadon, or blue-green; E flat Olive, or greenish yellow; F sharp Orange; A flat Crimson; and B flat Agate or Ruby. As you went up from one octave to the next, the same sequence of colours was repeated over again, only brighter.[8] Castel envisaged just twelve octaves, yielding nature's entire range of exactly 144 different colours.[9]

Castel was an inventor as well as a theorist and experimenter, with a special and obsessive interest in adapting keyboards to non-musical uses. He suggested, for instance, they could be attached to morsels of food or bottles of perfume, to provide the most variegated pleasures for the palate or the nose. Or they could be coupled with massage-machines, to impress a delightful range of sensations on the surfaces

7 Louis Bertrand Castel, 'Clavessin pour les yeux', pp. 279, 282, 284.
8 Castel expounded this theory in 'Nouvelles expériences d'Optique et d'Acoustique', published in six parts in the *Journal de Trévoux* (*Mémoires pour l'histoire des Sciences et des Beaux Arts*) between August and December 1735; the quotation is from the second part, p. 1666.
9 See 'Des Couleurs', in *Esprit, Saillies et Singularités du P. Castel*, p. 349.

of your body.[10] He told a story, too, of a German prince from Halle, who was sunk in a lethargy so profound that nothing could rouse him from it – until one lucky day he received a visit from a travelling musician equipped with a new kind of harpsichord, guaranteed to make even the saddest of melancholics cheer up. He had carefully selected a range of cats, with sonorous miaows of different pitches, 'finely diapasoned in accordance with all the rules'. Sharp needles were attached to the harpsichord-jacks, each one lined up with a cat's bottom. The performance on the cat-harpsichord was a triumph, of course: 'the prince consented to leave behind his melancholy: for who could fail to laugh at such a thing?'[11]

Castel's favourite keyboard project was for a colour-harpsichord, on which he hoped to be able to give Newtonian concerts, in the quick bright medium of light instead of the slow dull medium of sound. He announced the scheme in 1725, at first trying to make the keys operate glass prisms with light shining through them. When that failed he devised mechanisms for opening a shutter concealing a strip of dyed fabric with a light behind it. After ten laborious years, he was ready to exhibit this 'Harpsichord for the Eyes' in Paris in December 1734. Unfortunately, the inquisitive spectators who crowded in claimed that all they experienced was a sequence of coloured flashes, signifying nothing, and they left the performance before the end. Voltaire thought the failure both comic and inevitable, but Castel reproached the audience for their hasty reliance on first impressions. Colour-music, he said crossly, was not the sort of thing you could pass judgement on in a day. It required intelligence and conscientious cultivation. The public, he concluded, would have to be apprenticed in colour-music through graduated performances beginning with very easy pieces; but 'with time,' he affirmed, 'since light is faster than sound, colour-music will be performed faster than any sound-music.'[12]

Castel spent the rest of his life improving the colour-harpsichord: there was a version using a hundred candles in 1754, and it was announced that a vast instrument whose keyboard operated 500 lamps

10 'Clavessin pour les sens', in *Esprit, Saillies et Singularités du P. Castel*, p. 361.
11 'Clavessin pour les yeux', pp. 305–6.
12 'Clavessin pour les sens', pp. 297, 322, 325, 346. See also F. M. A. de Voltaire, *Élémens de la philosophie de Newton, mis à la portée de tout le monde*, Amsterdam, Desbordes, 1738, pp. 184–5.

behind 60 discs of coloured glass would be displayed at the Great Concert Room in Soho Square in London in 1757. But the light concert appears to have been cancelled, and Castel died that same year, success still just beyond his grasp.[13]

Castel was not the last inventor to be captivated by the dream of colour-music. At the end of the nineteenth century, Professor A. Wallace Rimington, a teacher of Fine Art at Queen's College in London, re-invented the idea of correlating a colour-wheel with a musical scale, believing that the result might generate progressive new styles for modern painting. He knew nothing of Castel's ocular harpsichord, but he too identified twelve colours in the spectrum corresponding to the twelve tones of the octave. His Colour Organ, first demonstrated in 1895, used electric lamps which lit up a huge screen of white drapery hanging in loose folds. Different colours could be projected onto different areas at the same time, though Rimington considered it more tasteful to use 'formless colour' filling the entire screen.[14] Musicians like Henry Wood were attracted by his work, and Alexander Scriabin wrote a part for a Rimingtonian light keyboard in his orchestral suite *Prometheus: Poem of Fire*.[15] Introducing an improved model of his Colour Organ in 1914, Rimington evoked the joys of waltzing to colour-music, and stressed the part the instrument might play in public education – strengthening the community's sense of colour, as he said, and so advancing 'its commercial prosperity as well as its aesthetic development'.[16] The Strand Electric and Engineering Company of London went on to manufacture 'light consoles' for many of the great theatres in England, as well as the opera houses in Ankara and Lisbon. Even the Royal Festival Hall in London boasted one when it opened in 1951.[17]

But despite all the technical improvements, the public still refused to take colour-music seriously. As far as its audiences were concerned,

13 See John Gage, *Colour and Culture*, pp. 233–5.
14 See A. Wallace Rimington, *Colour Music: The Art of Mobile Colour*, London, Hutchinson, 1912.
15 It was first performed in New York in 1915; for a full exploration of the background see John Gage, *Colour and Culture*, pp. 243–6.
16 'Music as Colour', *The Times*, 20 March 1914, p. 11.
17 See 'Colour and Music', in Percy A. Scholes, *The Oxford Companion to Music* (tenth edition), Oxford, Oxford University Press, 1970.

the revolutionary new art form kept regressing to the lowly craft of stage-lighting. Like Castel before him, Rimington concluded wearily that the philistine public was in need of further training.

But the real reasons for the failure of the art of colour-music were natural rather than cultural. What the colour-musicians all ignored – from Kircher and Newton to Castel and Rimington – is that music depends on the ways sounds combine with each other, and that the effect of mixing colours is quite different from that of mixing tones, and cannot provide any kind of analogue for it. The root of the difference – and one of the abiding riddles of physical thought[18] – is that beams of light pass chastely through each other without being affected at all, whereas soundwaves are constantly colliding and combining and mutually interfering.

Sounds therefore always have a special kind of complexity. In a way, in fact, there is no such thing as a simple sound. Even the pure tone of a tuning fork or an electronic bleep is different in a library, a bathroom, underwater, or in the open air. And the purest singing voice, or a musical instrument sounding a single note, emits a whole range of 'overtones' apart from its leading tone. These 'upper partials' were already noted in antiquity,[19] and in the seventeenth century Marin Mersenne claimed that he could hear no fewer than four of them when a string was plucked.[20] All the different qualities or timbres of different sounds – their particular 'colours' – depend upon their overtones, whether inharmonic (like tinkling cymbals), or harmonic (like sounding brass).[21] What is more, two tones sounding simultaneously can engender further ones – creating something out of nothing in what may seem a constant musical miracle. For instance there are 'difference tones', also known as 'Tartini tones' after the violinist who, when

18 Cf. Christiaan Huygens, *Traité de la Lumière*, 1678; see Shmuel Samebursky, ed., *Physical Thought*, London, Hutchinson, 1974, pp. 287–94.
19 The Aristotelian *Problems* includes the questions 'Why does the low note contain the sound of the high note?' and 'Why is it that in the octave, the concord of the upper note exists in the lower, but not vice-versa?' See Aristotle, *Problems*, Book XIX, No 8, 918a 19–20.
20 Marin Mersenne, *Harmonie Universelle, contenant la théorie de la pratique de la musique*, Paris, 1636, quoted in Alexander Wood, *The Physics of Music* (1944), revised by J. M. Bowsher, London, Methuen, 1962, p. 65.
21 Hermann von Helmholtz, *On the Sensation of Tone as a Physiological Basis for the Theory of Music* (1862), second English edition, translated by Alexander J. Ellis, London, Longmans, Green, 1885, pp. 69–74.

double-stopping in 1714, heard a 'third sound' whose tone corre-sponded to the difference between the two notes he was playing. There are also summation tones, and the beats you can hear when two musical instruments are slightly out of tune with each other.[22]

Wherever you are, you will always be surrounded by a symphony: the wind in the trees, the clock, the piano, the blackbirds, the conver-sation, the hum of traffic in the background – a medley of various sounds coming at you from different places, all with their particular colours and overtones, and all altering each other, mixing together, and making up new audible combinations. Every sound, you might say, is a complication of sound-effects. But with colours it is quite different. Of course a coloured cloth will not look the same in different lights or against different backgrounds, and your visual field is never filled with a single unvaried colour. You may see your reflection in a shop window at the same time as the objects behind it. You can take in a colourful scene at a glance, full of brinded, stippled, mottled, pied and dappled things. But even in a shimmering riot of colours, each colour is in itself simple, in a way that no sounds ever are. When different colours are combined – coloured beams projected at the same screen, for instance, or pigments mixed, or objects blurred together in the distance – the result is still just a simple colour. There is no intrinsic complexity in it, and the same colour could have been made from any number of different combinations of others.

The composition of colours is essentially invisible, whereas sounds contain specific mixtures of other sounds audibly within themselves. The various vowels, for instance, are distinguished by the fact that each of them carries a characteristic range of overtones – as Helmholtz established towards the middle of the nineteenth century.[23] And the same applies to sounds in general: to hear a sound is to hear the sounds of which it is composed. The objects of hearing are essentially multiple,

---

22 Alexander Wood, *The Physics of Music*, pp. 29, 20.
23 Helmholtz invited his readers to demonstrate it to themselves by singing different vowels on a particular note, say E flat, while sounding B flat a twelfth higher on the piano. 'By properly varying the experiment, it will be found possible to distinguish the vowels from one another by their upper partial tones,' Helmholtz explained, and with a bit of imagination one can convince oneself that he was right. See Hermann von Helmholtz, 'On the physiological causes of harmony in music' (1857), in *Popular Lectures on Scientific Subjects*, First Series, translated by E. Atkinson, London, Longmans, Green, 1893, pp. 83–4.

and the world of hearing has a kind of perceptible depth which has no equivalent in vision.

But if mixing sounds is unlike mixing colours, it is quite similar to mixing perfumes and flavours. When you add oil to vinegar, both of them are transformed; but even if the resulting smell and taste are quite unexpected, you will still be able to recognize the two ingredients and tell them apart within the mixture. It is the same with hearing. When you hear two people sing together, the combined effect may take you by surprise, but you will still be able to hear the two voices and even listen to each of them separately.

There is, you might say, something peculiarly sociable about sounds: they only come into their own in each other's company. Although their impermanence may make them a natural symbol of transience, the way they mingle to produce a fused unity makes them an emblem for companionable solidarity too. Pantheistic ideas of the unity of creation find a perfect illustration in communal singing: Mörike heard his chorus of nightingales singing with 'one voice', and for Schlegel, 'the whole is but a single choir, many a song from but one mouth.'[24] There is nothing like a whole crowd raising a concerted sound to symbolize unity of purpose, as the political, military and religious uses of music demonstrate. The audible complexity of sounds gives them a capacity for concord and disharmony which the world of colour could never possibly match. 'The eye,' as Helmholtz said, 'has no sense of harmony in the same meaning as the ear.' Unluckily for the colour-musicians, 'there is no music to the eye'.[25]

24 'Und eine Stimme scheint ein Nachtigallenchor' (Eduard Mörike, 'Auf eine Wanderung'), 'Und das All ein einzig Chor, Manches Lied aus einem Munde' (Friedrich von Schlegel, 'Abendröte').
25 Hermann von Helmholtz, 'On the physiological causes of harmony in music', p. 92.

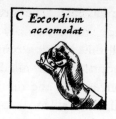

3

Metaphysics, idealism and the blind

It is often said, in accordance with a doctrine found in Aristotle, that the five senses fall into two groups.[1] First there are the contact senses – touch, taste and (probably) smell – whose objects have to impinge on your body before you can perceive them. And then there are the distance senses – sight and hearing (and just possibly smell) – through which you perceive things which are spatially separate from you. There is a suggestion that we can be detached and theoretical about what we see or hear, whereas we are always physically implicated in the things we feel or taste, and perhaps endangered by them too. The distance senses are nobler, purer, more detached, and perhaps – by some standards – more masculine than the contact senses. They are epistemologically and ethically more respectable, it seems, and their objects are dignified by that quality of impassivity and separateness from ourselves for which Bishop Berkeley coined the term *outness*.

But Berkeley thought that outness was an illusion. He devoted a lifetime's philosophical fervour to demonstrating the necessity of idealism, arguing that the very ideas of space and material substance are impossible, and – despite appearances and prejudices to the contrary – that all the senses are really contact senses. Outness, according to Berkeley, was nothing but 'a line directed end-wise to the eye', and

1 Aristotle, *Parva Naturalia*, 436b.

34

obviously it was therefore invisible. 'The ideas of space, outness, and things placed at a distance are not, strictly speaking, the object of sight,' he explained. It followed that anything a person could see was located only 'in his eye, or rather in his mind', and therefore must be 'as near to him as the perceptions of pain or pleasure, or the most inward passions of his soul'.[2]

The idea of seeing things at a distance was not only a mistake, according to Berkeley, but a threat to religion too: it encouraged belief in a materialist concept of matter – inert, independent, and unspiritual – and was therefore a step on the path to atheism. When he came to the other supposed distance sense, however, Berkeley's evangelistic fervour hardly stirred at all. It was not that he found the idea of hearing at a distance any more acceptable than that of seeing at a distance; but he thought the notion so thoroughly preposterous that even the most bone-headed materialist could never be tempted by it at all.[3] For everyone implicitly understands, he thought, that you do not really hear things at a distance, since 'bodies and external things are not properly the object of hearing; but only sounds'.[4]

Berkeley had a good point: it is indeed quite plausible to think of hearing as a contact sense. Sounds must physically reach your ears before you can hear them, just as textures must make contact with your skin before you can feel them. If you go out in wild weather, you may even hear sounds that actually originate in the play of the wind over the whorls and corrugations of your ears. In fact one might well think that the sounds we hear have even less 'outness' than the objects we touch: like flavours and perfumes, they must pass through openings in our bodies and brush against concealed interior surfaces before they can be perceived. It may not be what Berkeley had in mind, but it is not difficult to make something erotic of the idea that sounds have to enter into our bodies before they can be heard. (In *The Merchant of Venice*, for instance, Lorenzo invites Jessica to come and sit beside him – 'sit, and let the sounds of music Creep in our

2 George Berkeley, *An Essay towards a New Theory of Vision* (1709), §§2, 46, 41; see *Works*, edited by A. A. Luce, London, Nelson, Vol. 1, 1948, pp. 171, 188, 186.
3 Indeed even the materialistic Hobbes had rejected materialism about sounds: see above, p. 23.
4 *Essay towards a New Theory of Vision*, §§47; *Works*, Vol. 1. p. 189. See also *Principles of Human Knowledge* (1710), §43; *Works*, Vol. 2, 1949, p. 58.

ears.')[5] Sounds, to use a phrase of Berkeley's, are perhaps 'as near to us as our own thoughts',[6] and hearing might therefore be classified as another contact sense, alongside taste and touch.

There are some circumstances, indeed, in which the perception of sound is hardly distinguishable from touch at all. You can pick up the thunder of an avalanche in the mountains, or the hooves of galloping horses, the beat of a rock band, or the slamming of a door, by feeling them through your feet as much as hearing them with your ears. In *Émile*, Rousseau pointed out that you can tell whether a cello is playing a high note or a low one by laying a hand on its body. He even imagined that with practice you could learn 'to hear an entire melody through the fingers'.[7] And Pierre Desloges – a deaf contemporary of Rousseau and author of one of the earliest first-hand memoirs about living a 'deaf and dumb' life – concurred. 'In my room I can distinguish a passing coach from the beating of a drum,' he explained. He could hear loud noises at fifteen or twenty paces, although 'not through my ears'. He could also hear people speaking if he placed a hand on their throat or neck, or by holding an empty cardboard box in his hands and getting them to speak into it. He too claimed that 'if I put my hand to a violin or flute being played, I can hear them', and he could easily distinguish their tones, he said, 'even when I close my eyes'.[8]

Hearing is not always confined to the ears, any more than feeling is restricted to the fingertips. This means that deafness is never so absolute as blindness can be. ('Why was the sight To such a tender ball as the eye confined?', as Milton's Samson lamented – 'So obvious and so easy to be quenched, And not as feeling through all parts diffused, That she might look at will through every pore?')[9] Even those

5 Shakespeare, *The Merchant of Venice*, V. i. 54; see also W. H. Auden's 'Seascape' (1937).
6 Berkeley, *Principles*, §42; *Works*, Vol. 2, p. 58.
7 Jean-Jacques Rousseau, *Émile, ou de l'éducation* (1762), edited by François Richard and Pierre Richard, Paris, Garnier, 1957, Book Two, p. 147.
8 Pierre Desloges, *Observations d'un sourd et muet sur un cours élémentaire d'éducation des sourds et muets, publié en 1779 par M. l'Abbé Deschamps*, Amsterdam and Paris, B. Morin, 1779, Preface, pp. 8–10. Parts of the work are translated in *The Deaf Experience*, edited by Harlan Lane, translated by Franklin Philip, Harvard University Press, 1984, pp. 30–48; see pp. 31–2. In rather the same way, the deaf percussionist Evelyn Glennie has suggested that deaf people should be given balloons at concerts, to enable them to hear the music through their hands: see Evelyn Glennie, *Good Vibrations: My Autobiography*, London, Hutchinson, 1990, p. 46.
9 John Milton, *Samson Agonistes*, ll. 94–7.

whose auditory nerve has been totally destroyed can pick up sounds by other means, and people who lose their hearing suddenly may take some time to realize what has happened to them. There was a Cornish boy called John Kitto, for example, who was twelve years old when, in 1817, he fell from a roof where he was working with his stonemason father. He was carried home, and lay motionless for several days, surrounded by his anxious family. As he regained consciousness, Kitto saw his relatives talking to each other over his sickbed, and at first he was grateful for their quietness. 'I thought,' he recalled, 'that, out of regard to my feeble condition, they spoke in whispers, because I heard them not.' As he gained strength, though, their considerateness began to irk him, and he started to wish for conversation. 'Why do you not speak?' he cried out impatiently. In reply, they wrote upon a slate the awful words 'YOU ARE DEAF'.[10]

'No one inhabits a world of total silence,' according to the poet David Wright, who lost his auditory nerve through illness when he was seven. (He was encouraged in his vocation by the example of other deaf poets – Joachim du Bellay, Pierre de Ronsard, Jack Clemo.) Wright recalls that at first he did not realize what had happened. 'How was I to know?' he says. 'Nobody told me.' He had to 'deduce the fact of deafness through a process of reasoning'. He heard guns, motorbikes, lorries, crowds and drills by touch: 'there can't be much I miss,' as he said, 'of the normal orchestration of urban existence.' He could appreciate music too, resting his finger on a piano or a loudspeaker. And in a room with a wooden floor he would listen to drums and string instruments through his feet. There is no such thing as complete deafness, he concludes: and 'it is not necessary to be able to hear in order to hear'.[11]

The overlap between touch and hearing suggests that – contrary to my childhood ruminations on the question, and despite the opinion of Bishop Berkeley – hearing may actually be more earthy and materialistic than vision. At least it seems obvious that light is less solid, less grossly real, than sound – that it has 'less being', as Aristotle would have it, or is 'less substantial'.[12] There is an effortless superiority about

---

10 John Kitto, *The Lost Senses: Series I – Deafness*, London, Charles Knight, 1845, p. 11.
11 David Wright, *Deafness: A Personal Account*, London, Allen Lane, 1969, pp. 22, 10–11, 9, 104.
12 Aristotle, *Problemata* XI, 904b.

the way light travels – silently, instantaneously and in perfect straight lines. (It was these ideal and aristocratic qualities of light that led inventors like Castel and Rimington to think of colour as the medium for a higher music, freed from the material impediments of sound.) Sound, in contrast, is sluggish and laborious: it moves much slower, drifting aimlessly and letting itself get carried away by the wind.

On the other hand, sound possesses a kind of ponderous strength that light cannot rival: it can penetrate solid walls, boom through the depths of the ocean, go round corners, shatter delicate glasses, or force its way through the earth. It has a kind of gross clumsiness as well, and sounds which travel together through space get all tangled and messed up together, unlike rays of light. (This is part of what makes music possible, and it dashed the hopes of the colour-musicians.)

In many ways sounds are like material substances, though in a very fluid state. Prospero's island was 'full of noises, Sounds, and sweet airs, that give delight, and hurt not',[13] as if they were perfumes wafting from an incense-burner. 'My spirit like a charmed bark doth swim,' Shelley said, 'Upon the liquid waves of thy sweet singing'[14] – as if sound was gushing from his beloved's mouth like water from a fountain, or blood from a wound. And Marvell spoke complainingly of the fair singer, 'Whose subtle art invisibly can wreathe my fetters of the very air I breathe.'[15]

Some eighteenth-century scientists went so far as to argue that sounds consist of particles of 'sound-matter'.[16] Different kinds of 'phonic substance' resided within different materials – wood, flesh, or metal, for example – rather like seeds inside a pod, and they were gradually released when the object was struck or twisted or scraped. But the difficulty of tracing or weighing these hypothetical particles, or explaining where they came from and what they did when not actually sounding made the concept of sound-matter rather fatuous, and it did not survive for long.[17]

13 Shakespeare, *The Tempest*, II. iv. 147.
14 Percy Bysshe Shelley, 'Fragment: to one Singing', 1817.
15 Andrew Marvell, 'The Fair Singer', from *Miscellaneous Poems*, 1681.
16 According to M. J. Petry, the idea was given currency in Peter van Musschenbrock, *Introductio ad philosophiam naturalem*, 1762. See Hegel, *Philosophy of Nature*, edited by M. J. Petry, London, George Allen and Unwin, 1970, Vol. 2, p. 282.
17 Aristotle put forward an idea of potential sounds (*De Anima*, Book II, 419b5ff.) but he did not conceive of potentiality as a calculable force.

Contemplating this disarray in physical theory, Hegel concluded that sounds were intrinsically ambiguous. They belonged in part to the 'mechanical sphere', and he even described them as a kind of 'mechanical light'; but they also enjoyed a certain 'freedom from heavy matter', which made them 'soul-like rather than material'. And this ontological ambiguity was intrinsically edifying, according to Hegel, because it exhibited matter in its materiality aspiring towards an existence in 'a higher sphere', and trying to speak directly to our 'inner soul'.[18] Aristotle had been right to think that hearing is specially connected with character and morality,[19] for sound was nothing other than 'the plaint of ideal nature in the midst of violence', and an anticipation of something 'immaterial' and 'spiritual'.[20] It was not eyesight but hearing that was the true sense of the ideal, liberating us from our dependence on the visible material world.

Berkeley too had recognized a natural affinity between idealism and the experience of sound: that is why his campaign against materialism concentrated on vision, and especially on ridiculing the idea that our eyes can see the outness of things. And when the passionately materialistic young Diderot took up arms against idealism, he accepted the same equation: materialism was based specifically on visual experience, he said, and idealism was an 'extravagant system, which must have been invented by the blind'.[21] But experience was to deepen Diderot's sympathies for blind people, and, by his logic, for idealism too. In 1760 he met a young woman called Mélanie de Salignac, whom he was to describe as 'the most extraordinary blind person who has ever existed, or ever will'. She was just sixteen, but 'she had a great fund of reason', as Diderot recalled in his mellow and sentimental old age, 'a sweet charm, an unusual sharpness of ideas, and great simplicity.' Mélanie was exquisitely sensitive to sounds, conscious of auditory subtleties that eluded everyone else, and even expressed pity for her sighted friends, who were so distracted by the visible world that they could not thrill to music as she did – 'as if I were going to die for joy,' she claimed. Mélanie was high-minded, too: neither swayed by the charms

18 Hegel, *Philosophy of Nature*, §300, Addition, pp. 70–1.
19 'The objects of no other sense have any resemblance to moral qualities.' Aristotle, *Politics*, Book VIII, 1340a-b.
20 Hegel, *Philosophy of Nature*, §300, pp. 71, 72.
21 Denis Diderot, *Lettre sur les aveugles* (1749), in Diderot, *Œuvres Philosophiques*, edited by Paul Vernière, Paris, Garnier, 1964, p. 114.

of youth, nor shocked by the wrinkles of old age. The only qualities she set store by were those of the heart and the mind. This, according to the elderly Diderot, was yet another advantage of blindness, especially in women. 'I shall never have my head turned,' the virtuous Mélanie told him, 'by a good-looking man.'[22] Diderot was desolated when his sweet idealist died, at the innocent age of twenty-two.

David Hume also took an interest in the moral experience of the blind. Thomas Blacklock was an Edinburgh poet who had lost his sight in infancy through smallpox, and Hume once asked him to explain how he could include words referring to colours in his verses, when he had no ideas of the qualities they stood for. Blacklock replied that he managed on the basis of associations – 'false' associations of an 'intellectual' kind, as Hume insisted, since they were derived not from Blacklock's own impressions but from the conversation of his sighted acquaintances. What he lacked in sensations, he made up for with words. The implications of the case excited Hume's curiosity:

> I once said to my friend, Mr Blacklock, that I was sure he did not treat love as he did colours; he did not speak of it without feeling it . . . 'Alas!' said he, with a sigh, 'I could never bring my heart to a proper tranquillity on that head.' Your passion, replied I, will always be better founded than ours, who have sight: we are so foolish as to allow ourselves to be captivated by exterior beauty: nothing but beauty of the mind can affect you. 'Not altogether neither,' said he: 'the sweetness of the voice has a mighty effect upon me: the symptoms of youth too, which the touch discovers, have great influence.'

The touch? Hume was perplexed, so Blacklock went on to explain: 'the girls of my acquaintance indulge me, on account of my blindness, with the liberty of running over them with my hand,' so that he was able to 'judge entirely of their shape'. Hume was disappointed, and perhaps a little peeved. 'You may see from this conversation,' he concluded, 'how difficult it is even for a blind man to be a perfect Platonic.'[23]

22 Denis Diderot, *Additions à la lettre sur les aveugles* (1782), in Diderot, *Œuvres Philosophiques*, pp. 155, 157, 159.
23 Letter to Joseph Spence, 15 October 1754, in *The Letters of David Hume*, edited by J. Y. T. Greig, 2 Vols, Oxford, Oxford University Press, 1932, Vol. 1, p. 202. See also Ernest Campbell Mossner, *The Life of David Hume* (1954), second edition, Oxford, Oxford University Press, 1980, pp. 379–80.

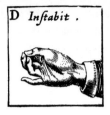

4

Grammar, sound and horror

Unfortunately, all these physical and metaphysical inquiries into the nature of light and sound seem to have led us nowhere. Colour-musicians like Kircher, Castel and Rimington may have convinced themselves of the ideality of light, consigning sound to the flesh if not the devil. But philosophers like Berkeley, Diderot and Hegel, though conceding that sound is in some ways more tangible and substantial than light, still maintained that it was more ideal and subjective, closer to the inner soul and less involved with the 'outness' of an objective material world. All their various reasonings seem, therefore, to point in opposite directions and cancel each other out.

In any case, none of this has much to do with my own starting point – my cheerful childhood preference for vision over the other senses. For what interested me was not the physics of light as such, nor the metaphysics of colours or visible forms. I cared for the *things* that I could see – my tricycle and my hammer, food and drink, paddling pools and pieces of wood, or my brother, my sister and our cats and chickens – all of which mattered to me much more than the objects of the other senses, whether tastes, smells, textures or sounds. About this, Berkeley was surely right: the sense of sight differs from the others in that – whether deceptively or not – it always holds out the promise of orienting us within a world of real material things. It seems to introduce us directly to objects as they really are, substantially and in

41

themselves. Of course, Berkeley regarded it as a false promise: if we were not careful, he warned, it would seduce us into believing in the existence of substantial independent physical objects. And who is to say he was wrong? The temptation was certainly too strong for me: I used to yield without a struggle, convinced that my eyes, far more than my other senses, led me straight up to the actual, unarguable bodily reality of *things*.

I am not sure quite what I would have meant by that word, but the thinghood of things seemed to me then, as it still does, an instinctive concept, primordial and perhaps indispensable. It covered all the every-day objects that I cared about, everything I could not avoid or ignore. Things (as opposed to nothings) included people, animals, plants, in fact all the items I could in any way be concerned with.[1] The weight and solidity of things, as revealed by touching, pushing or shoving, obviously contributed a lot to my idea of their thinghood; but it was through my eyes that I acquired most of my knowledge concerning them. My sense of things seemed to be the natural partner of my sense of sight. What horrified me about the idea of going blind was the thought of being cut off from this visible world of things. My eyes were uncompromising materialists, and I was just their loyal disciple.[2]

But why should ears be considered any less thing-centred than eyes? They are just as much part of the physical world, after all. Heidegger, for example, concluded that hearing has exactly the same architecture as vision, in that we hear things rather than qualities – 'never noises or complexes of sounds, but the creaking wagon, or the motor cycle . . . the column on the march, the north wind, the woodpecker tapping, the fire crackling.'[3] The idea of a 'bare sound' was a metaphysical abstraction. To hear sound as sound was to hear badly – to 'listen away from things, divert our ear from them, i.e. listen abstractly'.[4] When we hear truly, therefore, we hear things rather than sounds.

1 See Martin Heidegger, 'The Thing' (1950), translated by Albert Hofstadter in *Poetry, Language, Thought*, New York, Harper and Row, 1971, pp. 165–86.
2 The sort of perceptual experience described in the title essay in Oliver Sacks, *The Man who mistook his Wife for a Hat*, London, Duckworth, 1985, pp. 7–21, might perhaps be described as thingless seeing, and it would not be devastating in any perceptual field except vision, and perhaps touch.
3 Martin Heidegger, *Being and Time*, §34, p. 266.
4 '*Um ein reines Geräusch zu hören, müssen wir von den Dingen weghören.*' Martin Heidegger, 'The Origin of the Work of Art' (1950), translated by Albert Hofstadter in *Poetry, Language, Thought*, p. 26.

Or so Heidegger thought. But perhaps this realistic common sense about hearing was itself tainted by a metaphysical 'listening away'. Granted that what we see is things rather than qualities, it does not follow that the same applies to hearing; in fact this may be precisely the point where seeing and hearing part company.

When you wake in a bright dawn, what you see is your room and the things in it, not the sun which radiates the light in which you see them. But if a bustling market is taking place outside, you will hear the shouts of the traders and the murmur of the shoppers, not your room and its contents resonating to them. Even if they make a perceptible echo, what you attend to will be the original sound, not the surface from which it has been reflected. You do not hear your room crowded with street noises, as you see it flooded with sunlight; you do not hear things in the sound as you see them in the light.

If you wake up in the middle of the night, surrounded by utter darkness and absolute silence, you may perhaps sense a certain difference between them. The two null experiences are not the same: darkness is dense, thick and full, one might say, whereas silence is sheer expectant emptiness. Darkness signifies the temporary invisibility of things you would otherwise be able to see: it is impenetrable, because it prevents you from seeing them. Silence, however, does not impede your hearing, or muffle sounds that would otherwise be audible. It signifies a positive absence of sound: it is not opaque, but deathly.

These differences are not a simple consequence of the physical or metaphysical properties of light and sound, but rather of what might be called the grammar or semantics of perceptual experience – the principles that determine which categories of objects are placed in the foreground of sight and hearing respectively. Your eyes, in the main, reveal things more or less well illuminated; it is only in rare cases – if you are looking at the stars for instance, or a blazing fire, or the tail-lights of cars – that the objects you see are the origin of their own illumination. In other words, light and its sources are not, as a rule, the *objects* that you see: you look at the things light makes visible, rather than at the light itself. But the grammar of hearing is quite different: the objects which concern your hearing are always either sounds or sources of sound.

It is this grammatical fact which explains, more satisfactorily than physics or metaphysics, why the objects of hearing are elusive and insubstantial wraiths compared with those of vision. We do not really hear wagons, motorbikes, woodpeckers, or fires; rather we hear them creak, roar, and clatter, or whistle, crackle and hiss. Ordinary language has an astonishing abundance of names for the fleeting, unthinglike events which constitute sounds, not to mention its huge vocabulary for actions defined through the noise they make, such as flapping, slurping, coughing, slapping, bonking, juddering, beating, or hooting. It is no wonder that Hegel, who deplored all kinds of luxury and wastefulness, worked himself into a lather of indignation at the 'completely superfluous richness' of the lexicon used for describing sounds, and the profligacy with which feckless poets keep adding to it.[5] With the possible exception of obscenities – which may not really be a separate field anyway – there is no sector of our vocabularies which is so uninhibited and extravagant, or so open to popular improvisation and inventiveness, as that which represents the world of sound.

One reason for the proliferation of sound-words must be that language itself exists in the form of sounds, and therefore automatically calls sounds to mind. But the phenomenon is also grounded in the grammatical fact that hearing is concerned with qualities that are exclusively audible – sounds or sound effects – whereas vision is more at home with objects that can also be identified in non-visual terms – with solid, durable, material things. There is not even any special word for visual sensations in general, or for directly visible qualities – no word which covers everything that can be seen, in the way that 'sound' serves for the entire range of what can be heard. (*Sights, visions, views, light* and *appearances* come quite close, but none of them has the simple aptness or neutral generality of the word *sounds*.) It is also very unusual to express visual experiences in purely visual language – in terms of hues or flashes or gleams – rather than referring them directly to material things. The vocabulary for describing specifically visual aspects of experience is comparatively sparse, even colourless: popular coinages are dully iconic (with a remarkable affinity for exotic fruit, flowers and vegetables – *pistachio, olive* and *aubergine* for example, or Newton's *orange* and *violet*); and after that the language of colour

5 Hegel, *Philosophy of Nature*, §300, Addition, Vol. 2, p. 71; Petry's editorial note on pp. 282–3 refers to an authority who cited no fewer than 53 words for sounds in early nineteenth-century German.

is professional, technical and scientific (*cyan, magenta,* or *strontian yellow*).

Hearing has to be content to live in a world of sounds – floating, ungraspable, and weightless nothings that they are; unlike vision, it cannot pretend to deal only with real solid things. Wordsworth, hearing an early cuckoo, was aware of a song, a mystery – 'a wandering voice', but not a bird.[6] What your ears catch first is the tumult, not the crowd, the tune before the orchestra. When you listen to music, you hear compound structures of harmony and melody, rather than the separate strings, pipes, reeds or throats which collaborate to produce them. Or, to put it differently, the things that occupy your auditory experience are sounds rather than material objects. Considered physically or metaphysically, light may or may not be less material than sound; but considered as an experience, hearing is decidedly less materialistic than seeing.

The materialism of vision – its implicit promise to place us directly in the midst of a world of things – makes it peculiarly liable to illusions, and that is why the so-called 'optical' illusions are dramatic, tenacious and universal. No one can help thinking that the sun or moon looks bigger and closer when near the horizon than when high in the sky. Everyone is liable to be tricked by the devices of classical architecture, where columns are tapered to make them look taller, or galleries narrowed towards the end to make them seem longer. Similar effects are manipulated in experimental psychology, with its Muller-Lyer arrows and the Ames room, whose sloping ceiling and slanting back wall create bewilderingly paradoxical perspectives. Even after we have realized that our eyes are deceiving us, and even if we have understood exactly how they do it, we will still be subject to the illusion – even though, as Kant says, we may eventually learn not to be deceived by it.[7]

What makes optical illusions peculiarly disturbing, apart from their cussed persistence, is that they confuse us about the dimensions of physical objects and their positions and spatial relations. They perplex our assumptions about how the space in which we move and act is organized; in fact they threaten them with catastrophic meltdown.

6 William Wordsworth, 'To the Cuckoo,' 1807.
7 Immanuel Kant, *Critique of Pure Reason*, A 297, B 354, translated by Norman Kemp Smith, London, Macmillan, 1933, p. 300.

Hearing, however, is not much bothered by such perceptual glitches. The reason is not that it is particularly reliable – you can easily mistake birdsong for a telephone, or confuse two people's voices. But auditory mistakes are never more than isolated errors: unlike optical illusions they do not systematically threaten your sense of how things fit together in space. When your ears mislead you, you have simply failed to recognize a sound. It is like seeing people in the distance and hailing them as old friends, only to discover, when you get closer, that you have never met them before – a visual illusion, one might say, but not an optical one. Of course you may be tricked by the effect of echoes into thinking that a shout has come from in front of you when it really came from behind, and ventriloquists are supposed to 'throw' their voices so that they appear to be coming from a different direction. Or you may think a band is drawing closer or going further away, when it is really only playing louder and softer, or the wind has changed. But none of us sets much store by our capacity to establish distances, directions, or locations through our sense of hearing; we can always be far more certain that there was a sound than we can of what made it or where it came from.

The fundamental difference between auditory and optical mistakes arises from the fact that we are less tempted to attribute 'outness' to what we hear than to what we see. Hearing does not presume as much as vision. It is not so arrogant, and it is willing to refer its experiences to evanescent qualities without insisting, as sight does, that they have to be tethered unambiguously to definite things in the material world. The ear is not hung up on the reality of things: it is happy to live modestly in a world of sounds which, as Proust wrote, 'have no position in space'.[8] Thanks to its spatial agnosticism, hearing suffers from no perceptual paradoxes to parallel the optical illusions.

On the other hand, the spatial indeterminacy of sounds means that auditory illusions can be even more disconcerting than either optical or visual ones. If you wake in the middle of the night to see frightful half-human forms stalking your bed, you can always switch on the light in the hope that they will resolve themselves into a bedpost or a

8 See the extended discussion of sound in Marcel Proust, *Le Côté de Guermantes: A la recherche du temps perdu*, Vol. 2, pp. 74–8; *The Guermantes Way: Remembrance of Things Past*, Vol. 2, pp. 73–5.

jumble of clothes on a chair. If your first visual impressions do not tally with your later investigations, they can be discounted and attributed to your imagination instead. But sounds are not amenable to that kind of reality-testing and cross-checking, since they do not make any such definite claims to spatial location. If you think you hear something strange – your whispered name as you stand alone in a susurrating wood, or footsteps in a deserted house – you have no reliable way of reassuring yourself that it was only an illusion. You may be able to establish that there was no one there, but that does not prove that you heard no sound. It must be for this reason that the conscience, considered as an intensely personal but also fiercely peremptory source of morality, is always thought of as calling and speaking to us – a voice or summons that comes to each of us individually from nowhere and everywhere at the same time.[9] How could you ever prove the unreality of the call, and show that it was only imaginary? And what would make a sound unreal anyway?

Vision differs from hearing in that it permits a far tidier separation between illusion and reality. In fact most of the vocabulary in which the distinction is customarily framed – beginning with words like *ideal*, *imaginary* and *fantastic* – is rooted in the theory of visual experience, and it gets confused when transplanted to the less substantial world of sounds. Your vision may be disturbed by after-images, or opacities inside your eyeballs, or as a result of a migraine; but these effects are too unsteady to be scrutinized like ordinary visible objects. If you suffer from tinnitus, however, or if the sound of your breathing or your pulse disturbs you, then you can hear the ringings, whistles and thumps, and listen to them just as objectively as any other sounds. The fact that they originate inside you does not make them seem at all unreal.

Theorists of dreams often treat them as if they were largely or even exclusively visual. But in fact it is often the 'contact' senses which provide the stuff that dreams are made of, and when we dream of tastes or smells or bodily sensations, we experience them as if they were really affecting us physically. Often enough, in fact, we rouse ourselves to find that they are genuine perceptions, forming a kind of bridge into the waking world: the same experience figures in both

---

9 On the call of conscience, see Heidegger, *Being and Time*, §§55–59, pp. 315–41.

fading dream and dawning reality. But whilst the linking events are sometimes tastes, smells or sensations, they are more usually sounds. Sounds in dreams are always dreamt as if they were actually resonating in our ears; and we will often wake to find that in fact they are doing so in reality: it was with good reason that Freud called these half-real dream-experiences 'alarm clock-dreams'.[10]

Sounds are the perfect material not just for dreams, but for madness too: for systemic uncertainty about the dividing line between reality and imagination, or indeed life and death. Hallucinations and paranoid delusions, in particular, take advantage of the peculiar unarguability of the experience of hearing. In the celebrated memoir he wrote in 1902 in order to prove his sanity and secure his release from an asylum in Leipzig, Dr Daniel Paul Schreber explained how his troubles had begun several years before, as he found himself assailed by scratching and crackling noises whenever he tried to get some sleep. At first he thought they were caused by mice behind the walls. But then he established that there were certainly no mice in his house; and yet he could still hear the crackling and scratching when he went to bed. Dr Schreber kept hold of his scientific objectivity however. 'Having heard similar noises innumerable times since then . . . I have come to recognise them as undoubted divine miracles,' he wrote coolly. There were mysterious patterns in the sound too, which he concluded must be fragments of speech in '*nerve-language*', repeated over and over again inside his head: he was reminded, he said, of 'a child learning a poem by heart'. And then there were the 'wandering clocks, that is to say souls of departed heretics . . . preserved for centuries under glass in medieval cloisters . . . who announced their survival by a vibration connected with an infinitely monotonous and doleful humming noise'. For seven years Schreber had to put up with this racket, night and day, but it only strengthened his resolve that 'God must never succeed in his purpose of destroying my reason'.[11]

Schreber's superhuman efforts to defend his rationality in the face

10 Sigmund Freud, *The Interpretation of Dreams*, (1900), I (C)(1), translated by James Strachey, *Standard Edition of the Complete Psychological Works of Sigmund Freud*, Vol. IV, 1953, pp. 27–9.
11 Daniel Paul Schreber, *Denkwürdigkeiten eines Nervenkranken*, Leipzig, 1903, pp. 37–8, 46, 96–7, 288; translated by Ida Macalpine and Richard A. Hunter, *Memoirs of my Nervous Illness*, London, William Dawson, 1955, pp. 64, 69, 100, 211.

of this unrelenting barrage of sounds impressed his judges, and they granted him his freedom. It is possible that he would not have been so lucky if he had claimed to be seeing things: in that case the judges might have decided that he was subject to dangerous illusions. But with sounds it is different: how could they argue with the authenticity of the sounds he heard, or expect him to treat them as mere hallucinations? The miraculous foreign languages and the monotonous humming sounds were as much part of his everyday auditory experience as his conversations with his wife or doctor, and there was no valid way of persuading him that they were any less real. Sounds, being intangible and unverifiable, make ideal raw material for the 'work of delusion-formation' (as Freud called it) on which Dr Schreber laboured unstintingly for so many years.[12]

Story-tellers, too, like to exploit the uncanny insubstantiality of sound and its affinity with the work of delusion-formation. In Jules Verne's *Carpathian Castle*, for instance, a group of drinkers gathers one evening at the inn of a little Transylvanian village, where an intrepid young man is planning to climb up to the mysterious ruin which lies a few leagues off through the forest. Suddenly a voice reverberates through the room: 'Do not try to approach the castle,' it intones. But none of the company has spoken, and no one can tell where the voice can have come from. The inference is unavoidable: a ghost, a supernatural manifestation, a message from the other side. Eventually, despite this warning from the 'voice of shadows', the villager sets off, accompanied by a young Count who has recently returned from a sojourn in Italy. Once in the vicinity of the castle, the Count swoons, and it seems to him he can hear the most ravishing sound in the world – the voice of the great soprano La Stilla, with whom he had fallen in love on his travels, attending every single night of her triumphant season in Naples. She had eventually consented to forsake her operatic career and become his wife; but at her farewell performance he watched in horror as she collapsed and died in the full flood of her greatest aria. Its phrases were sculpted in his heart, and naturally they returned to haunt his dreams. But now, outside the mysterious castle, the sounds do not disperse as he surfaces from

---

12 '*Wahnbildungsarbeit*': see Sigmund Freud, *Psychoanalytic Notes on an Autobiographical Account of a Case of Paranoia (Schreber)* (1911), translated by James Strachey, *Standard Edition of the Complete Psychological Works of Sigmund Freud*, Vol. XII, 1958, p. 38.

unconsciousness. The voice of La Stilla echoes through the crumbling vaults as unmistakably as ever it did through the auditorium of the San Carlo opera house. The young lover cannot doubt what he is hearing, and has no choice but to trace the sound back to its source, and reunite himself with the voice that sings to him from beyond the grave.[13]

Edgar Allan Poe also understood the unique power of auditory experience as a means of undermining our sanity: the inventor of the horror story was always an orchestrator of unattributable sounds. The narrator of 'The Tell-Tale Heart', for instance, tells us that he is endowed with exceptionally sharp sensory powers, above all a remarkable sense of hearing. He has entered the pitch-dark room of an old man he plans to kill, but his thumb has slipped on the fastening of his lantern, making a slight noise. The old man has woken, and tried to convince himself it was only a mouse crossing the floor, or a cricket which has made a single chirp. But all in vain: the old man cannot master his terror, and the murderer's ears are now filled with the throbbing of the old man's frightened heart. It beats a 'hellish tattoo . . . quicker and quicker and louder and louder every instant . . . amid the dreadful silence of that old house', until at last he is impelled to leap up and suffocate the old man, and put an end to the horrible thundering. Afterwards, he dismembers the body and stashes it underneath the floor. When the police arrive he feels no fear; but then a dull thudding starts up again in his ears. It grows clearer and more definite . . . 'until, at length, I found that the noise was *not* within my ears'. Is he mad then? Certainly not: 'I heard all things in the heaven and in the earth,' he explains. 'I heard many things in hell. How, then, am I mad?' The sound grows louder and louder, and in the end he tears up the planks to reveal its source – the dead man's heart, still beating out its awful tattoo. The murderer was merely gifted with a terrible sharpness of hearing: 'What you mistake for madness,' he says, 'is but over-acuteness of the senses.'[14]

---

13 Jules Verne, *Le château des Carpathes*, Paris, Hetzel, 1892.
14 Edgar Allan Poe, 'The Tell-Tale Heart' (1843), *Collected Works*, edited by T. O. Mabbott, Harvard University Press, 1978, Vol. 3, pp. 792–7.

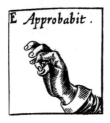

5

Listening with the voice

When I was a child, I used to love playing about with my visual world. I would spend hours shutting first one eye then the other, making things move from left to right and back again, or watching distorted people through old-fashioned irregular windowpanes, or making faces at my misshapen reflection in the back of a shiny spoon. I held pieces of paper with the edge against my nose, so that I could see both sides at the same time; strained my eyes downwards trying to catch sight of my lips and tongue; and moved my eyeballs with my hands to get them to look in two different directions at once. I was intrigued too by the way I could still see a kind of red luminosity when I shut my eyes in the sunshine, and I enjoyed staring at bright lights and then looking away, and trying to inspect the darting after-images. And so on and on and on: the visual field was a playground to me, an endless source of experimental diversions.

But there were not many such games to be played with my hearing. I had no real control over my ears, for a start. They could not be closed or swivelled, and though I might block them with my fingers, I could not shut out external sound completely; in any case there was the ceaseless internal concert of my breathing and swallowing, and the eerie continuo of my beating heart. All I could do with my ears was take them with me to different places, like a pair of buckets, and wait for them to collect whatever sounds happened to drop into them.

Visual perception, in contrast, is distinctly voluntary and subject to intellectual control. Often it takes the form of deliberately *looking*, rather than merely seeing – looking *at* what is present, or *for* what is absent. It is as if the visual field were overlaid with a target-shaped view-finder, with a bull's-eye in the middle and concentric circles of diminishing attention shading off towards the outermost horizon. Looking, as opposed to seeing, means training one's eyes on this focal point, and concentrating one's gaze upon it.

It is natural to suppose that listening is the auditory counterpart of such concentrated looking: listening is to hearing, it might seem, as looking is to seeing. But the parallel is not exact. Although you may cup an ear with a hand, or put your ear to the ground, hearing is not intrinsically spatial: there is no auditory 'field' to compare to the visual one. Listening to or for a given sound – a specific instrument in the orchestra, a certain kind of birdsong in the dawn chorus – means analysing the total sound-effect and picking out some aspect of it; it is more like attending to some particular element of a smell or flavour than focusing your gaze on a visible object. You may well find it simpler if you can have a look – it is far easier to separate the sounds of the different instruments of an orchestra if you can see the musicians playing them – but listening is not itself a matter of homing in on a definite zone or object in a spatial field. It is only by a precarious analogical extension that the idea of concentration gets transferred from looking to listening.[1]

Vision is for the most part sheer self-commanding voluntariness compared with hearing, which appears to be little more than supine passivity. The ideas of visual concentration and freewill are closely similar, and they may indeed be somehow connected. Some psychoanalysts would even align the eyes with masculinity and the ears with femininity – vision being rigid, detached, and demanding, whilst hearing is fluid, responsive and selfless. According to many of them, in fact, sexual differentiation is itself rooted in visual experience, starting with the traumatic ocular proof that the little boy has something 'strikingly visible' which the little girl lacks.[2] (This is supposed to explain

1 For a superb discussion of auditory attention, see Don Ihde, *Listening and Voice: A Phenomenology of Sound*, Athens, Ohio University Press, 1976.
2 Sigmund Freud, 'Some Psychical Consequences of the Anatomical Distinction between the Sexes' (1925), translated by James Strachey, *Standard Edition*, Vol. XIX, 1961, p. 252.

why masculinity is typically identified with a stern, objectivizing gaze, and femininity with a warm and obedient embrace; but it stumbles when confronted with the fact that girls can see the difference as well as boys, and that sexual differentiation does not take particularly unusual paths in those born blind.)

Some apprehension of the lowliness of hearing compared with the lordliness of vision can be found sedimented in the depths of our vocabularies. The German language suggests that hearing or hearkening is related to belonging (*hören/gehören*); and, in Latin, obedience (*ob-audire*) appears as a kind of listening. In several languages, including English, many verbs designating different modes of sensory perception can be turned round and applied to the activity of their objects. You look at something, to find out how it looks; you smell how it smells, feel how it feels, and taste how it tastes. But the verbs 'listen' and 'hear' cannot be reversed out in the same way: you do not listen to how things listen, or hear how they hear. All you can listen to or hear is how they *sound*. Hearing, it seems, has nothing active in it: it is mere supine susceptibility. Hearing, as Theodor Adorno once put it, appears 'unconcentrated and passive . . . dozy and inert'.[3]

The idea that auditory perception is passive compared with seeing and looking seems to forget, however, that hearing and listening may also, in their way, be means of active inquiry, and methods of orienting oneself in the world. Doctors specialize in it and call it auscultation: investigating a patient's internal organs by means of the ear, perhaps assisted by a stethoscope (literally: chest viewer). But auscultation is part of common experience as well. Becoming acquainted with buildings or landscapes is partly a matter of getting to know their acoustic profiles – listening to the sounds they produce, and the echoes they give back. You are not really at home in a place until you have made yourself familiar with how it sounds and resounds. Part of the special personality of the limestone landscapes of Yorkshire, for instance, derives – as Ruskin once noted – from the watery whispers, murmurs, patters and gushes emitted by intermittent underground streams.[4] And

3 Theodor Adorno and Hanns Eisler, *Komposition für den Film*, Munich, 1969, pp. 41, 43, cited in Adorno, *In Search of Wagner*, translated by Rodney Livingstone, London, New Left Books, 1981, pp. 99–100.
4 John Ruskin, *Praeterita* (1885–9), Oxford, Oxford University Press, 1978, p. 151.

Wordsworth, when he recalled the lakeland hills where his early feelings were formed, spoke of their 'audible seclusions, dashing lakes, Echoes and waterfalls, and pointed crags That into music touch the passing wind'.[5]

On the whole, though, exploratory listening attends to artificial sounds deliberately produced, not natural ones that are occurring anyway. Doctors drum on the patient's chest with their fingers and listen to how it responds; or you may drop a stone down a well and count how long it takes before you hear it plop into the water, or locate the struts in a hollow wall by tapping along it. 'Suppose you are stuck in a building in the middle of the night,' Rousseau says in *Émile*. 'Just clap your hands: you will be able to tell, from the resonance, whether the space you are in is large or small, whether you are in the centre or in a corner.'[6]

William Gilpin, the eighteenth-century English traveller who is credited with inventing the taste for the picturesque, cultivated a particular interest in how landscapes appeared to the ear. The traveller in the Lake District should pay great attention, he said, to the differences in aural scenery between Derwentwater, Windermere and Ullswater. On Ullswater, in fact, the Duke of Portland had obligingly equipped a boat with several brass cannon which could be fired one after the other to awaken the local echoes – an amenity which later became available to tourists in the Alps as well.[7] 'Such a variety of awful sounds, mixing and commixing, and at the same moment heard from all sides, have a wonderful effect on the mind,' Gilpin told his readers; and the performance was instructive from a geographical point of view too, providing 'a sort of aerial perspective' on the entire valley. But a small wind-band worked even better than the Duke's cannon. A few French horns and clarinets could send their harmonious sounds dancing round the lake to produce a thousand symphonies, and a quantity of notes that would amaze the most musical ear: 'in short, every rock is vocal,

5 William Wordsworth, *The Prelude* (1850), edited by Ernest de Selincourt, second edition, Oxford, Clarendon Press, 1959, Book Eight, ll. 636–8.
6 Jean-Jacques Rousseau, *Émile*, p. 139.
7 As one traveller recorded in 1838: 'Half a mile from Bonneville – to the Café at Balme, where I paused on my own account to honour the grotto with a cannon shot; the grotto returned the compliment with a thunderous rumbling.' See Henriette d'Angeville, *My Ascent of Mont Blanc*, translated by Jennifer Barnes, London, HarperCollins, 1991, p. 7.

and the whole lake is transformed into a kind of magical scene; in which every promontory seems peopled by aerial beings, answering each other in celestial music.'[8]

Travellers who were not equipped with a boatload of cannon or a consort of wind instruments could presumably achieve much the same effect by shouting, singing or hallooing to the lakes, rousing the local echoes by the power of their own voices. Gilpin did not canvass this possibility, however: no doubt he would have found it rather indecorous. But Rousseau, who was less prone to embarrassment, or at least less averse to it, was fascinated by the part the voice could play in our auditory exploring. He admitted that hearing might be lazy, inert and beyond our voluntary control; but he pointed out that it had a unique advantage over all the other bodily senses, since it alone was paired with an 'active organ'. 'We have an organ which corresponds to hearing, namely, that of the voice,' he said. (He was in fact taking his cue from Buffon, who argued in his *Natural History* that an animal's sense of hearing is a 'passive property', whereas the human faculty of hearing 'becomes active through the organ of speech'.)[9] The pivotal position of vocalization in the experience of sounds meant that in their case active production and passive perception grew up in the closest possible connection: the voice was educated through hearing, and hearing through the voice. 'We have no such thing corresponding to vision,' Rousseau observed, because 'we cannot give forth colours as we can sounds.'[10]

The special bond between hearing and the voice is so obvious that it is easy to miss both its oddity and its significance; but Rousseau's observation deserves to rank amongst the key theorems in any philosophy of sensory experience. You can use your voice to populate your auditory world at will, and nothing remotely comparable applies to the other senses. You cannot make your body emit colours for the entertainment of your eyes, nor smells or tastes or tactile surfaces to please your nose, your tongue or your fingertips. Artists like Leonardo da Vinci – who sustained a constant inquiry into the way things look

8 William Gilpin, *Observations, relative chiefly to picturesque beauty, made in the year 1772, of several parts of England*, London, 1786, Vol. 2, pp. 59–62.
9 Georges-Louis Leclerc, Comte de Buffon, *Histoire Naturelle*, Vol. 3, Paris, 1749, p. 347.
10 Rousseau, *Emile*, p. 161.

by making sketches in little notebooks – are perhaps trying to get into the same relation to their visual world that every hearing person already enjoys with sounds simply by virtue of possessing a voice. But making drawings will always be at a disadvantage compared with vocalizing, because it needs a supply of inks, chalks, and paper, not to mention light, and hands free from other work. You cannot draw while walking, cooking, digging or dancing. In any case, you cannot fill your surroundings with your drawings as you can fill them with the sound of your voice. The analogy between drawing and vocalizing would be much closer if we were able to make pictures appear on our palms at will; or even better, if we could turn ourselves into magic lanterns, or natural colour-harpsichords, effortlessly beaming illuminated images onto our surroundings at will. Only then would vision have an active counterpart corresponding to the voice in relation to hearing.

Ice-skating on the lakes with his boisterous friends, the young Wordsworth noticed how the din of their voices would smash against the crags and precipices, making them ring and tinkle like iron, and then roll back from distant hills with 'an alien sound Of melancholy'.[11] Later, he would sing out greetings to the empty fields and groves and bowers, intermixing the strains of his voice with their own melodies; and so, as he experienced it, he taught the hills the sounds of poetry, and discovered to his delight that 'they lacked not voice to welcome me in turn'.[12]

Such attributions of voices to nature may of course be mere poetic artifice, if not sentimental projection – typical, we may knowingly say, of the bad old romanticist habit of painting human emotions onto mountain scenery. When Coleridge, inspired by Mont Blanc, imagined how 'Earth, with her thousand voices, praises God',[13] or Wordsworth, under the influence of the same landscape, noticed 'The rocks that muttered close upon our ears,/Black drizzling crags that spake by the wayside/As if a voice were in them',[14] they were of course proposing analogies, even allegories. But when Coleridge described 'the brook's

---

11 Wordsworth, *The Prelude*, Book One, ll.438–444.
12 Wordsworth, *The Prelude*, Book Thirteen, ll.133–6 (see also the 1805 text, ll.139–40); Book Five, ll.173–6.
13 Samuel Taylor Coleridge, 'Hymn: Before Sunrise, in the Vale of Chamouni' (1802).
14 Wordsworth, 'The Simplon Pass' (1799).

chatter', or 'the breeze, murmuring indivisibly', it is less certain that he was abandoning literal statement in favour of metaphorical evocation.[15] If the very same sounds can be made by a natural process and a human voice, why insist that the epithets describing them have been transferred from humanity to nature? Might it not just as well be the other way round? May not chattering, singing, or murmuring be the proper activities of brooks and breezes, or birds and bees, as well as human beings? Who is to say that such a perception is only ever figurative, and never literal? Similarly, when Wordsworth heard the 'loud/Protracted yelling' of the ice-break on Esthwaite, or the 'roar of waters, torrents, streams' as he looked down at the Atlantic from the top of Snowdon, he could have been offering a direct description, not just a metaphor. You may suspect that he crossed the line into figuration when he spoke of them 'roaring with one voice', or when he portrayed the brooks as 'muttering along the stones';[16] but how could you ever be certain? The desire to segregate metaphorical from literal uses of words tends to overreach itself at the best of times, and it very soon becomes mere pedantry when applied to the description of sounds.[17]

The noisy vociferousness of nature as depicted in poetry – the endless murmurs of romantic streams, together with the yells, shouts, chatterings and mutterings of the mountains and lakes – are not blatant figurations, comparable to a smiling sun or a chaste moon. They need not be put down as relics of a 'pathetic fallacy', a transfer of epithets from humanity to nature: when it comes to sounds there is no clear and unbroken boundary between the two. For our voices are the radiant centre of our auditory world. We can use them like torches, as a means of exploration; but whilst a beam of light can only touch the surfaces of things, our voices go out and mingle with all the other sounds we hear. We use them as a probe for sounding out the world, and they draw us into it, and anchor us there. We hear with our voices as well as our ears, and it should therefore be no surprise if nature often turns out to sound uncannily familiar – in fact, very much like ourselves.

15 Coleridge, 'Lines written in the Album at Elbingerode' (1799).
16 Wordsworth, *The Prelude*, Book One, ll.539–43; Book Fourteen, ll.59–60; Book Twelve, ll.18–19.
17 Cf. Heidegger's observation that the idea of conscience as issuing a 'call' or having a 'voice' is more than just a 'picture' (*Being and Time*, §55, p. 316).

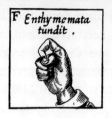

F *Enthymemata tundit .*

6

Voice as expression

It is hard to get away from the idea that we all have a concealed inner life as well as a public, outer one: our own secret garden where we can be alone with our thoughts, our private memories, hopes and fears, behind the wall of appearances that we present to the outside world. Such images of spiritual seclusion are probably the most constant and universal element in every variety of folk metaphysics. Each of us, we imagine, is essentially a self or soul, contained by our bodies like wine in a bottle, or cooped up inside our heads like a poor bird in its little cage. We think that we are essentially an inner self, and conceive our emotions as accumulations of energetic animal spirits which, if we do not discharge them regularly, will build up inside us until the pressure can no longer be contained. Or we picture ourselves as vulnerable little creatures who can either stay cowering apprehensively within our bodies, or stiffen their resolve and step out boldly into the dangerous traffic of the real objective world.

Traces of these ideas of private inwardness as opposed to outward expression can also be found all through the vocabulary of folk morality. Every contrast between sincerity and hypocrisy, for instance, or between what you are and what you do, every dramatic confrontation between your impulses and your attempts to keep them under control, suggests some kind of imaginary diagram of yourself as a world within the world, a soft subjective kernel inside a hard objective shell. In scientific psychology and physiology, too, it has been hard to escape the assumption that the nervous system must, like the well-ordered classical political state, have a single centre of command, to which incoming information is ultimately referred and which is finally responsible for all external actions. The same kind of imagery is usually implicated in beliefs about the possibility of surviving bodily death: a bubble of plasma, perhaps, slipping out of our mouths with the last breath, to be whisked away to an absolute elsewhere. And of course it also affects the movements of love: what is lurking there, I wonder, behind those dark shining eyes? And of anxiety and loss: is the one I love still in there, beneath that cold impassive mask?

The living of a human life, according to this way of imagining it, is a two-way process: there are perceptions or passions going in towards the centre, and expressions or actions coming back out. As far as the inward traffic is concerned, the basic facts have always seemed quite straightforward: the senses are so many gateways to the soul, supplemented perhaps by inner faculties such as fantasy, conscience or reflection. And the opposite process – self-mastery and the controlled outward expression of inner states – will be familiarly compared to a pilot steering a ship, a sovereign controlling the machinery of government, or a shepherd calling a dog to heel. But as Plato observed, the whole idea of self-mastery appears to be thoroughly contradictory. 'There is something ridiculous in the phrase *master of oneself*,' he says: 'for the master must also be the servant and the servant the master, since in all these modes of speaking the same person is denoted.'[1]

Hegel was characteristically undismayed by these old difficulties, and undertook to demonstrate that there was a deep truth implicit in the tangle of folk doctrines about inwardness and outwardness, expression and self-control. He decided to raise these instinctive insights to the level of a science of the bodily actions of the soul, or what he called *psychic physiology*. The task of this science would be to explain how inward sensations become objectified within the 'circle of corporeity', and for this purpose it was necessary to interpret the human body not as a biological organism, but as the 'systematic embodying of what is spiritual'.

1 Plato, *Republic*, translated by Benjamin Jowett (adapted), 430e-431a.

The most interesting aspect of a psychic physiology would be
... the ... specific investigation of the embodiment assumed
by spiritual determinations, especially as affects. One would
have to comprehend the connectedness involved in anger and
courage being sensed in the breast ... in the same way as
meditation, spiritual activity, is sensed in the head.[2]

The basic principle behind the localization of psychic functions in
different parts of the body was that when inner sensations 'form themselves from the soul' and find outward expression, they are not just
made public, but physically extruded or 'expelled'. Weeping provided
the most vivid example of the process, because it transforms stunned
inward grief into 'a real material being'. It may be only a poor thing
in itself, but still it is a genuine and tangible trophy, distilled from
bodily or spiritual pain: a droplet of salty water, that is to say – a tear,
or even on occasion a flood of them.

But weeping is a rather special case, and Hegel noted that expression
is based, for the most part, on the element of air rather than water:
inner feelings acquired objectivity, that is to say, primarily through the
expulsion of air from the lungs. The simplest form of this affective
exhalation was the 'vigorous and intermittent expulsion of the breath'
in laughter, which enabled the soul to rid itself unreflectively of any
feelings that happened to be causing irritation. A similar process under-
lay the convulsions of crying, sobbing and sighing. But the best and
highest way of exhaling or expressing inner sentiments was by means
of the sustained sounds of the voice in singing, wailing and moaning.
A sentiment which has been vocalized in this way, Hegel says, 'dies
away as fast as it is uttered' – a point which he thought was well
understood by the women of ancient Rome, when they wept and
yelped at funerals in order to transform, externalize, and hence elimin-
ate their inward pain. 'It is primarily through the voice that people
make known their inwardness, for they put into it what they are,'
according to Hegel. The human voice was the most perfect instrument
for giving expression to the inwardness of the soul and thus accomplishing an 'objectification of subjectivity'.[3]

2 G.W.F. Hegel, *Philosophy of Mind* (1830), §401; see *Hegel's Philosophy of Subjective
Spirit*, translated by M. J. Petry, 3 Vols, Dordrecht, Reidel, 1978, Vol. 2, pp. 171, 163,
183–4.
3 Hegel, *Philosophy of Mind*, §401; Petry, pp. 195, 193, 199, 181, 201.

In making the voice the key instrument for the outward expression of inner emotion, Hegel was keeping close to common sense. Ordinary language is littered with fragments of the idea that you can relieve emotions by 'outing' or 'uttering' them, and with words like *spirit* or *expression*, which are historically connected with the idea of breathing out. For centuries, *pneumatology* was philosophy's formal name for the systematic study of the soul. These linguistically attested connections, according to Hegel, 'cannot very well be explained away as an age-old error'.[4] Like all such persistent patterns in ordinary language, he thought, the association between breath and the soul must contain an element of truth.

In any case it would be absurd to imagine that our sense of ourselves could be unaffected by images that pervade our entire everyday vocabulary. It may be hard, too, to get away from the child's familiar conundrum, as to where exactly the voice comes from. Is it the lips or mouth? Or the throat? the head? the chest? Clearly none of these answers is quite satisfying, so it may be better to accept the mystery of it and say that your voice comes straight from your self, from deep inside you, from your soul. Where else should it come from, indeed? And perhaps the converse is equally true: how else could we imagine the soul, except as the source or the seat of the voice?

The Renaissance metaphysician Francis Mercury van Helmont was probably the most dogged and systematic theorist of the link between the glory of the voice and the mystery of life. Part of his theory, as elaborated in conversations taken down by a disciple in London in 1685, was that the voice is carried by air from the belly, which was itself a 'true living fiery Essence' – as could be seen, he explained, when 'wanton Children that are in health, let a fart through their shirt . . . into the flame of a Candle', thus producing 'a great blaze much like that of Brandy or Brimstone'.[5]

But, Helmont continued, there was more vitality in the voice than could be accounted for by the brimstone in the breath. The voice was also controlled and articulated by our inmost soul, by the 'central Spirit' located in our heart, at the nerve-centre where the body's active,

---

4 *Philosophy of Mind*, §401; Petry, pp. 187–8.
5 Francis Mercury van Helmont, *The Paradoxal Discourses Concerning the Macrocosm and Microcosm, set down in writing by J. B.*, London, 1685, Part Two, p. 47.

masculine, 'out-flowing' faculties meet up with its passive, female, 'in-working' ones. Whilst the spirit's female side welcomed and nurtured the 'images' which entered the body through the senses, the male side busied itself making decisions about them, and despatching 'out-going Spiritual Ideal Beings' to carry its orders to every part of the body, and also beyond it in the form of vocal utterances.[6] These airy messengers were infused with a special 'reproductive power' extracted, Helmont maintained, from semen held back from physical emission so that it could be 'consumed and dispersed in a spiritual force' instead.[7] (Those whose voice was troubled with a cough are, as he observed, 'at the same time indisposed for the act of generation.') The mouth, Helmont concluded, 'was chiefly given to man for this end, that he might (through his voice) bring forth the Issues and Births of the other Senses'. And these, once expressed in the sublime form of vocal sounds, could be consecrated to God, before freeing themselves from our bodies and flying off heavenwards to participate in the bliss of 'endless and everlasting Being'.[8]

In Amsterdam about five years later, Helmont made the acquaintance of a young Swiss physician called Johann Conrad Amman, soon to become famous for his specialized work in the treatment of vocal disorders. With the help of Helmont, Amman was able to adorn his empirical practice with an ostentatious metaphysical superstructure. What possible explanation could there be, he asked, for the universally acknowledged centrality of the voice to all of human life?

> I have oftentimes heard from some Persons, that it was little beneath a Miracle, that God should give Men, to express the Thoughts of the Mind, rather by Motions, which are effected by the Lips, the Tongue, the Teeth etc., than otherwise, and that so universally, that there is no Nation so Barbarous, no not excepting the Hottentots, which cannot speak in a Language.[9]

6 Francis Mercury van Helmont, *The Paradoxal Discourses*, pp. 13, 34, 7.
7 Francis Mercury van Helmont, *Alphabeti vere naturalis Hebraici brevissima delineatio*, Saltzbach, 1667, pp. 56–7. See also Allison Coudert, 'Some Theories of a Natural Language from the Renaissance to the Seventeenth Century', in *Magia Naturalis und die Entstehung der Modernen Naturwissenschaften*, *Studia Leibnitiana* Sonderheft 7, 1978, pp. 56–118, p. 63. Coudert reports that the equation between speech and the ejaculation of semen was a 'standard renaissance theory'.
8 Francis Mercury van Helmont, *The Paradoxal Discourses*, pp. 51, 49, 63.
9 Johann Conrad Amman, *Surdus Loquens*, Amsterdam 1692; translated by Daniel Foot, *The Talking Deaf Man*, London, 1694, p. 3.

In a later presentation of his theory, Amman extended his discussion by means of a historical speculation:

> Let us suppose the inhabitants of the globe to be in absolute ignorance of any kind of language, yet equally gifted with the same sympathies as ourselves, and consequently possessing an intense desire to discover the thoughts of others and to communicate their own; it is very likely that they would leave nothing untried to effect this object, and eventually . . . they would have recourse to the voice.

The voice has the notable advantage of being detectable 'at a considerable distance, in the dark also, and by the blind', and it is exceptionally easy to articulate at will, and 'without the interruption of other work'. All of this makes it 'a really wonderful convenience', and a natural choice as the principal means of human self-expression.[10]

But the selection of the voice for its special place in human life was, Amman thought, more than just a practical convenience. The substance of the voice is breath, after all, and it was metaphysically fitting that breath should be the means by which people enjoy the solace of conversation.

> They desire to open the most inward Recesses of the Heart, yea, and to transfuse their own proper Life into others, which thing cannot be more commodiously done, than by Speaking; for there is nothing which floweth forth from us, which carrieth with it a more vivid Character of the Life, than our *Voice* doth; yea, in the Voice is the *Breath* of Life, part of which passeth into the Voice; for indeed the voice is the child of the Heart, which is the Seat of the Affections, and of Desire . . . Thus, when we desire something in ourselves, and yet are afraid to express it, the Heart labours like a Woman with Child, and becomes Anxious; but if we can pour it forth into the Bosom

---

10 Johann Conrad Amman, *Dissertatio de Loquela*, Amsterdam, 1700, pp. 5–6; translated by Charles Baker, *Dissertation on Speech*, London, 1873, pp. 6–7. This way of explaining the origins of language was by no means original to Amman: see for instance Locke's comments on how, in order to communicate our thoughts, which by nature are 'invisible, and hidden from others', we resorted to 'articulate Sounds', nothing else being 'so fit, either for Plenty or for Quickness'. John Locke, *Essay concerning Human Understanding*, III, II, §1, p. 405.

of a Friend, there presently ariseth great Tranquility, and we
say, that we have emptied our Hearts.

Words themselves might be arbitrary human institutions, but the voice
that animated them was a gift from God – 'an Emanation from that
very Spirit, which God breathed into Man's Nostrils, when he created
him a living Soul'.[11] God himself, furthermore, had created the world
by means of his voice. ('By pronouncing the Ideas of things to be
created he commands them to become creatures,' Amman said.) Our
own voices, properly used, were 'luminous emanations from the source
of light, and therefore God has given to man the power of propagating
by his living voice effective rays of his own life into the creatures subject
to him'.[12] The human voice, in other words, placed us above the rest
of God's earthly creatures, and allowed us to participate directly in the
power of the Creator.

Amman, Helmont, and Hegel, therefore – the physician, the metaphysician, and the dialectician – all agreed in endorsing the traditional
link between spirituality and the voice. And their unanimity is hardly
surprising: the basic human experiences of hearing and vocalizing provide the clearest possible illustrations of the idea that perceptions enter
into the body and pass through it on their way in to the soul, whilst
actions push past them in the opposite direction, heading out towards
the objective world. Vocalizing is one of the most voluntary kinds of
activity, after all, and hearing the most passive form of perception. The
voice, it seems, is not only the centre of the world of sound, but also
the expressive secret of the soul.

11 Amman, *The Talking Deaf Man*, pp. 5, 6.
12 Amman, *Dissertatio de Loquela*, p. 14; *Dissertation on Speech*, p. 15.

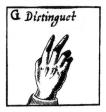

7

Speech and repetition

In Weimar at the end of the eighteenth century, Johann Gottfried Herder was also moved to praise the miraculous powers of the human voice. He suggested that if anyone were to claim to have invented a technique for 'making colour sound, sound thought, and thought a depicting voice', then the notion would strike us all as absurd and incredible. But on reflection we would realize that we unthinkingly perform this miracle all the time, in our everyday use of language. Whenever we speak, that is to say, 'the breath of our mouths is the picture of the world, the type that exhibits our thoughts and feelings to the mind of another'. Exactly how this feat is executed was a complete mystery – a 'divine problem', as Herder said. But he was certain that all the distinctive achievements of humanity depended on this mysterious 'movement of a breath of air', and that 'if this divine breath had not inspired us, and floated like a charm on our lips we should all have still been wanderers in the woods'.[1]

It may sound as if Herder was simply perpetuating the vocal super-naturalism propounded by Helmont and Amman a hundred years before, especially when he argued that the origins of human vocalizing

1 Johann Gottfried Herder, *Ideen zur Philosophie der Geschichte der Menschheit* (1784–91), 2 Vols, Leipzig, Johann Hartnock, 1841, Vol. 1, pp. 295–6. Translated by T. Churchill, *Outlines of a Philosophy of the History of Man*, London, J. Johnson, 1800, pp. 232–3.

could be traced to an instinct that we share with the apes: a drive to play with the affinities of sounds and imitate them with our voices, as thoughtlessly as birds calling to each other, or strings resonating in spontaneous harmony. This inborn 'organic sympathy', Herder said, was the sole law of human infancy, and it still prevailed amongst the 'savage nations, the children of nature'.[2]

But Herder went on to argue that the ears and voices of human beings are by nature more finely tuned than those of other creatures, and that we are 'more peculiarly formed, to repeat the tones of all other beings and sympathise with them'. It was this natural advantage in the art of repetition that enabled the first generations of humanity to break out of the closed circuit of instinctive vocal copying, and eventually 'attain the artificial characteristic . . . of reason'. The fateful transition from instinctive animal nature to rational human artifice was accomplished when elements of the playful, imitative, infantile vocal world began to crystallize out into standardized, repeatable units. As this occurred, perceptions ceased to be scattered, dissipated and meaningless, each one isolated in its separate spot of time, and experience began to gather itself into significant regular patterns. It must have been through vocal repetition, then, that our distant ancestors first developed a sense of themselves as continuous entities – as consciousnesses which manage to retain their personal identity through all the instabilities of an ever-changing world. The 'divine gift of speech' had equipped them with a sense of past and future, and thus changed them from animals into cultured and sociable beings. The ultimate basis of 'the whole history of man', in short, and the source of 'all the treasures of tradition and cultivation', was simply the exceptional ability of human beings to repeat sounds with their voices.[3]

This idea that speech is a precondition for human consciousness, and not just an expression of it, enabled Herder to open a gap between two themes that had always been thoroughly intertwined in ordinary folk metaphysics, and which the theories of Helmont and Amman had completely fused together. Vocality and speech, to Herder, were not one and the same phenomenon: they belonged at opposite poles, speech being what happens when the voice takes on the artificial inflec-

---

2 Herder, *Ideen zur Philosophie der Geschichte*, Vol. 1, pp. 294–6; *Outlines*, pp. 232–3.
3 Herder, *Ideen zur Philosophie der Geschichte*, Vol. 1, pp. 294–5; *Outlines*, p. 232.

tions of a human institution, whilst the voice in itself was simply the medium for the spontaneous animal exuberance of shouts, exclamations, and song. 'Speech alone awakens slumbering reason,' as Herder put it, not mere 'voice'. It was only when the artificial sounds of speech had become a kind of second nature that coherent experience could begin:

> By speech alone the eye and ear, nay the feelings of all the senses, are united in one, and centre in commanding thought, to which the hands and other members are only obedient instruments . . . The delicate organs of speech, therefore, must be considered as the rudder of reason, and speech as the heavenly spark, that gradually kindles our thoughts and senses to a flame.

It was not the sounds of voices, but the words of language, that were the essence of humanity. 'Man did not attain the artificial characteristic of his species, reason, by . . . mimicry: he arrived at it by speech alone.' The human voice does not vocalize any longer; it speaks, and 'speech alone has rendered man human'. By 'setting bounds to the vast flood of his passions, and giving them rational memorials by means of words' spoken language had created human memory and continuity, and was thus the source of human society and history, as well as human individuality. For it was only by articulating the words of a human language that human beings became participants in a community – members of a people, holders of a nationality, and possessors of a tradition. 'The loveliest imagination remains an obscure feeling, till the mind finds a character for it, and by means of a word incorporates it with the memory, the recollection, and lastly the understanding of mankind, tradition: a pure understanding, without speech or language, upon earth, is an utopian land.'[4] The voice could speak as well as sing; it could say things, because the sounds it repeated were no longer sounds, but signs. Flesh had become word, and a prodigious novelty was born.

In working out this idea of speech as distinct from voice, and treating it as the basis of understanding and tradition, Herder moved away from

4 Herder, *Ideen zur Philosophie der Geschichte*, Vol. 1, pp. 296–7, 295; *Outlines*, pp. 233, 87, 233, 232.

the old philosophical interpretation of vocal experience as expression. Speech was not the airy exhalation of an original inwardness. It had nothing in common with the expulsive processes of ejaculating, sneezing, laughing, or shedding tears: it was not so much an instrument of the human soul as its creator. If the speaking voice made a journey of some kind, the path it took led from sound to sound (wherever that might be), rather than from inner subjectivity to an objective outside world. Where Helmont and Amman had seen a movement from silent inner depth to outer public speech, Herder heard a movement from speaker to speaker, from voice to voice. Where they had celebrated the voice as a means of expressing the inner state of the soul, he praised it for its ability to speak, and to repeat the speech of others. The essence of language was not utterance, but iteration; not action but reaction; not expression, but response. In short, Herder had begun to conceive the virtue of the human voice in terms of *repetition*.

Now repetition is not at all the same thing as recurrence. The reappearance of the sun every day is not a case of repetition, nor is printing multiple copies of a document, duplicating images in mirrors, or playing the same recording over and over again. Recurrence is mindless and mechanical, whereas repetition – as the Latin meaning of the word suggests – involves deliberate seeking, demanding, or questing, in other words an element of selective intention. A repetition, unlike a copy, is not meant to mimic its original in every possible respect: only structures that are taken to be salient get repeated, and everything else is ignored. Repetitions essentially involve variation. A musical score may instruct the performer to repeat a passage, but this does not mean that it should sound identical the second time round. The same material can be repeated over and over again, without any two versions being exactly similar. Things get transformed – clarified, with luck, and enhanced, even perfected – in their repeats, whereas they are at best preserved, but more likely degraded and obscured, in copies, imitations and reflections.

And that is the vital difference between speech and the voice: speech by its nature can be repeated, whereas voices can only be imitated. The repetition of people's words signifies something very different from the imitation of their voices. Imitating what people say conveys either mockery or incomprehension; repeating it, in contrast, is a way of opening a dialogue and participating in their language: it is the beginning of conversation. Repetition attempts to ignore outward appearances in order to focus on essential forms: it is interested in identity, not similarity. It presupposes the recognition of an underlying structure, and an ability to hold it constant in the midst of change: it is an attempt to identify a sameness in difference, a one in the many. There is, you might say, *no repetition without abstraction*. And, as Herder saw, it is only when the voice has become a faculty of repetition as distinct from imitation that it is capable of language or speech. Repetition is the element in which language lives: a speaking voice is always intrinsically an infinitely redoubled echo.

So it was that the young Wordsworth, out walking on his own in the lakeland hills in the very years when Herder was working out his theory of language in Weimar, used to lift both hands to his mouth and fill the valleys with his 'mimic hootings to the silent owls', to be enchanted by the long halloos and screams with which they answered him, their 'echoes loud redoubled and redoubled'.[5] And then he would recite poetic compositions to the open fields, to be cheered by the resoundings of his own voice, and heartened yet again by 'the mind's Internal echo of the imperfect sound'.[6]

This experience of the echoed speaking voice suggests a rather different interpretation of selfhood than that inspired by psychic physiology and the traditional metaphysical shuttling between insides and outsides. In ancient Greek, the word *echo*, apart from referring to the phenomenon of reflected or redoubled sound, had a secondary career as the name for a mythological figure, a mountain nymph whose fate became tragically entwined with that of the more famous Narcissus. The story, in the form given it by Ovid, is of a gloriously beautiful boy, sixteen years old, and proud; everyone falls for him, but he is never moved in turn. Understandably, one of his heartbroken admirers prayed that Narcissus himself might be smitten with the same pain he was inflicting so carelessly on others: he was to fall in love with the first creature he saw, and then learn for himself what it was like to be scorned. And so, as Narcissus was hunting through the forest in the heat of the day, he became separated from his companions and dis-

5 Wordsworth, *The Prelude*, Book Five, pp. 364–79.
6 Wordsworth, *The Prelude*, Book One, pp. 55–6.

covered an enchanting clearing: a grassy sward beside a perfect pool; a silvery spring; and all shaded and secluded by trees. The spell was about to do its work. This is how the story comes out in an Elizabethan translation:

> The stripling wearie with the heate and hunting in the chace,
> And much delighted with the spring and cooleness of the place,
> Did lay him downe upon the brimme: and as he stooped lowe
> To staunch his thurst, another thurst of worse effect did growe.
> For as he dranke, he chaunst to spie the Image of his face,
> The which he did immediately with fervent love embrace.
> He feedes a hope without cause why. For like a foolish noddie
> He thinks the shadowe that he sees, to be a lively boddie.

Poor Narcissus, not realizing that it was only a reflection of his own beauty, drove himself to despair as he tried to kiss the lips of his beloved and clasp him in his arms: in the end, he was so worn out by yearning that he wasted away. His body was never found, only a flower in its place.

But Narcissus had a loyal and helplessly devoted admirer, the nymph Echo, who was condemned never to say anything of her own, but only repeat the words of others. She watched in impotent despair as the light of her life grew dark. Her body wasted like his, and slowly merged with the trees and the rocks, as she gave Narcissus his own words back in return:

> Although in heart she angrie were, and mindefull of his pride,
> Yet ruing his unhappie case, as often as he cride
> Alas, she cride alas likewise with shirle redoubled sound.[7]

The tragic pair, it would seem, stand for opposite moral types: Narcissus the perfection of self-centredness and self-ignorance, and Echo the last extreme of receptivity, to the point, indeed, of servility and self-starvation. Perhaps one could say that the difference between their moralities corresponds to the fact that Narcissus inhabits a world of pure vision – a world of visible beauty, ocular concentration, and optical illusion – whereas Echo lives in the ambiguous qualitative world of hearing, voice, speech and sound. Her element is outside herself,

---

7 Ovid, *Metamorphoses*, translated by Arthur Golding (1567), edited by John Frederick Nims, London, Macmillan, 1965, Book III, p. 73, pp. 514–22; p. 75, pp. 621–3.

redoubled. She was a mouth as well as an ear, but he was only an eye.[8]

Diderot, it will be remembered, was of the opinion that the absurdities of idealism must have been invented by the blind, who were simply unable to see for themselves the overpowering reality of physical objects in the material world. But it may be that idealism – at least if it means taking the inner life of the soul to be self-evident and self-sufficient – really involves an opposite and subtler neglect. Diderot's gibe against idealists might have been more effective if he had criticized them for too much ocularity, not too little – for visualizing the world, that is to say, instead of listening to it. Perhaps the self-centred doctrines of folk metaphysics are really the philosophy of those who will not hear – of those who do not understand that the speaking voice is an instrument of repetition rather than expression, and who do not realize that the human soul is not so much narcissistic, as echoic.

8 See John Hollander, *The Figure of Echo: A Mode of Allusion in Milton and After*, Berkeley, University of California Press, 1981.

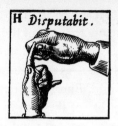

8

Spiritual etymology

These two aspects of the voice – the voice as natural expression or sound, and the voice as artificial repetition or language – may not have been explicitly separated before the work of eighteenth-century theorists such as Herder. But everyone must always have been aware, at least subliminally, of a certain doubleness at the core of vocal experience. Young children adjusting their instinctive babbling to the forms of their first human language provide an obvious and inescapable model for a distinction between spontaneity and training, nature and convention, instinct and culture. And from there it is only a small step to the idea that the human voice is divided against itself, like human life itself: riven by a gap between the animal and the spiritual, the narcissistic and the echoic.

Once the rift between the artificial speaking voice and the natural expressive voice has been noticed, attempts will inevitably be made to bridge it by means of historicist speculations – by metaphysical stories, that is to say, purporting to show how languages in their present state are descended from an archaic and presumably universal repertoire of natural vocal sounds. Perhaps, indeed, the wish to close this gap is the origin of historical curiosity as such.

Herodotus, known since antiquity as 'the Father of History', paid tribute to a peculiar piece of linguistic research conducted 200 years before him, in the seventh century BC, by Psammetichus I, King of

72

the Egyptians. Psammetichus wanted to find out whether the Egyptians were the most ancient people on earth, or whether the Phrygians were right to claim the honour for themselves. The matter would be settled, he thought, if he could discover what language children speak by nature. He therefore abducted two new-born babies and arranged for them to be brought up without ever being exposed to the sound of speech. According to one version of the story, Psammetichus entrusted them to some women whose tongues had been cut out; according to another, which Herodotus preferred, he gave them to an old peasant who promised that they would be raised with his goats in an isolated hut, away from all human company. The assumption was that when the children eventually 'left off their childish cries and began to prattle and speake plainly', the language that they thus discovered for themselves could be identified as the natural language of humanity, and the race which spoke it would be vindicated as the oldest race.

Two years later, when the peasant was making one of his regular silent visits to the hut where the children were kept, he found 'both the little brats sprawling at his feet, and stretching forth their hands', and shouting out: 'Beccos, Beccos.' He was indifferent at first, and 'made no words' of what he heard. But after a while he realized that the children were not vocalizing, but speaking; and they 'spake the same word' whenever he visited them. He therefore carried them off for an audience with King Psammetichus, at which they continued to 'chat in the same manner'. After further investigations, the King discovered that 'Beccos' was the Phrygian word for bread, and so – with some disappointment, but great scientific probity – he acknowledged that the Phrygians must, after all, be a more ancient race than the Egyptians.[1]

The general name for this kind of verbal archeology – the quest for deep historical truths preserved in current linguistic practices – is *etymology*, which literally means, in Greek, the search for the pristine truth or *etymon* of words. But the attractions of etymology often outstrip its theoretical and empirical controls, and it sometimes turns out to be little more than an excuse for untrammelled intellectual fantasy.

---

1 Herodotus, *Histories*, Book 2, §§ 2–3, translated by Barnaby Rich (1584), edited by Charles Whibley, London, Constable, 1924, pp. 138–9.

Plato himself drew attention to the dangers of etymology in a dialogue which stages a debate between Cratylus, who holds that words (*onomata*) are natural, and Hermogenes, who believes that they are artificial or conventional. Socrates presides, and at one point gets quite carried away by the idea of an original inventor of language – the *onomata*-poet, or the first maker of words – who presumably had no hesitation in choosing the sounds which best imitated the true natures of the things they were to represent. (He suggests for example that conditions like shivering, seething, shaking and shock all call for words which are pronounced with 'a great expenditure of breath', and hence are naturally expressed by the consonantal sounds *phi*, *psi*, *sigma* and *zeta*.)

But the *Cratylus* as a whole, far from endorsing etymological speculation (or 'Cratylism' as it is sometimes called) is actually a kind of comedy at its expense. After indulging his fancies for a moment, Socrates immediately deprecates them as 'truly wild and ridiculous', and claims that the desire to discover ancient natural names, undistorted by convention, is the product of an insane and contradictory hunger. Even if natural resemblances could account for the matching of certain sounds to particular meanings, they would always need to be 'supplemented by the mechanical aid of convention' before they could amount to a genuine language with a valid claim to 'correctness'. Languages were obviously conventional, after all – otherwise there would be only one language in the world – and the whole idea of true and original names was intrinsically implausible. For how could there ever have been a first name? How could the original poets have set about inventing a language, unless they already had some words at hand to start working with? 'How,' as Socrates put it, 'can we suppose that the givers of names had knowledge, or were legislators, before there were names at all, and therefore before they could have known them?'[2]

The idea of languages as arbitrary human institutions was a commonplace of ancient and medieval philosophy, but the Platonists of the Renaissance were to revive Cratylus's dream of a naturally expressive vocal language, and his infatuation with the idea of etymology as a

2 Plato, *Cratylus*, translated by Benjamin Jowett, 383a, 427a, 426b, 435c, 438b.

path to linguistic truth.[3] But they knew enough about the variety and mutability of human languages to realize that any search for an original 'natural language' would have to face some formidable difficulties. The 'divine manner of speaking', as Johann Conrad Amman observed at the end of the seventeenth century, would seem to have 'almost perished from the earth'. As a result of our stubborn sinfulness and prevarication, human speech was no longer capable of 'vividly uttering the very essences of things', or performing miracles and magic as of old.[4] 'Speech', as he reflected regretfully, was no longer 'natural to us, but a Habite, contracted by long Use or Custom.'[5] Yet there was still hope: a few traces of 'genuine pronunciation' survived amidst the artificial conventions of modern speech and the ritualized intonations of priests; and these 'very rude remnants . . . of the lost natural language' could, Amman thought, be used to reconstruct the original form of human speech, and perhaps even to recapture some of its old supernatural power.[6]

Renaissance etymology could also draw support from the Bible, where the existence of an original name-maker was presented not as a metaphysical hypothesis but a plain historical fact. When God created the world and placed Adam in the Garden of Eden, he made all the different birds and beasts and then, according to Genesis, 'brought them unto Adam to see what he would call them: and whatsoever Adam called every living creature, that was the name thereof'. Adam's language survived for several generations, and even after the Flood the whole earth was still 'of one language, and of one speech'. But then the descendants of Noah conceived a great plan: 'Go to,' they said; 'let us build us a city and a tower, whose top may reach unto heaven.' This ambition was not pleasing to God, however, and he resolved to 'go down, and there confound their language, that they may not understand one another's speech'. As a result, the great city was never completed, and 'therefore is the name of it called Babel; because the

3 See E. J. Ashworth, ' "Do Words Signify Ideas or Things?": The Scholastic Sources of Locke's Theory of Language', *Journal of the History of Philosophy*, Vol. XIX, No 3, July 1981, pp. 299–336, esp. p. 304.
4 Johann Conrad Amman, *Dissertatio de Loquela* (1700), pp. 14–15; *Dissertation on Speech*, p. 16.
5 Amman, *Surdus Loquens* (1692), *The Talking Deaf Man*, p. 16.
6 Amman, *Dissertatio de Loquela*, p. 41; *Dissertation on Speech*, p. 46.

Lord did there confound the language of all the earth'.[7] Our ancestors were reduced to babbling, and we have been plagued by linguistic strife and diversity ever since.

The seventeenth-century Cratylists proposed to sift through the 72 different languages which, according to tradition, had grown up after the catastrophe of Babel, and identify archaic fragments from which they might piece together the 'root' words of the language of Adam. In the Middle Ages it had been assumed that Latin, Greek and Hebrew were the closest to this original source, but in the Renaissance the field was enlarged, with Leibniz intermittently supporting the claims of German, whilst his English contemporary John Webb preferred Chinese.[8]

Francis Mercury van Helmont, however, was still convinced that the language of Noah was pure Hebrew. In 1667, in his *Very short delineation of the Natural Hebrew Alphabet*, he went so far as to claim that the sounds which 'the tongue . . . naturally forms . . . in the Mouth' were identical with those uttered by Adam in the Garden of Eden.[9] He even argued that natural Hebrew was older than Adam, indeed older than the first creation, having originally been used by God himself for summoning his creatures into existence. (Was it not written in the original Hebrew Bible that 'God said: Let there be light . . . And God called the light Day, and the darkness he called Night'?)[10]

Helmont went on to suggest that the very sequences of sounds that made up God's natural language could be reconstructed on the basis of the letters of the Hebrew alphabet. For according to him, the Hebrew characters were originally pictorial; and they depicted not the objects or ideas they referred to, but the configuration of the vocal organs required for producing their sound. Thus they functioned rather like the tablature notations used for medieval instrumental music, which directly indicated how the musician was to touch the strings, frets or keys.[11] Hebrew letters, according to Helmont, were diagrammatic instructions for their own pronunciation, having 'the

7 Genesis 2:19; 11:1–9.
8 See Allison Coudert, 'Some Theories of a Natural Language from the Renaissance to the Seventeenth Century', pp. 108, 101.
9 Francis Mercury van Helmont, *The Spirit of Diseases, or Diseases from the Spirit*, London, Sarah Howkins, 1694, p. 109.
10 Genesis 1:3–5.
11 See C. F. Abdy Williams, *The Story of Notation*, London, Walter Scott, 1903, p. 146.

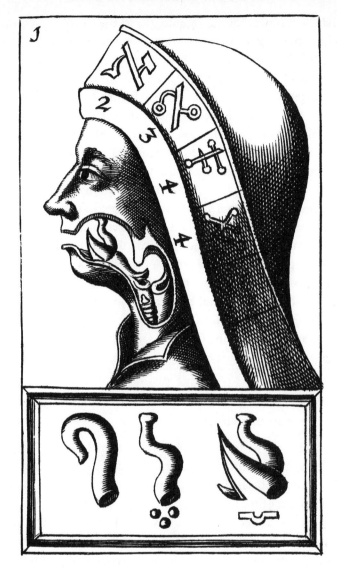

FIG 1. The letter ALEPH: Helmont's demonstration that
Hebrew characters depict the vocal organs

same figure and form as they are shaped and formed by the Tongue
in the Mouth.'[12] (See Figure 1)

Despite being persecuted by the church, and imprisoned and tortured

12 Helmont, *Paradoxical Discourses*, p. 57; see also *Alphabeti vere naturalis Hebraici
brevissima delineatio*, pp. 5–6.

by the Inquisition in Rome, Helmont persevered with his etymological researches, studying the shapes of the characters in conjunction with the workings of the vocal organs, and the frontispiece to his *Alphabet of Nature* shows him at work in his prison cell, measuring his mouth with a pair of calipers in front of a mirror. (See Figure 2) By carefully arrranging his lips and tongue in accordance with the shapes of the Hebrew letters, Helmont thought, he should surely be able to reproduce the very same speech sounds once uttered by Adam and by God himself: eventually he might even manage to steal away some of God's creative virtue.[13]

Helmont's argument was not without supporters. In 1679, Athanasius Kircher's *Turris Babel* gave further arguments in favour of Hebrew as the language used by Adam and authorized by God.[14] And Leibniz appears to have endorsed Helmont's entire theory of the Hebrew alphabet, even venturing that 'the Figures of the Letters, and their Tone or Sounding do indicate the nature of things'. He also supported Helmont's idea that speech could be an act of generation or creation, and that words rightly pronounced might bring their objects into real existence – as, for instance, when God had said 'Let there be Light'.

> Constituting to himself an Object of Thinking, into which he might send forth his inward Power, in so doing, I say, he outed or produced the same, and gave Existence to something separate from himself.

Furthermore – so Leibniz speculated – if it had not been for man's disobedience in the Garden of Eden, human reproduction itself could have been accomplished through the pleasant, dignified and convenient medium of speech, instead of the humiliating physical activities to which we are obliged to resort now that our souls are 'coated with gross earthly shell'.[15] For reasons one can perhaps guess at, Leibniz published these thoughts not under his own name, but under that of his friend Francis Mercury van Helmont.[16]

13 Coudert, 'Some Theories of a Natural Language', pp. 57–9.
14 Paul Cornelius, *Languages in Seventeenth- and Early Eighteenth-Century Imaginary Voyages*, Geneva, Droz, 1965, pp. 8–11.
15 See Francis Mercury van Helmont, *Cogitationes super Genesis*, Amsterdam, 1697, pp. 2, 16, in a contemporary English translation (*Thoughts on Genesis*, London, 1701, pp. 9, 34–5), cited in Coudert, pp. 60, 61.
16 See Anne Becco, 'Leibniz et François Mercure van Helmont', in *Magia Naturalis und die Entstehung der Modernen Naturwissenschaften, Studia Leibnitiana* Sonderheft 7, 1978, pp. 119–41. The attribution is accepted by Coudert at n. 6, p. 58.

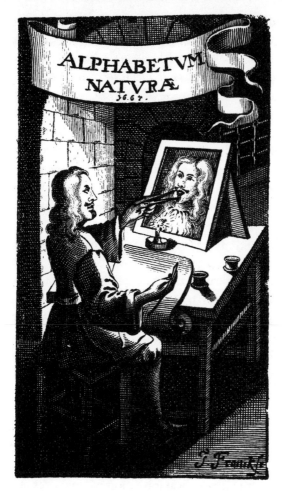

FIG 2. In search of the alphabet of nature:
Helmont in prison

In spite of all Helmont's heroic efforts, however, it was still impossible
to ascertain how language had actually sounded, hundreds or thousands of years ago. And according to Marin Mersenne, it did not
matter much anyway: etymologists ought to forget about ancient languages and linguistic history and fantastic experiments such as that
conducted by Psammetichus. He adhered to the traditional commonplace that languages are essentially conventional. Like Socrates in the
Cratylus, he held that every sound is 'indifferently able to signify whatever anyone chooses', concluding that even Adam's choice of the

original names of God's creatures was entirely arbitrary and insignificant.[17]

But Mersenne still believed in a single natural linguistic source or
mother-language – *une Langue Originaire et Matrice* – to which all
human languages ultimately owed their meanings.[18] The units of this
original natural language were not words, but smaller and more
elementary expressive sounds, corresponding to the letters of the alphabet. Take the vowels, for instance: *a* is pronounced with the mouth
wide open, and naturally signifies things that are wide and open; *e*
signifies delicate or doleful matters, because the mouth narrows when
uttering it; *i* implies diminutiveness; *o*, a great suffering, and *u*, conceal-
ment and obscurity, just as it is pronounced.[19]

Thus etymology, for Mersenne, ought to concentrate on showing
how words are built up out of monosyllabic, sub-verbal vocal sounds.
It was in this same spirit that Leibniz offered the following explanation
of why *Aelohim* was the true name of God. The sound *El*, he wrote
– which is also 'framed with a topping Eminence in Writing' – signifies
strength; *O* is the highest sound; *Hi* signifies breath, growth and
heavenly influence; *I* has a shrill sound 'and signifies the strong Life
that produceth the manly Member', whilst *M* denotes 'Mother, the
Womb, and the multiplicity of Births'. From all of this, Leibniz claims,
'we understand that *Aelohim* is the Creator'.[20]

Eighteenth-century linguistics as a whole took up with enthusiasm the
idea of an 'archeology' of the natural one-syllable proto-words from which
all human languages were supposed to have sprung. Charles des Brosses's
researches into 'the mechanical formation of languages and the physical
principles of etymology', for instance, identified nearly 400 'original
roots' – basic inflections of the human voice, common to the whole of
humanity and providing 'the true and original physical sense of words'.[21]

The culmination of the tradition of natural etymology came about

17 Marin Mersenne, *Harmonie Universelle, Traitez de la voix et des chants*, 1636, Prop.
XLVII, p. 65.
18 Mersenne, *Traitez de la voix et des chants*, Prop. XI, pp. 11–12.
19 Mersenne, *Traitez de la voix et des chants*, Prop. L, pp. 75–6.
20 Francis Mercury van Helmont, *Cogitationes super Genesis*, pp. 4–5, *Thoughts on
Genesis*, pp. 13–15, cited in Coudert, p. 60.
21 Charles des Brosses, *Traité de la formation méchanique des langues et des principes
physiques de l'étymologie*, 1765. See Ronald Grimsley. 'Some aspects of "nature" and
"language" in the French Enlightenment', *Studies on Voltaire and the Eighteenth
Century*, Vol. 56, 1967, pp. 659–77.

in France in 1808 with the publication of a *Dictionary of Onomato-poeias* by the enthusiastic amateur scholar Charles Nodier, who had traced the physiological roots of basic words across fifty different languages. The naturally significant sounds that most fascinated Nodier were what he called *mimologisms*. These were words that had grown out of natural vocalizations – sighs and shrieks, for instance – and which were therefore used to designate something about the situations that typically give rise to them. There were, in the first place, simple 'mechanical' mimologisms, as when parts of the vocal apparatus are named in accordance with the sounds they make – for instance, nasal consonants (/m/, /n/, /z/) are typically used to designate the nose; dentals (/d/, /t/, /l/) for the teeth; and gutturals (/g/, /h/) for the gullet. And then there were the still more significant mimologisms of infancy, derived from the moment when children first start to articulate their simple cries by opening and closing their lips and producing the range of labial consonants (/p/,/b/,/m/,/f/,/v/,/w/). Naturally, these sounds furnish the names for all the most salient items in a child's world – notably *mama* and *papa*. 'In every age and every land,' Nodier says, 'lip-consonants, or failing that dentals, or a combination of the two, are used to construct the child's words for mother and father.'[22]

But Nodier was interested above all in the etymological origin of the idea of the soul. Like Socrates in the *Cratylus*, he described his hypothesis as bizarre, but elaborated it all the same. His idea was that the root of words like *âme* or *anima*, and indeed of *amour* and *amitié*, was a vivid mimology of expiration:

> In forming this word [*âme* – soul], the lips, slightly parted to let out the breath, close again upon each other. In the word *vie* [life], in contrast, they open gently and seem to breathe in: a mimologism of respiration. In English, the word *be* has the same character and is produced in the same way; and what is truly remarkable is that in the declension of the same verb, the first person is *I am*.[23]

22 Charles Nodier, *Dictionnaire Raisonné des Onomatopées Françoises* (1808), second edition, Paris, Delangle, 1828, pp. 15–16, 18. Some of Nodier's conclusions are refined and endorsed in Roman Jakobson, 'Why "Mama" and "Papa"?' in *Studies on Child Language and Aphasia*, The Hague, Mouton, 1971, pp. 21–9.
23 Charles Nodier, *Examen Critique des Dictionnaires de la Langue Françoise*, Paris, Delangle, 1828, pp. 33–4.

Reverse the sound, however, and you get the root *ma*, which is the natural expression for matter, man, mother and mortality. Nodier admitted that his explanation might not yet be correct in all its details, but one thing was established to his complete satisfaction: every word is a modification of the breath, and the words most suited to describing the soul are mimologisms of breathing. Thus the paths of etymology turned out to converge, like those of Renaissance metaphysics, on an essential bond between the voice and the human soul. The soul was the source of all speech, and every spoken word a natural metaphor for the soul.

TWO

VISIBLE SPEECH
AND THE FATE
OF THE DEAF

A history of science

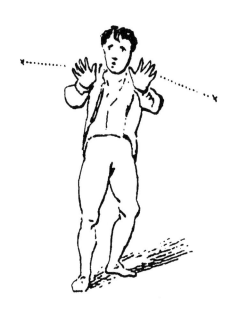

Such are the webs we spin for ourselves when we start to reflect on the five-fold world of the senses and the significance of the human voice. But our conclusions may often seem too obvious for words, or too foolish or inane, and it will be understandable if we decide to give up on metaphysics and turn our attention to concrete practical matters instead: for example the predicament of those who have a faulty sense of hearing and therefore cannot speak.

Few groups in history have suffered such sustained and uncomprehending cruelty as the so-called 'deaf and dumb'. In most civilizations they have been treated like animals, if not worse: their sensory disadvantage has not only deprived them of the natural experience of sound, but also shut them out from the human world of language.

It was not till after the Renaissance that remedies for the linguistic handicaps of deafness began to be explored. Most of the early educators of the deaf, subscribing to some notion of the human voice as an image of the divine soul, wished above all to teach their pupils to use their voices. But vocal training for the deaf was a long and arduous process, tiresome for children as they underwent it, and not much use to them in later life. Before long various rival policies on deaf education were coming forward to challenge the 'method of speech'.

Since deaf children could not absorb language through their ears, it was clear that it had to be instilled through another sense instead: touch perhaps, or even taste, but most likely vision. The obvious way of presenting language to the eyes was of course writing, whether alphabetic or pictographic, but the pioneers of deaf education recognized several other methods too: you could spell out letters with your hands ('manual alphabets'); you could, at least in theory, see words on people's faces as they talked ('lip reading'); or, more controversially, you could communicate by gestures and pantomimes that bore no relation to spoken language at all ('signs').

Of all the numerous overlapping debates over deaf education, the most bitter were those that divided partisans of the spoken word from advocates of visible gestures. 'Oralists' appealed to the notion of speech as the source of civilization or as God's special gift to humankind; but they were opposed by 'gesturalists' who contrasted the evident arbitrariness and obscurity of spoken languages with the naturalness, universality and lucidity that they saw in gestural signs.

There was one commonsense assumption, however, on which most oralists and gesturalists could agree: that speech, being audible, is essentially transient and temporal, whereas gestures, being visible, belong to space rather than time. The oralists concluded that true spirituality depends on speech, which forces us to consider ideas deliberately, one after another in time; whereas the gesturalists argued that true intelligence depends on signs, which allow us to consider different ideas simultaneously, side by side in space.

The same metaphysical assumptions about vision and space, and hearing and time, also guided theoretical investigations into the nature of language, and especially the relationship between writing and speech. On the one hand, there were earnest spelling reformers devising new alphabets which they thought would revolutionize human communication by permitting exact visible records of the fleeting sounds of speech; and on the other, antiquarians and anthropologists whose researches into the writing systems of Egypt, China and North and South America seemed to suggest that the original purpose of writing was not to portray spoken words, but to represent visible objects, or to depict manual gestures or the shapes of a speaker's lips.

These notions were overtaken in the course of the twentieth century by two complementary developments. First there was the rapid progress made by scientific linguistics once it got beyond describing the outward forms of language and began trying to give explicit formulation to abstract principles which are unconsciously followed by every language user – an approach which led before long to the realization that writing systems are not so much portrayals of our linguistic behaviour as codifications of our linguistic knowledge. And secondly there was the growth of defiant deaf communities, using sign systems which, from the point of view of the new linguistics, turned out to embody exactly the same kinds of structural principles as speech.

The belated vindication of sign languages upset the natural assumption that pictures, writing systems, lip movements, manual alphabets and gestural signs must – since they are all 'addressed to the eye' – be essentially similar forms of representation; and it showed that the differences between vision and hearing have nothing much to do with the relations of gestural communication to speech. What had always been perfectly obvious proved in the end to be deeply mistaken.

The story of deaf education has three great lessons to teach us: the banality of ignorant cruelty, the tenuousness of scientific progress, and – last but not least – the stubborn persistence of folk metaphysics.

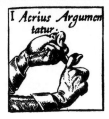

9

Mutism and mythology

The sounds of voices – mingled, diverse, echoing voices – give us some of our earliest inklings about our existence amongst others. Redoubled voices, you might say, form the natural cradle of human selfhood and personal relatedness. Our childish babblings, when we attack the same sounds over and over again, letting them mix with the talk of adults who return them to us refined and redefined, must be amongst our most elementary experiences of society and sociability. Consciousness dawns, it might be said, on a primal sea of sounds, when the child first learns to respond to the voices of others with an answering voice of its own.

But if the voice is really the breath of human life, then vocal impediments such as stammering or lisping must, conversely, be an appalling spiritual calamity. And the task of treating and curing diseases of the voice will be not so much a medical speciality as a spiritual calling. That was certainly how Johann Conrad Amman justified himself when he embarked on his career as the world's first voice-doctor in 1690: even God, he pointed out, had to make use of his voice in order to create the world, and Christ too was obliged to use vocal means when performing his miracles. Since the voice was the embodiment of divine power, Amman said, 'creatures formed in God's image ought, of necessity, to be able to speak, and in this respect resemble their Creator'.[1]

---

1 Johann Conrad Amman, *Dissertatio de Loquela*, pp. 15, 11; *Dissertation on Speech*, pp. 17, 12–13.

On the other hand, anyone who was altogether incapable of speech or vocalization must, it would seem, be quite beyond reach of spiritual comfort and assistance. Mutism, in short, was a state of utter spiritual dereliction, the atrophy and death of the soul. So it would seem probable that the eulogies to the voice that keep surfacing in the history of metaphysics are really just covers for a corresponding fear: the fear of being struck dumb. Dreams or tales about terrible and irreversible dumbness are surprisingly rare, however. There is a common nightmare about trying to scream and not being able to, but if you scan literary sources looking for paralysed gullets or throats gouged out, or tongues tied, cut, or pulled up by the root, you will probably come back with a rather small and disappointing collection. Echo may have been reduced to servile mimicry, for example, but she certainly was not dumb.

The great exception is another female figure from Ovid, the extra-ordinarily pathetic Philomela – an exquisite virgin, abducted by her sister's husband Tereus, raped and imprisoned in a high-walled grange overgrown by an ancient forest. When she threatens to denounce his crimes – 'my voyce the verie woods shall fill, and make the stones to understand' – he makes as if to kill her, but, thinking of future pleasures, attacks only her tongue, pulling at it with pliers and cutting it off with his sword, leaving her to watch it expiring in slow agony at her feet.[2]

But the fate of Philomela is quite unusual. When dumbness becomes a theme in stories, it is far more often comic than serious. Low characters are temporarily silenced, as a punishment for their garrulousness – like Papageno, for instance, whose mouth was padlocked to prevent him telling any more lies. But even then, he could still hum his tune, and anyway the punishment was brief and did not do him much harm, or much good for that matter.[3]

In 1719 an imitator of Daniel Defoe wrote a flippant account of a certain Dickory Cronke, who was 'born Dumb' but somehow managed to produce a stream of 'Prophetick Observations', together with fine

2 Ovid, *Metamorphoses*, trans. Golding, Book VI, pp. 150–9, esp. ll.695–715. The story is echoed in Shakespeare's *Titus Andronicus*, II.3.42–4: 'His Philomel must lose her tongue today, Thy sons make pillage of her chastity.'
3 In Mozart's opera *The Magic Flute*, to a libretto by Emanuel Schikaneder, first performed in 1791.

metaphysical meditations on the transitoriness of earthly life. The story of this 'Dumb Philosopher' was offered up 'to a wicked and degenerate Generation' to act as a 'proper Emblem of Virtue and Morality';[4] a year later another silly book in Defoe's name returned to the same theme, with a eulogy of a real individual called Duncan Campbell, who is praised as a gentleman mute with a notable 'presaging Power' and 'prophetical Genius'. Although the silent prophet is said to have been 'adored by all the beautiful women' on account of his 'Dumb, yet oracular, Majesty', he apparently suffered sadly from the hordes of 'virgins and widows' who harassed him with requests for the names and natures of their future husbands.[5]

The contrast with blindness is stark: dreams about it are numerous, and poems and stories too. And literary blindness is a dignified condition – a favoured theme of high tragedy, in particular, where it is usually paired with a compensating spiritual insight. There are no noble literary mutes to set alongside the terrible eyeless figures of Oedipus, Tiresias and Samson.

Dumbness may never be tragic, but it can be sad and affecting. Hans Christian Andersen's little mermaid, for example, was foolish and devoted enough to insist on having her tongue cut out by the sea-witch so that she could become a mortal woman, and offer herself to the handsome prince she loved. Kvapil and Dvořák's wood-nymph Rusalka also sacrificed her voice in order to acquire a human body and be possessed by a gorgeous prince.[6] But if these tales are touching, they are also decidedly abject: dumbness is merely pitiful, and lacks the redeeming spiritual depths associated with blindness. And to add insult to injury, neither Rusalka nor the nameless little mermaid finally got her man.

Literary dumbness, it seems, afflicts victims rather than heroes,

4 Daniel Defoe (?), *The Dumb Philosopher, or Great-Britain's Wonder*, London, 1719, pp. 49, viii. On the inauthenticity of this attribution and the next, see P. N. Furbank and W. R. Owens, *Defoe De-Attributions*, London, The Hambledon Press, 1994, pp. 121, 126.

5 Daniel Defoe (?), *The History of the Life and Adventures of Mr Duncan Campbell – A gentleman, who tho' Deaf and Dumb, writes down any Stranger's name at first Sight; with their future Contingencies of Fortune*, London 1720, pp. 125, 39. The *Dictionary of National Biography* gives Campbell's profession as 'charlatan'.

6 Hans Christian Andersen's 'The Little Mermaid' (1837) was one of the sources for Jaroslav Kvapil's libretto (1899) for Antonin Dvořák's *Rusalka* (1901).

others rather than self, females rather than males. It affects them most especially in their capacity as sexual consorts of men. For although mutes may not be appropriate objects of fear or veneration, it would seem that they can still make excellent brides: ideal recipients of a husband's jealous pity, protectiveness and watchful care. Ben Jonson's unpleasant play *Epicoene* describes a gentleman called Morose, who hates noise and chatter, and has therefore refrained from taking a wife. But at last he is introduced to an irresistible freak, a prodigy, a marvel of nature: nothing less than a quiet woman. Incredulous at first, then overjoyed, he marries her according to the full rites of the church; but as soon as the ceremony is over, he finds he has been duped: beneath the skirts and wig, the perfect wife turns out to be a raucous boy.[7] The hero of Anatole France's *The Man who Married a Mute*, in contrast, had the good fortune to have a true-born mute for a wife. He loved her deeply and they enjoyed great happiness together; but then the foolish man decided to try and improve perfection, and sent for a surgeon to untie her tongue. The surgeon operated, and the operation succeeded. But now the husband found himself yoked to an unstoppable chatterbox, and it drove him to the edge of despair. The surgeon was summoned a second time; another operation was performed; and again it was a success. But on this occasion the patient was the husband, not the wife: the surgeon turned him stone deaf – the only sure remedy, apparently, for a man afflicted with a talkative wife.[8]

The archives of anthropology and natural history contain numerous accounts of people supposedly born incurably dumb – males as much as females. These congenital mutes are always unattractive: idiotic, ugly, inert, atheistic and amoral. Buffon, for example, recounted the case of a young man from Chartres who began to speak for the first time at the age of 24, having previously been completely dumb. His parents were respectable Catholics, and trained him in all the rituals of their church – prayer, confession, mass – but theologians were appalled to discover, once he began to speak, that he had never attached any spiritual meaning to them at all. He had no conception

7 Ben Jonson, *Epicoene; or, the Silent Woman*, 1609 (later adapted by Stefan Zweig to form the libretto for Richard Strauss's *Die schweigsame Frau*, 1935).
8 Anatole France, *La comédie de celui qui épousa une femme muette*, Paris, Calmann-Lévy, 1919.

of the soul or salvation or the significance of Christ's suffering, and despite his outward piety he had led 'a purely animal life', wholly preoccupied with his present sensations and the immediately visible world.[9]

Herder, too, maintained that the dumb were doomed to remain 'like children, or human animals'. Lacking any words to organize their experience, he said, they had no chance of raising themselves above their 'brutal state', and becoming capable of ordinary humanity or morality. He was not surprised when he read about a dumb boy who, having watched a butcher slaughtering a pig, went off and killed his own brother, tearing out his bowels 'with tranquil pleasure, merely in imitation of what he saw' and showing no twinge of remorse afterwards. Herder regarded the report as a confirmation of his theory of language and culture. It was not the only instance, he claimed, of a mute who became a serene murderer, and it served as 'dreadful proof of how little man's boasted understanding, and the feelings of the species, can effect of themselves'.[10] For speech was the source of civilization; and, as Immanuel Kant put it at about the same time, the dumb could never attain the faculty of Reason itself, but only, at best, a mere 'analogy of Reason'.[11]

Such stories and parables about the inhumanity, irrationality, stupidity and depravity of the dumb are numerous and quite well attested, and for centuries they have circulated as if they were plain and unassailable facts. And yet the accounts cannot possibly be true, not even metaphorically and approximately. For the physiological reality is that no one is born without a voice, and there are practically no instances of long-term loss of voice through injury, mutilation or disease. Perhaps the rarity of literary myths about the dumb is misleading, therefore: there are numerous fictions about mutism, but they are to be found not in works of imaginative literature, but in the archives of natural history and philosophical anthropology.

However, significant numbers of children (perhaps one in 3–5,000) are born profoundly deaf. They are obviously not dumb: they will

9 Georges-Louis Leclerc, Comte de Buffon, *Histoire Naturelle*, Vol. 3, Paris 1749. pp. 348–9.

10 Johann Gottfried Herder, *Ideen zur Philosophie der Geschichte*, vol. 1, pp. 111, 296; *Outlines*, pp. 87, 233.

11 Immanuel Kant, *Anthropologie* (1798), *Gesammelte Schriften*, Vol. VII, Berlin, 1917, p. 155.

laugh and cry, or groan and shriek as loudly and expressively as anyone else – in fact rather more so, since they are not inhibited by any direct awareness of the noise they may be making. But they are unable to hear the speech of others, and in the natural course of things will never learn to speak a language. Traditionally, therefore, the prelingually deaf have been categorized as 'deaf and dumb', as if vocal incapacity were somehow intrinsically connected with an inability to hear. Aristotle taught that those born deaf are 'always dumb too',[12] and Pliny the Elder held that 'there are no persons born deaf who are not also dumb'.[13] Indeed in some languages, such as Hebrew and Latin, the same word can be used to cover both conditions. The social connotations of the Latin *surdus* are manifest in its use as a translation of Euclid's *alogos*, meaning an irrational number, and in the formation from it of the idea of absurdity, utter deafness and irredeemable madness. Galen, the leading authority in European medicine for one and a half millennia, attributed deafness and dumbness, along with stupidity, to a single and incurable abnormality of the brain.[14] It is common for words for hearing (such as *entendre* in French) to cover intellectual comprehension as well as auditory recognition, so nothing has been easier than the presumption that the deaf are bound to be dumb as well – in every sense of the word. For in ordinary language, the word *dumb* – like *eneos* in Greek or *stumm* and *dumm* in German – is often used as a casual insult, implying mere idiocy, even by tender-hearted people who would never abuse the name of any other afflicted sector of humanity.

Congenital deafness therefore entailed not just sensory deprivation, but exclusion from language as well, and hence from social and cultural achievement. But deafness is not usually detectable in children until they are well over a year old – too late, in most societies, for the exposure or infanticide that might well have been their fate if the abnormality were apparent at birth. In ancient Greece and Rome, it was permissible to kill deaf children up to the age of three. On the other hand, Mosaic law went out of its way to protect them: 'Thou

12 He notes, however, that the dumb are capable of making vocal sounds: see Aristotle, *History of Animals*, IV, 9, 536b.
13 Pliny the Elder, *Natural History*, X, LXXXVIII.
14 See Thomas Arnold, *Arnold on the Education of the Deaf*, revised and rewritten by Abraham Farrar, London, Simpkin Marshall, 1901, p. 2.

shalt not curse the deaf', as it says in Leviticus.[15] They were permanently childlike, and the Jewish legal tradition did not grant them the responsibilities or rights of adults – they were neither liable to punishment, nor competent to own property, particularly buildings and land.[16]

Under Roman law, too, there were strict limits to the legal capacities of the 'deaf and dumb'. They certainly could not make a will,[17] and might also be barred from marriage, and even from access to the protection of the law. This ruling was sustained in the Christian church. Paul had laid it down that 'faith cometh by hearing' and that 'with the mouth confession is made unto salvation',[18] and it was therefore debatable whether the deaf could ever be validly received into Christian communion, since they could neither show that they understood and accepted the creed, nor confess their sins. Their inability to swear an oath also debarred them from the proceedings of civil courts, and from most feudal rights and duties; and there was also doubt as to whether they could ever be validly married.

This combination of logical, religious, legal and medical principles made the predicament of the 'deaf and dumb' seem hopeless: nothing in the ordinary course of nature could unstop their ears, unlock their tongues, and allow them to enter the circle of human language. Even in the sphere of miracles, remedies were exceptionally rare. Reporting that Christ had actually cured a dumb man, Matthew says that 'the multitudes marvelled, saying, It was never so seen in Israel'.[19] A similar exceptional miracle is attributed to St John of Beverley, who in 685 took pity on a scabby peasant boy who was completely dumb. According to Bede, writing some fifty years after the event, John held the boy by the chin, got him to stick his tongue out, and made the sign of the cross on it. Then he instructed him to say *gae*, or yes, which he did, and to repeat all the letters of the alphabet, so that in a short space of time all the bonds that tied his tongue were broken. Now that he was ungagged, the boy talked without pause for the whole day and through the following night, giving voice to a lifetime of pent-up thoughts and wishes that had never been expressed before.

15 Leviticus, 19:14.
16 See Kenneth W. Hodgson, *The Deaf and their Problems*, London, Watts, 1953, pp. 69–71.
17 Justinian, *Corpus Iuris Civilis*, VI, xxii, 10; *Institutionum sive elementorum*, II, xii.
18 Romans, 10:17; 10:10.
19 Matthew, 9:32–3.

As a result of the miracle, the boy 'gained a clear complexion, ready speech, and beautiful curly hair, whereas he had once been ugly, destitute and dumb'.[20]

Apart from Christ and John of Beverley, though, miracle workers steered clear of the deaf: their dumbness put them not only outside the pale of humanity, but beyond the range of magical and spiritual help as well.

---

20 *Bede's Ecclesiastical History of the English People*, edited by Bertram Colegrave and R. A. B. Mynors, Oxford, Clarendon Press, 1969, Book 5, Chapter 2, pp. 456–9.

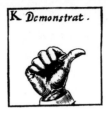

10

'Seeing words' and the beginnings of deaf education

There had always been some loopholes in the prison walls that closed in around the deaf and condemned them to perpetual dumbness. For one thing, deafness is relative rather than absolute, and many children who appear deaf have sufficient residual hearing to learn to speak, provided people around them make an effort to talk to them slowly and distinctly. For another, those who lose their hearing later in life may continue to speak even if they can no longer hear anything at all, demonstrating conclusively that deafness does not immediately entail an inability to speak. Of course, their speech will tend to deteriorate over time, and after some years may be lost altogether; but even then, provided they are literate, they will still be able to communicate by reading and writing. And they may well display a further and (as it was thought) even more astonishing skill, using their eyes to recognize the speech they could no longer hear with their ears. In Cornwall at the end of the sixteenth century, for instance, there was a celebrated old man called Grisling, 'deafe from a longe time', but, it was reported, gifted with 'a strange quality', his astonishing ability 'to understand what you say by marking the moving of your lips . . . so as (contrary to the rules of nature, and yet without the help of arte) he can see wordes as they pass forth of your mouth'.[1]

1 Richard Carew, *The Survey of Cornwall*, London, 1602, Book II, p. 113.

There were clear indications, then, that the predicament of the deaf might not be entirely hopeless. But these clues were persistently ignored, and for centuries no one challenged the assumption that it was physically impossible for those born deaf ever to participate in language. It was not till the middle of the sixteenth century, at least in Europe, that a concerted effort was made to rescue some of them from their isolation. The path was opened in Spain in about 1550 by a Benedictine monk, Pedro Ponce de Leon, who was dismayed by the thought that the 'deaf and dumb' would have to go to their graves without absolution, merely because they had no language in which to make confession of their sins. His proposal was simple and radical: in the absence of a sense of hearing, language could be taught through the other senses, especially vision, aided to some extent by touch. Deaf children should be encouraged to watch people speaking, that is to say, and perhaps use their fingers to feel the resonances in their throats; and then, he argued, they had only to imitate them with the help of a mirror in order to produce sounds themselves and thus to speak.

Before long Ponce de Leon's theory came to the attention of a Castilian aristocrat who had two young sons, Pedro and Francisco de Velasco, both of whom were deaf. Their disability threatened to exclude them not only from heaven, but also from their inheritance, and their father was determined to find some way to teach them to speak. When Pedro Ponce was first introduced to them, he found to his dismay that they 'knew nothing, like a stone',[2] so instead of setting to work immediately on their voices, he decided to reverse the usual order, and teach them visible language – that is to say, writing – before requiring them to tackle speech.[3] The boys did exercises in associating everyday objects with their written names, and also learned to trace out the shapes of written words for themselves. As Pedro de Velasco himself was to recall later: 'I started to learn by writing down the things my master taught me.' Next he was trained, through vision and touch, to copy his teacher in vocalizing each letter of the alphabet,

2 The achievement of Pedro Ponce de Leon is acknowledged in most histories of deaf education, but there are conflicting versions of it. The account which seems to keep closest to original sources is in Abraham Farrar's introduction to Juan Pablo Bonet, *Simplification of the Letters of the Alphabet and Method of Teaching Deaf-Mutes to speak*, translated by H. N. Dixon, Harrogate, Abraham Farrar, 1890, pp. 21–9.
3 Franciscus Vallesius, *De Sacra Philosophia, sive de iis quae physice scripta sunt in Libris Sacris* (1588), Frankfurt, 1600, pp. 60–1.

mastering the five vowels first and then proceeding to the consonants. He could then return to the written words he had learned, and spell them out loud, letter by letter, until eventually he was in a position to make a stab at pronouncing whole words, 'though with much saliva'. By the time Pedro Ponce died in 1584, he had earned the gratitude of several 'notable people whom I have taught to speak, read, write and reckon, to pray, to assist at the mass, and to know how to confess themselves by speech'.[4]

The remedy was not perfect, but it seemed pretty miraculous all the same: thanks to Pedro Ponce, it became imaginable that the deaf might eventually learn to participate in language, both written and spoken, and therefore in legal and religious ceremonies, as well as everyday human affairs. A monk with a special skill for 'making the deaf and dumb hear and speak after a fashion, and for curing madness' would appear before long in a story by Cervantes,[5] and Mersenne cited Pedro Ponce's use of writing with his deaf pupils as further proof of the old Platonic principle that language is 'arbitrary' and entirely dependent on 'human institution'.[6]

Half a century after these epoch-making cures, another deaf child was born into the same family. He was Luis de Velasco, great-nephew of Francisco and Pedro, and his father entrusted him to a follower of Ponce de Leon for training according to the same method: visible writing first and then audible speech. By 1623 the young man could express himself quite clearly, and he was presented to the Prince of Wales (the future Charles I), who was in Madrid to seek the hand of the Infanta in marriage. As it happened, the Prince found Luis de Velasco to be quite as interesting as the prospective bride, and far more responsive to his attentions. A member of Charles's retinue, Sir Kenelm Digby, left an influential account of what they heard and saw.

> The spanish lord, was borne deafe; so deafe, that if a gunne were shott off close by his eare, he should not heare it: and

4 See Abraham Farrar, Introduction to Bonet, *Simplification of the Letters of the Alphabet*, pp. 21–9.
5 Miguel de Cervantes, 'The Glass Graduate', in *Exemplary Stories* (1613), translated by C. A. Jones, London, Penguin Books, 1972, p. 145.
6 Marin Mersenne, *Traitez de la voix et des chants*, Prop. LI ('Si l'on peut faire parler les muets'), pp. 78–9.

consequently, he was dumbe ... The lovelinesse of his face and especially the exceeding life and spiritfulnesse of his eyes, and the comelinesse of his person and whole composure of his body throughout, were pregnant signes of a well-tempered mind within. And therefore all that knew him lamented much the want of meanes to cultivate it, and to imbue it with the notions which it seemed to be capable of in regard of its selfe; had it not been so crossed by this unhappy accident.

Physicians were called in, but to no effect. Then at last, as Digby relates, a priest came forward and undertook to teach him. It was not easy; but eventually,

after strange patience, constancy and paines; he brought the young Lord to speake as distinctly as any man whosoever; and to understand so perfectly what others said that he would not loose a word in a whole dayes conversation.

Like his great-uncle, Luis was taught first to read, then to write, and then to pronounce words on the basis of their spelling. And in learning to articulate, he had also developed an ability to 'heare by his eyes', or 'see' words on a speaker's face, almost as well as he could on a printed page. This 'seeing of words' was impossible in the dark, of course, or when the speaker's face was out of sight; on the other hand, Luis had the advantage of being able to decipher a whispered conversation at a distance, which would be quite lost on his hearing friends. What is more, so Digby reports, he was a remarkable mimic: the Prince of Wales tested him by getting some of his servants to talk to him in Welsh, and – despite the fact that their words were mostly guttural, formed more in the throat than on the lips – Luis 'so perfectly echoed, that I confesse I wondered more att that, than att all the rest'.[7]

Luis de Velasco, then, appears to be the first 'deaf and dumb' person to learn to participate fully in the conversations of hearing people – not only producing vocal sounds in accordance with his knowledge of a written language, but also recognizing the words of others simply by watching their faces as they spoke. Digby implies, probably falsely, that the worker of this unprecedented double cure was Juan Pablo

7 Kenelm Digby, *Two Treatises*, Paris, 1644, pp. 253–5.

Bonet, whose book of 1620 on *The Simplification of the Letters of the Alphabet* was the first ever published on the art of teaching language to the deaf.[8] Like Ponce de Leon (whom he did not acknowledge however), Bonet taught reading and writing as a preliminary to speech. But he added a powerful new technique as well, making language visible in the form of a 'finger alphabet', based on a method of silent communication already in use in various religious communities. The art consisted simply in using a different handshape to represent each letter of the alphabet, which enabled the master and his deaf pupil to spell out words to each other by making gestures in the air, without the encumbrance of chalks, slates or pieces of paper.[9] (See Figures 3 and 4 overleaf)

Having mastered reading, writing and finger-spelling, Bonet's pupil would be ready to learn to speak. Bonet used a leather model of a tongue to provide an ocular demonstration of its various positions, and a well-lit room, so that the inside of his mouth could be easily seen. His task was then comparable to teaching a musical instrument: the deaf child simply had to memorize the positions of tongue, lips and teeth required for producing various vocal sounds, rather as an apprentice guitarist had to learn the fingering for different chords.[10]

This raised the question of which vocal sounds the child should be taught, and Bonet's proudest boast was that he had solved the problem by means of a new doctrine of the alphabet. He took it for granted that the purpose of written alphabetical characters was to symbolize different vocal sounds, so that 'as the voice of the writer is absent, they represent this voice, supplying entirely the place it would have taken'. The art of the written word was therefore 'nothing more than joining together as many different letters as the sounds which compose the word pronounced, keeping the correct order'. In practice, however,

8 Juan Pablo Bonet, *Reducción de las Letras, y arte para enseñar à ablar los mudos,* Madrid, 1620. It has often been assumed that the education of Luis de Velasco was started in 1615 by E. Ramirez de Carrión, and taken over by Bonet a year later: see Jean-René Presneau, 'Le son "à la lettre": l'éducation des sourds et muets avant l'abbé de l'Épée', in Alexis Karacostas, ed., *Le Pouvoir des Signes*, Paris, Institut National des Jeunes Sourds, 1989, pp. 20–32, p. 26. But for a juster appreciation of the work of Ramírez de Carrion, see Susan Plann, *A Silent Minority: Deaf Education in Spain 1550–1835*, Berkely, University of California Press, 1997, p. 66.
9 Juan Pablo Bonet, *Simplification of the Letters of the Alphabet*, pp. 69, 154.
10 *Simplification of the Letters of the Alphabet*, pp. 152, 156–7.

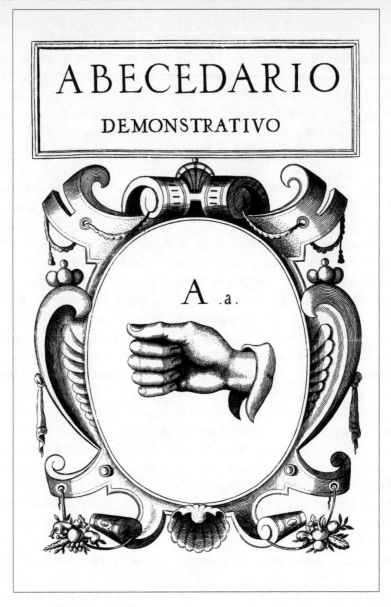

FIG 3. The letter A in Bonet's one-handed finger alphabet

matters were not so simple, because the letters of the alphabet were traditionally known by arbitrary names, like *aleph* or *alpha* for A. Bonet's reform was to call the letters by names which were identical to their sounds when pronounced as part of a word, and to reduce their

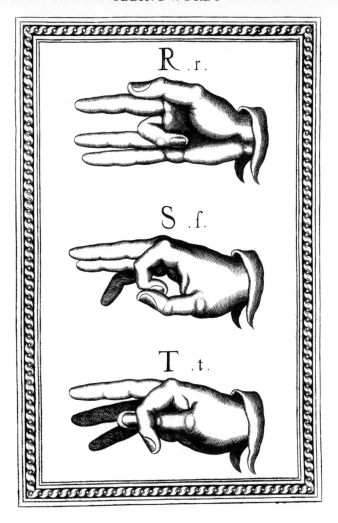

FIG 4. R, S and T in Bonet's finger alphabet

number to twenty-one basic 'natural letters'. (Bonet was susceptible to the attractions of etymology, and claimed to have discovered the 'primitive names' of the letters, the names they had been given 'by their first inventors' – a claim which may well have inspired Francis Mercury van Helmont in his obsessive quest for the true pronunciation of Hebrew letters.) With the help of the model tongue, Bonet then taught his deaf pupils how to produce for themselves the twenty-one sounds corresponding to the letters of his alphabet; then, once they had mastered a language in its written form, they would automatically be able to speak it as well.[11]

Reports about the deaf Spanish nobles who had been taught reading, finger-spelling and writing, and then learned to speak and understand the speech of others, spread rapidly throughout Europe, exciting a mixture of curiosity, compassion and incredulity. In 1660, Anton Deusing of Groningen published an account of several deaf contemporaries in Holland who, if they could not speak, could communicate visually by reading and writing, and also follow sermons by seeing words directly on the lips of the preacher: 'it will be no absurdity to say that tis probable they take the Word in at their eyes, they are so intent, which others use to do by the ear.' Referring to St Paul's doctrine that 'faith cometh by hearing', he was moved to exclaim:

> Oh this is indeed a very hard saying, which shipwracks the Soul! Truly since those that are born deaf are no more guilty of neglecting the means of their Salvation, than Infants . . . what reason can there be why we should think God less merciful to them?

Surely, he argued, these deaf and dumb creatures had the same capacity as any other children for learning language and acquiring the 'saving knowledge' of religion. What justice could there possibly be in shutting them out from happiness and 'knowledge of the Invisible mysteries'?[12]

Another indignant campaigner in the cause of the deaf was George Dalgarno, a Scot who ran a grammar school in Oxford and published a *Deaf and Dumb Man's Tutor* in 1680. He was not very interested in the Spanish art of teaching the deaf to speak, and he dismissed Digby's story about Luis de Velasco imitating the sounds of unfamiliar foreign words as 'hyperbolical' and 'impossible'. He was also wary of claims about the deaf being able to 'read the Speaker's words from his face' and to do so 'as readily as from permanent Characters upon paper'. But all these activities were superfluous anyway, according to Dalgarno: the only thing necessary was that the deaf should be taught to 'speak by the eye' – in other words, to write. His advice to the educator of the deaf

11 Bonet, *Simplification of the Letters of the Alphabet*, pp. 93, 79, 84, 70–1.
12 Antonius Deusingius, *De Surdis ab Ortu; Mutisque*, in *Fasciculus dissertationum selectarum*, Groningen, 1660, pp. 184–6, 177, 175; the essay is best known in an English version which has often been mistaken for an original work: George Sibscota, *The Deaf and Dumb Man's Discourse*, London, 1670, see pp. 44–6, 36–7, 34.

was simple: 'Keep your scholar close to the practice of writing.'[13]

Dalgarno's cautious comment about the possibility of 'reading' words by looking at the movements of a speaker's face is probably the first occasion when the concept of reading was extended from the recognition of written characters to include what would eventually be called 'lip-reading' as well. And he also tried to expand the concept of 'writing', so that it would cover all possible ways of making language visible – not only the traditional 'grammatology' but also 'dactylology', or the fluent spelling of words in space, using a manual alphabet. Deaf children could, he suggested, be given a glove for the left hand, with the five vowels written on the tips of the fingers and thumb, and all the single consonants, together with several double or triple ones, displayed on the palm. (See Figure 5 overleaf) They could then 'write' in fluent two-handed 'hand-language' by pointing to the appropriate place on the glove with their right hand, using a finger for vowels and the thumb for the consonants. Eventually they would be able to communicate without the glove, much faster than by grammatological writing, and almost with the speed of speech.

Dalgarno was apparently unaware of Bonet's one-handed dactylology. Nevertheless, he said that when confronted with a deaf man who had lost an arm he had devised a one-handed version of his own system, using the thumb to indicate parts of the same hand. With a touch of the whimsy that has often appealed to teachers of the deaf, he suggested that the hand then functioned so much like a mouth that it really began to look like one, with the thumb figuring as the tongue, and the fingers and hollow of the hand as the lips, teeth and palate. The one-handed dactylology could also be a boon to busy public men: a modern Julius Caesar might use it, Dalgarno mused, to 'keep up discourse with 3 several persons, upon several subjects, talking to two with his two hands, and to a third with his Tongue'.[14]

The education of the deaf was now becoming something of a fad, but Dalgarno chose to neglect the most spectacular part of it: the production and comprehension of speech. This development, though, presupposed some theorization of the nature of language, along the

13 George Dalgarno, *Didascalocophus, or the Deaf and Dumb Man's Tutor*, Oxford, 1680, pp. 45, 32, 40, 25.
14 George Dalgarno, *Didascalocophus*, pp. 84, 86, 88.

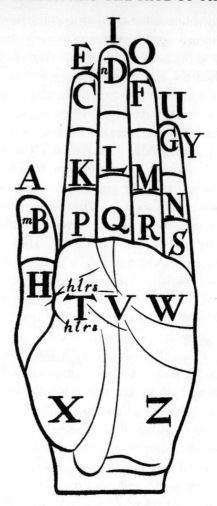

FIG 5. Dalgarno's Dactylological Glove

lines already suggested in Bonet's theory of the alphabet. John Wallis, Savilian Professor of Geometry at Oxford and an acquaintance of Dalgarno's, had already laid down some of its principles in 1653. His brief essay on 'the formation and true sound of letters' was, he claimed, 'a new attempt, never before undertaken'.[15] In conformity with the usage of his time, Wallis used the word 'letters' to refer not so much to the

15 See Christopher J. Scriba, 'The Autobiography of John Wallis, FRS', *Notes and Records of the Royal Society of London* 25, 1970, pp. 17–47, p. 41.

elements of the written alphabet, as to the corresponding sounds of speech.[16] (The practice parallels the use of 'note' to mean a musical tone rather than its graphic notation.) Letters, Wallis wrote, are 'simple, incomposite sounds, not divisible into simpler', and should not be confused with characters, the elements of writing. Ideally, letters and characters would correspond to each other, but in practice they often diverged. For example, both *ph* and *th* were pronounced as simple sounds in English, though written with two characters; and he identified nine distinct vocal or vowel letters in English, with only five characters to represent them in writing.[17]

Six years later, in 1659, a deaf and dumb child named Alexander Popham was entrusted to William Holder, Rector of Bletchington near Oxford. It appears that Holder managed to teach the boy reading, writing and some version of 'an Alphabet upon his fingers', but he was not satisfied with that. Although he acknowledged that it was possible to use many different kinds of '*Signes* for communication', he was convinced that none were so excellent as 'the variety of instructive expressions by *Speech*, wherewith *Man* alone is endowed'. He therefore undertook what was to be the first reliably attested cure of 'dumbness' in England. Like Dalgarno, he was sceptical about accounts of deaf people 'who could discern Speech by their Eye'. He realized that many significant differences of vocal sound depended on movements of the vocal organs that had no visible effect on the speaker's face at all. For this reason he constructed a full plaster model of the upper jaw and palate, together with a tongue made of stuffed leather, which he used for showing his pupil how to produce these more sequestered sounds. Then – drawing, it would seem, on Wallis's recent work on the 'letters' of English – he distinguished between the visible characters used in writing, printing and engraving, and the audible letters themselves, 'the natural Elements of Speech'. He also devised ingenious charts –again following Wallis – showing how the various sounds of language were 'differenced and defined', and used these as a basis for a new simplification of the English alphabet. Thus equipped, he set out to

16 See 'What is a letter?' (1949), in David Abercrombie, *Studies in Phonetics and Linguistics*, Oxford, Oxford University Press, 1965, pp. 76–85.
17 John Wallis, *De Loquela, sive Sonorum Formatione, Tractatus Grammatico-Physicus*, printed as a preface to his *Grammatica Linguae Anglicanae*, Oxford, 1653, pp. 2, 5, 12.

remedy 'the calamitous and Deplorable Condition of persons Deaf & Dumb'.[18]

Within a year, Alexander Popham was able to speak, apparently rather well. Various members of Oxford University, including Wallis, went out to visit Holder in Bletchington and observe the young deaf man, and they marvelled at his capacity 'to pronounce plainly and distinctly, and with a good and graceful tone, whatsoever words were shewn him in Print or Writing, or represented to him in several other ways'.[19]

Soon after that, Wallis decided to emulate Holder's success. He found another deaf boy, Daniel Whaley, and began trying to train him to an even higher level than Holder's pupil Popham. In May 1662, Wallis exhibited Whaley to Charles II at Court, and also to members of the Royal Society, where Whaley was observed to 'pronounce distinctly enough such words as by the Company were proposed to him; and though not altogether in the usual Tone or Accent, yet so as easily to be understood'.[20] Later that year, Wallis claimed, he 'did the like for Mr Alexander Popham . . . with like success'.[21]

Alexander Popham? But surely Popham was Holder's prodigy, not Wallis's?

It would seem that Wallis was stealing Holder's pupil, and trying to steal his reputation as well. In due course Holder retaliated by reclaiming Popham for himself, and also attacking Wallis's claims about Daniel Whaley. He did not deny that Whaley had been taught to speak by Wallis. But he disclosed that Whaley was not born deaf, and had already learnt to speak before losing his hearing, so that Wallis was lying when he claimed to have trained him to speak for the first time. Holder also stated, perhaps correctly, that the same applied to the celebrated Luis de Velasco. That, he thought, left his own pupil, Alexander Popham as the first clear case in history of a child born profoundly deaf and finally brought to speak through assiduous training:

18 William Holder, *Elements of Speech: an Essay of Inquiry into the Natural Production of Letters, with an appendix concerning Persons Deaf & Dumb*, London, Royal Society, 1669, pp. 151, 3, 5, 125, 137, 9, 37, 40, 52, 53, 62, 126, 110.

19 William Holder, *A Supplement to the Philosophical Transactions of July 1670, with some Reflexions on Dr John Wallis*, London, Henry Brome, 1678, p. 5.

20 See *Philosophical Transactions of the Royal Society of London*, Vol. 5, No 61, 18 July 1670, p. 1098. See also J. F. Scott, *The Mathematical Work of John Wallis*, London, Taylor and Francis, 1938, p. 85.

21 'The Autobiography of John Wallis, FRS', p. 42.

and that achievement was the work not of Professor Wallis, but of Dr Holder.

This kind of petty rivalry was to occur over and over again amongst educators of the deaf. But behind it all there lay one of the greatest scientific advances of the entire seventeenth century, and one of the most beneficial medical and educational discoveries of all time. It was now established beyond doubt that the deaf – contrary to the traditional principles of metaphysics, medicine, theology and law – could, after all, be taught to understand language, and even to speak. By using their eyes in place of their ears, it seems, they were exploding the ancient common sense which amalgamated deafness and dumbness into a single indissoluble category. The deaf were displaying skills of the most paradoxical kind – reading and writing before they could speak, speaking with their fingers, hearing with their eyes, and reading words that were not even written; not to mention speaking out with their own voices. After centuries of neglect, the deaf were turning into a curiosity, a spectacle, a wonder.

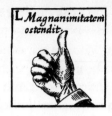

11

Writing, meaning and parroting

Apart from the talking deaf, another of the great marvels of seventeenth-century Europe was the 'rational parrot' – in particular, a bird that belonged to Johan Maurits, otherwise Prince Maurice of Nassau, when he was Governor of the Dutch colony in Brazil between 1636 and 1644. According to Sir William Temple, there was 'a common, but much credited Story' about Prince Maurice's parrot, which 'spoke, and ask'd, and answer'd common Questions like a reasonable Creature'. The Prince's followers were convinced that the bird was bewitched or possessed, and one of his chaplains went in fear of parrots ever after, because 'they all had a Devil in them'. When questioned by Sir William in 1668, the elderly Prince Maurice corroborated the story, recalling that when it was first introduced to him, the parrot said: 'What a company of white men are here?' Asked who it thought the Prince was, it answered, 'Some general or other,' and so on through a short but coherent conversation – a creditable diplomatic audience, then, if not a rich human dialogue.[1]

John Locke, who recounted the story in what is sometimes said to be the most memorable paragraph of his *Essay concerning Human Understanding*, regarded it as 'sufficient to countenance the suppo-

---

1 William Temple, *Memoirs of what past in Christendom, from the War begun 1672 to the Peace concluded 1679*, London, 1691, pp. 57–60.

sition of a rational Parrot'. In Locke's opinion it was probable, in fact, that the bird could 'discourse, reason, and philosophize' with rather more intelligence than many an ordinary 'dull, irrational *Man*'.[2]

A comparison with the talking deaf could have suggested itself too, since their intellectual range was turning out to be sadly limited, and their conversation in some ways less adaptable and natural than that of Prince Maurice's parrot, which at least had the advantage of being able to hear what was said to it and monitor the sound of its own voice. Take Wallis's description of his prize pupil Daniel Whaley for example:

> I had taught him to pronounce distinctly any words, so as I directed him (even the most difficult of the Polish Language, which a Polish Lord then in Oxford could propose to him . . .) and in good measure to understand a Language and express his own in writing. And he . . . read over to me distinctly (the whole or greater part of) the English Bible; and did pretty well understand (at least) the Historical part of it.[3]

As spectacular cures go, this treatment of Whaley's dumbness is distinctly disappointing. He could imitate the sounds of Polish, and read out passages of written English when told to do so; but the spiritual aspects of the Bible were definitely unintelligible to him, and he was quite unable to speak and argue on his own account. Despite having learned to read, write and speak, Daniel Whaley seems to have remained pretty dumb in every other sense of the word – not much better than the talkative old parrot, in fact, and in some respects rather worse.

The problem was that even if the deaf could be taught to pronounce words tolerably well, their relationship to language remained so strange and irregular that it was never certain that they could understand it as others do. Ordinary hearing children, after all, progress spontaneously from echoing the sounds of others in infancy, to forming word-like sounds, then words and structured sequences of words, so that in the first four or five years of life they acquire a whole language – both a system of sounds and a corresponding system of meanings, not to

2 John Locke, *An Essay concerning Human Understanding* (fourth edition, 1700), Book II, Chapter XXVII, §8, p. 333.
3 'The Autobiography of John Wallis, FRS', p. 42.

mention some grammar and a wealth of information picked up by casually listening to people talking around them.

Eventually, they may begin the arduous process of adding a third element to their linguistic skills, by learning to read and write. Of course they will never acquire literacy without the help of a teacher; but on the other hand the teacher will always have the extensive groundwork of the child's untaught linguistic knowledge to build upon. Literacy is imparted to hearing children, therefore, as a kind of supplementary technique – an auxiliary method for representing spoken forms which they can already recognize and repeat, and whose meanings and grammatical relations they already implicitly understand. If for some reason they never learn to read it will do no harm to their ability to speak. The triangle of their linguistic ability – linking the fields of audible sound, intelligible meaning, and visible script – rests on a base of sound and meaning, and their literacy is little more than an optional superstructure, an afterthought.

But it was obvious that deaf children are shut out from this way of experiencing language. The early beneficiaries of the new art of educating the deaf – from Pedro and Francisco de Velasco in Spain in the 1570s to Alexander Popham and Daniel Whaley in England in the 1660s – were well beyond childhood by the time they started to learn their first language; physically they were healthy enough, but culturally they were so backward that they appeared to be mere idiots.

Moreover, their teachers – Ponce de Leon, Bonet, Holder and Wallis – all found it necessary to start them on their linguistic education exactly where their hearing brothers and sisters would have finished: with reading and writing, that is to say, not meaning and sound. If, after many years of study, a deaf pupil could match vocal sounds to written characters one by one, and thus manage to speak from a written text and give formulaic responses in church, then it was a remarkable and praiseworthy achievement, even a noble one; but their general linguistic knowledge would still be lagging far behind that of an ordinary uneducated child.

It is true that certain teachers – including Ponce de Leon and John Wallis – tried to remedy the difficulty by writing words on cards and attaching them to simple objects so that their pupils could guess at their meanings. But it would obviously never be possible to explain more than a few hundred words by this method, and then only the kind of words that stand directly for mundane physical realities: hats and shoes, tables and pens, or hands and feet. With such a lopsided vocabulary, it is hardly surprising that Daniel Whaley had difficulty with the spiritual meaning of the Bible. John Wallis warned, therefore, that the deaf might never learn to read and write with real comprehension. Instead they would be acting 'like a Scrivener':

> a Scrivener, who understanding no language but English, transcribes a piece of Latin, Welsh or Irish; or like a printer of Greek or Arabick, who knows neither the sound nor significance of what he printeth.[4]

Indeed the intellectual prospects for the deaf were even worse than that: the scriveners and printers of Oxford might not know much Latin, Welsh, Irish, Greek or Arabic, but at least they understood their native English. The talking deaf, in contrast, had no prior linguistic knowledge whatsoever, and they would be lucky if they could learn to speak at all, even 'to speak like a Parrot'. It was rather like teaching portrait-painting to the blind, or training the deaf to sing by following a musical score: even if they eventually attained some proficiency, the meaning and point of the whole exercise was bound to elude them. They were, it seemed, being forced to act a part in a ridiculous and alien masquerade, bringing possible amusement to others, but no benefit whatever to themselves.

To the spiritual etymologists, of course, the apparent limitations on the linguistic understanding of the talking deaf were not particularly worrying. When Francis Mercury van Helmont boasted that he had taught speech to several patients who were 'deaf and dumb from birth', he only meant that he had got them to pronounce his Natural Alphabet of pristine, pre-Babelian Hebrew letters. They had not learned the words of any actual human language, and even if, as he maintained, they were deriving profound spiritual benefit from taking part in the God-like activity of vocalization, it still gave them no access whatever to ordinary human conversation.[5]

His follower Johann Conrad Amman opened his practice as a vocal

---

4 John Wallis, Letter to Robert Boyle, dated 14 March 1661/2, *Philosophical Transactions of the Royal Society*, Vol. 5, No 61, 18 July 1670, p. 1087.
5 Francis Mercury van Helmont, *Cogitationes super Genesis*, 1697, pp. 2–3, and Johann Conrad Amman, *Dissertatio de Loquela*, Preface; *Dissertation on Speech*, p. xxi.

therapist in the Netherlands by working with hearing patients who suffered from disorders such as stammering or Hottentotism (defined as 'being able to distinguish and understand the sounds of others but not being able so to elaborate sounds . . . as to be intelligible to others'), and teaching them articulation on the basis of a conventional written alphabet.[6] And when he began to treat various 'deaf and dumb' children, he took exactly the same approach, training them to chant the alphabet and then drilling them in speech, without making any allowance for the fact that, unlike his previous patients, they had no knowledge of language. An English doctor named Charles Ellis visited Amman in 1699 and was very taken with one of his pupils, a young girl of seventeen who was 'born Deaf and Dumb, yet taught by Dr Amman to speak very intelligibly'. Ellis was entranced by her ability to read out texts in both Latin and Dutch, and did not worry about her inability to understand them, or to devise any conversation of her own.[7]

No doubt the parents who were paying Amman's fees urged him to teach their deaf children the meanings of words as well as their sounds, and Amman decided to accept the challenge, though he still insisted that pure vocalization in accordance with the Natural Alphabet must come first. 'When my pupil, a born mute, is able to read and to imitate me a little in speaking, I treat him as a *tabula rasa*, a sheet of white paper or a new-born child,' he wrote. 'First I teach him the names of the most obvious things . . . as also the more necessary verbs and adverbs . . . and not till last, the peculiar construction of the language.'[8]

When Helmont eventually came to Haarlem to observe Amman's practice, he was amazed to find that he had

> found out a way whereby such as are born deaf may with a certainty, scarce inferiour to that of a Mathematical Demonstration, learn to read readily, and to take in the Sense of others, not at their Ears, but at their Eyes, and to express their Minds with an articulate Voice; of which to pass by other Instances, I myself have been an Eye-witness at Haarlem.[9]

6 Amman, *Dissertatio de Loquela, pp. 106–7; Dissertation on Speech*, p. 119.
7 Letter from Charles Ellis, 1699, *Philosophical Transactions of the Royal Society*, Vol. 23, No 46, July–August 1703, p. 1416.
8 Amman, *Dissertatio de Loquela*, pp. 102, 103; *Dissertation on Speech*, pp. 114, 115.
9 Francis Mercury van Helmont, *The Spirit of Diseases, or Diseases of the Spirit*, Preface to the Reader.

Helmont was introduced to Amman's prize pupil, Esther Kolard, a young woman who had originally been able to say nothing except 'Pappa', but who after her training 'speaks upon any subject whatever without awkwardness, and though deaf . . . hears others speak with her eyes, and promptly replies to their questions'. Confronted with this charming prodigy, Helmont had to admit that, for everyday human purposes, as distinct from spiritual and divine ones, his own method of sticking to the true Natural Alphabet left something to be desired, and Amman triumphantly recalled his master's recognition 'that I had greatly surpassed him in practical results'.[10]

John Wallis did not learn of Amman's work until 1699, and then wrote a dry letter congratulating him for reinventing in the 1690s what he himself had already achieved thirty years before.[11] But while Wallis agreed with Amman's policy of starting with reading and writing, he was now firmly opposed to his emphasis on getting the deaf to speak with their voices and 'hear' with their eyes. For Wallis, speech might be useful for certain practical purposes, but it did not have any special metaphysical virtue. Spoken forms of language, like written ones, were 'purely Arbitrary', and 'there is nothing, in the Nature of the Thing it self, why Letters and Characters might not as properly be applyed to represent Immediately . . . what our conceptions are'. It was a waste of time to bother with speech: 'we may as well make use of that Character, or Collection of Letters, to express the Thing to the Eyes of him that is Deaf, by which others express the Sound or Name of it to those that Hear.' After all, children who can hear will automatically learn the form of language that is easiest for them to perceive, picking up grammar and meaning at the same time. According to Wallis, there was no reason at all why deaf children should not do exactly the same: the visible forms of writing could play the same role in their linguistic education as the audible forms of speech in the development of those who can hear. As far as Wallis was concerned, there was no great mystery about teaching articulation to the deaf, but there was not much point in it either – certainly not

10 Johann Conrad Amman, *The Talking Deaf Man*, p. 73; *Dissertatio de Loquela*, Dedication and Preface, n.p.; *Dissertation on Speech*, pp. xviii, xxi.
11 Wallis's letter was reprinted in *Dissertatio de Loquela*, Preface; *Dissertation on Speech*, p. xxii.

before they had understood linguistic meanings on the basis of reading. Speech for deaf children was like writing for those who could hear: a potentially useful adjunct to their basic linguistic knowledge, but not an essential part of it.[12]

In 1698, in response to an inquiry from a correspondent called Thomas Beverley who had five 'deaf and dumb' children, Wallis remarked that the deaf could learn '*marks. . . by the eye*' just as pain-lessly as other children learn 'sounds by the ear'. Written marks and spoken sounds, after all, 'do equally signify the same Things or Notions, and are equally . . . of meer Arbitrary Signification'.[13]

As a mathematician, indeed, Wallis considered that written marks could be distinctly preferable to spoken sounds. The arabic numerals, and the symbols of alchemy and algebra, had the great virtue of signify-ing the same meanings to everyone, though expressed by different vocal sounds in different languages. The fact that the deaf could learn to understand marks on paper without having to worry about how to pronounce them could therefore put them at a positive advantage. Writing would have much the same function for them as it apparently had amongst 'the Chineses, whose whole language is said to be made up of such characters as to represent Things and Notions, independent on the Sound of Words, and is therefore differently spoken, by those who differ not in the Writing of it'.[14]

Leibniz too, despite his affection for Helmont's metaphysics of the voice, was beginning to wonder if the deaf should not be considered fortunate rather than cursed in being confined to visible forms of language. In a letter of 1706, he speculated that there was no reason why the deaf should not become superb inventors and scientific inno-vators, 'without recourse to speech, but simply using equivalent written characters'. He too likened the situation of the deaf to that of the Chinese, who, he thought, would have little to lose if they all became deaf and dumb: their speech was acknowledged to be impoverished and

---

12 John Wallis, Letter to Robert Boyle, pp. 1091–2.
13 John Wallis, 'A letter to Mr Thomas Beverley, concerning his Method for Instructing Persons Deaf and Dumb', *Philosophical Transactions of the Royal Society*, Vol. 20, No 245, October 1698, pp. 354–5.
14 John Wallis, Letter to Robert Boyle, p. 1091. Wallis's view of Chinese script is hardly accurate (the characters in fact represent words or syllables, rather than 'things and notions'), but it was widely credited by Western philosophers and metaphysicians till the nineteenth century, and even by some in the twentieth.

barely articulate, but their writing system compensated, he claimed, by being 'abundant, and independent of languages'. It was even conceivable, Leibniz mused, that if an entire nation were congenitally deaf and dumb, it could raise itself to the highest levels of civilization through vision alone, on the basis of a writing system like that of the Chinese.[15]

As the novelty of the talking deaf wore off, and harsh doubts arose as to whether they could really understand speech as opposed to parroting it, an intriguing new possibility began to suggest itself. Far from languishing in linguistic idiocy, the deaf could be enjoying the privileges of a special etymological truth. Being confined to visible means of communication, they might be formulating and communicating their thoughts with a vividness and precision inconceivable to those who content themselves with the conventional forms of speech. The stream of metaphysical speculation about the deaf would now plunge down to an even more mysterious level of meaning – to a deeper etymology, beyond both voice and sound.

15 Gottfried Wilhelm Leibniz, Letter to the Dowager Duchess of Orléans, 9 February 1706, *Die Werke von Leibniz*, edited by Onno Klopp, Vol. IX, Hanover, 1873, pp. 163–9, p. 167.

12

Muscular etymology and
the language of signs

Until the Renaissance, the idea of educating the deaf had always seemed impossible: they had no language, so how could they ever be taught? But when Ponce de Leon and the other early pioneers of deaf education eventually embarked on the task, a simple solution presented itself, so obvious that at first it was not even noticed or discussed. Since deaf children could not be given their first lessons through audible words, their teachers would have to make use of visible deeds instead, or 'little Actions and Gestures', as John Wallis was to put it in 1661.[1] These gestures would of course have to be self-explanatory and independent of the conventions of spoken language, unlike ordinary manual alphabets. To construct their first bridgehead of communication to deaf children, therefore, teachers would need to learn how to 'signify . . . by Signes',[2] that is to say by naturally meaningful bodily movements.

In order to achieve this direct form of visible communication, the educators of the deaf would have to forget their dignity and turn themselves into actors – miming, playing parts, pointing things out, and expressing reactions with exaggerated smiles, stares and grimaces. Performances like these, as Wallis said, had 'a kind of Natural signific-

1 John Wallis, Letter to Robert Boyle, p. 1092.
2 John Wallis, 'A Letter to Mr Thomas Beverley', p. 359.

ancy',[3] and deaf children with no knowledge of language should be able to understand them without much difficulty. Then, Wallis said, the teacher should simply take up a pen or a piece of chalk and write out the linguistic equivalent of what had been indicated or acted in gestures. Deaf pupils would thus come to associate gestural signs with written words, and at length they would learn to understand a conventional language, at least in its written form.

In his earlier discussions of gestural communication, Wallis assumed that there were very few signs whose meaning would be obvious to the deaf pupil from the outset; but he hoped that, if the teacher was very patient, this foundation might be enlarged and elaborated by small degrees, until at last it would be extensive enough to provide 'the explication of a compleat Language'.[4] Many years later, however, Wallis realized that there was also a far more interesting possibility: uneducated deaf children might already have their own repertory of signs, which owed nothing to any lessons from their laborious hearing tutors. 'Deaf persons,' as he observed in 1698, 'are often very good at . . . signifying their mind by Signes.' Their skill would obviously develop best where groups of them were brought up together, and Wallis advised his correspondent Thomas Beverley, who had five deaf children, to learn signs from them, rather than making up new ones of his own: 'We must endeavour to learn their language (if I may so call it) in order to teach them ours.' The deaf could then be shown 'what *Words* answer to their *Signes*', and it would be as if they were learning their second language, not their first.[5]

Wallis's idea that the deaf might already have an effective substitute for language in the form of gestural signs was not entirely new. Indeed the possibility had been mentioned in Plato's *Cratylus*, where Socrates – before setting off on his comical search for the 'original names' whose sound was a natural expression of their meaning – paused for a moment to follow up another line of thought:

> I will ask you a question. Suppose that we had no voice or tongue, and wanted to indicate objects to one another, should

3 Wallis, Letter to Robert Boyle, p. 1092.
4 Letter to Robert Boyle, p. 1092.
5 Wallis, 'A Letter to Mr Thomas Beverley', p. 359

we not, like the deaf and dumb, make signs with the hand and head and the rest of the body? . . . We should imitate the nature of the thing; the elevation of our hands to heaven would mean lightness and upwardness; heaviness and downwardness would be expressed by letting them drop to the ground; if we were describing the running of a horse, or any other kind of animal, we would make our bodies and their gestures as like as we could to them.[6]

Socrates referred to the use of signs by the 'deaf and dumb' as if it were a matter of common experience in ancient Athens, and there is a passing reference in St Augustine too.[7] But it was not till the beginning of the sixteenth century that the phenomenon began to be noticed again in Europe.[8] Leonardo da Vinci was apparently the first to suggest that painters might learn how to give authentic expressiveness to their depictions of the human body 'by copying the motions of the dumb, who speak with movements of their hands and eyes and eyebrows and their whole person, in their desire to express that which is in their minds'.[9] And Rabelais's Pantagruel speculated that the 'gestures and signs' of a deaf man might be blessed with a kind of pure prophetic validity, innocent of equivocation or obscurity. (Deaf women, he suggested, were less reliable, as they would always see obscene implications even in the most innocent of gestures.)[10]

About sixty years later, in 1608, François de Sales, Bishop of Geneva, encountered a 'deaf and dumb' boy called Martin who was able to 'explain himself by signs'. Having learned to communicate with the boy by

6 Plato, *Cratylus* translated by Jowett 414c, 422e-423a.

7 'Have you never noticed how men converse, as it were, with deaf people by gestures and how the deaf in turn use gestures to talk and answer questions, to teach and to make known to each other their wishes . . . ?' See Augustine, *De Magistro*, translated by Robert P. Russell as *The Teacher*, Washington, Catholic University Press of America, 1968, p. 13.

8 For an optimistic account of gestural language and the situation of the deaf in medieval Europe, see Aude de Saint-Loup, 'Les sourds-muets au Moyen-Age: Mille ans de signes oubliés', in Alexis Karakostas, ed., *Le Pouvoir des Signes*, pp. 11–19.

9 See Nicholas Mirzoeff, *Silent Poetry: Deafness, Sign and Visual Culture in Modern France*, Princeton, Princeton University Press, 1995, pp. 13ff., where this comment is cited from Leonardo da Vinci, *Treatise on Painting*, translated by Philip McMahon, Princeton, Princeton University Press, 1956, Vol. 1, p. 105.

10 In the event, the deaf Nazdecabre's gestured advice proved difficult to interpret: see François Rabelais, *Le Tiers Livre des Faicts et Dits Heroiques du bon Pantagruel* (1546), XIX-XX, in *Œuvres Complètes*, edited by Pierre Jourda, Paris, Garnier, 1962, Vol. 1, pp. 479–87. A disputation in signs is also described in *Pantagruel, Roi des Dipsodes* (1532), XIX, *Œuvres Complètes*, Vol, 1, pp. 319–24.

this means, François adopted Martin as a servant, and is said to have taught him the rules of morality and the mysteries of faith, all by means of gestures.[11] And in Holland, in the middle of the century, it was observed that 'those that are originally Dumb, and Deaf, do by certain gestures, and various motions of the body, as readily and clearly declare their mind . . . as if they could speak'.[12] In London, too, there was a 'Dumb boy' working in the service of Lord Downing, and when Samuel Pepys saw them conversing together in signs he was astonished by the 'many things they understood but I could not'. Downing encouraged Pepys to learn some signs for himself, saying that 'it is only a little use, and you will understand him and make him understand you, with as much ease as may be', but Pepys never bothered to take up the challenge.[13]

Meanwhile philosophers were also becoming interested by the idea that gestural signs might provide an alternative to spoken language. In 1580, Montaigne claimed that the deaf were able to 'argue, dispute, and relate stories by means of signs', and that they were 'nothing short of perfect' at making themselves understood in this way. According to Montaigne, in fact, the deaf shared this skill with animals, who were also capable of 'full and entire communication with each other' by the use of gestures.[14] On the other hand, Descartes was of the opinion that the 'signs' used by those 'born deaf and dumb' constituted a fully human language and had nothing in common with the purely mechanical communicative behaviour of lowly animals.[15]

Francis Bacon also interested himself in the use of gestures to express meanings, especially 'in the practice of divers that are dumb and deaf'. Although such signs would never, he supposed, be so exact as words, they could still be good enough to 'serve the turn', and as such they disproved the traditional view that language must essentially take the form of speech. ('Whatsoever is capable of sufficient differences, and

11 The event occurred in about 1608; see Maryse Bézagu-Deluy, *L'abbé de L'Épée, Instituteur gratuit des sourds et muets*, Paris, Seghers, 1990, pp. 135, 312.
12 Antonius Deusingius, *De Surdis ab Ortu*, pp. 181–2; George Sibscota, *The Deaf and Dumb Man's Discourse*, p. 41.
13 Samuel Pepys, 9 November 1666; see *The Diary of Samuel Pepys*, edited by Robert Latham and William Matthews, London, George Bell, 1972, Vol. VII, p. 363.
14 Michel de Montaigne, 'Apologie de Raymond Sebond' (1580), *Essais*, II, xii, edited by Pierre Michel, Paris, Gallimard, 1965, Vol. 2, p. 157.
15 René Descartes, *Discours de la méthode* (1637), Part Five, in *Œuvres de Descartes*, edited by Charles Adam and Paul Tannery, Paris, Cerf, 1897–1913, Vol. VI, pp. 57–8.

those perceptible by the sense, is in nature competent to express cogitations,' as Bacon put it.) He also linked the use of signs with the mysterious linguistic practices of Antiquity and the Orient, arguing that the signs used by Europe's deaf and dumb were a living equivalent of the non-alphabetic writing systems with which (as it was supposed) ancient and exotic peoples were able to communicate directly, without reference to spoken language. They had something in common, for example, with the celebrated Chinese characters, which (Bacon thought) 'express neither letters nor words in gross, but Things or Notions', so that in China those who 'understand not one another's language, can nevertheless read one another's writings'. But, Bacon went on, gestural signs were even closer to the yet more primitive 'Hieroglyphics' of the ancient Egyptians, which, unlike Chinese characters, had a visible 'similitude or congruity' with the objects they stood for. 'Gestures,' Bacon wrote, 'are as transitory Hieroglyphics, and are to Hieroglyphics as words spoken are to words written, in that they abide not; but they have evermore, as well as the other, an affinity with the things signified.'[16] Gestures, in other words, were the primitive original of language, the source of all linguistic sources, and the prelinguistic root of etymology itself.

The idea that gestures had an affinity with exotic civilizations was soon confirmed by a report, published in Holland in 1660, about a retinue of 'mutes' maintained by the Sultan of the Turks. The Sultan employed mutes because they would not be able to betray court secrets to outsiders; but they could communicate amongst themselves through 'a kind of Speech shadowed out by gestures'. The Dutch jurist Cornelius Haga, who served as Ambassador to the Court in Constantinople from 1611 to 1639, was so intrigued by the Sultan's mutes that he invited them all to a banquet, where 'there was not a syllable heard, yet they did exchange several discourses'. Some of their gestures were quite easy to understand, 'as when they close one hand, and move it up towards the nostrils, thereby to signifie a flower'. But on the whole their 'significations ... proceed not from nature but from their own institution', and the Ambassador had to call upon two interpreters,

16 Francis Bacon, *Of the Advancement of Learning* (1605), in *Philosophical Works*, edited by John M. Robertson, London, George Routledge, 1905, pp. 121–2; cf. *De Augmentis* (1623), vi, 1.

'by whose assistance he himself did discourse with the mutes upon all subjects'.[17] Thereafter, the spectacle of gesticulating mutes at the Ottoman court or harem became a commonplace in European travellers' tales, removing some of the humiliating stigma from deafness and lending it an allure of oriental glamour.[18]

But the summit of the seventeenth-century fascination with gestures or signs was the work of a young English doctor named John Bulwer, who decided in the 1640s to dedicate his life to the service of the 'virgin Philosophie of Gesture'.[19] Bulwer's affection for his 'Darling study' was inspired by a belief in occult correspondences amongst the five senses, illustrated by an engraving which showed people enjoying music through the eye and the mouth – by gazing at musical instruments or sucking them – and monstrous human heads with eyes looking out of their ears, a tongue in place of a nose, or an ear instead of an eye.[20] (See frontispiece.) Having postulated the interchangeability of the senses, Bulwer reasoned that audible speech had no special affinity with the expression of meaning, and indeed that it was inferior to other methods, particularly that of visible gestures.

Gestures, as Bulwer explained them, could be divided into two groups, according to the 'amphitheatre' in which they were performed: that of the hands, and that of the head. They could also be divided into two fundamentally different kinds of action: artificial and natural. Bulwer discussed artificial manual gestures first – that is to say the art of 'manual rhetoric', or *chironomia*, meaning 'the artificiall managing of the Hand'.[21] He realized that this was not altogether a new discipline,

---

17 Antonius Deusingius, *De Surdis ab Ortu*, pp. 182–3; George Sibscota, *The Deaf and Dumb Man's Discourse*, pp. 41–3.
18 See for example Paul Rycaut, *The Present State of the Ottoman Empire*, London, 1668, pp. 34–5: 'The language of the *Mutes*. . . is made up of several signs in which by custom they can discourse and fully express themselves; not only to signifie their sense in familiar questions, but to recount stories, understand the Fables of their own Religion, the laws and precepts of the *Alchoran*, the name of *Mahomet*, and what else may be capable of being expressed by the tongue.'
19 John Bulwer (Chirosopher), *Pathomyotomia, or a Dissection of the significative Muscles of the Affections of the Minde*, London, Humphrey Moseley, 1649, Epistle Dedicatory, p. A11R. For a general account of Bulwer, see H. J. Norman, 'John Bulwer, the Chirosopher', *Proceedings of the Royal Society of Medicine*, 36, 1943, pp. 589–602. His work is examined from a very different and somewhat uncomprehending point of view in B. L. Joseph, *Elizabethan Acting* (1951), second edition, Oxford University Press, 1964.
20 John Bulwer, *Philocophus: or the Deafe and Dumbe Mans Friend*, London, 1648, p. A3.
21 John Bulwer (Philochirosophus), *Chironomia, or the Art of Manuall Rhetorique*, London, 1644, p. 24.

since rhetorical training in ancient Greece and Rome had also covered the use of appropriate bodily gestures to enhance the effect of a speech.[22] Still, manual rhetoric had fallen into neglect since then, and Bulwer meant to revive it, offering some simple graphic tables or 'chirograms' to illustrate the basic range of rhetorical handshapes, and correlating them with letters of the alphabet so that they could also be used for the purposes of manual spelling. (See Figure 6 opposite.) Bulwer had high hopes that his canons of chironomy would before long become an accepted part of the basic University arts course, alongside those of ordinary verbal rhetoric.

But Bulwer's chief enthusiasm was the second aspect of manual theory – *chirologia* as opposed to *chironomia*. For the object of *chirologia* was not artificial rhetoric, but natural language itself – specifically the 'Naturall Language of the Hand' which was 'the only speech and generall language of Humane Nature.'[23] The excellence of chirological communication, Bulwer claimed, was confirmed in

> that wonder of necessity which nature worketh in men that are born deafe and dumbe; who can argue and dispute rhetorically by signes, and with a kind of logistique eloquence overcome their amaz'd opponents; wherein some are so ready and excellent, they seeme to want nothing to have their meanings perfectly understood.

The natural language of the hands was also in regular use amongst mimes, jesters and comedians on the stage, and merchants engaged in international trade were familiar with it too, prizing it as a means of circumventing 'the crafty Brocage of the tongue'.[24]

The purpose of chirology was to describe all the different natural 'dialects' of the hand, and trace them back 'to their spring-heads and originall, even to the finding out their *Radicall Derivations* and *Muscular Etymologies*'.[25] As well as describing the 25 roots in the natural

22 The only extended classical treatment of gesture as a part of rhetoric to survive is in Quintilian, *Institutio Oratoria*, XI, 3, §§68–184, especially §88. See also Fritz Graf, 'Gestures and Conventions: the gesture of Roman actors and orators', in *A Cultural History of Gesture*, edited by Jan Bremmer and Herman Roodenburg, Oxford, Polity Press, 1991, pp. 36–58.
23 John Bulwer, *Chirologia, or, the Natural Language of the Hand*, London, 1644, 'To the Reader'.
24 *Chirologia* p. 5.
25 Bulwer, *Philocophus*, pp. A3–4.

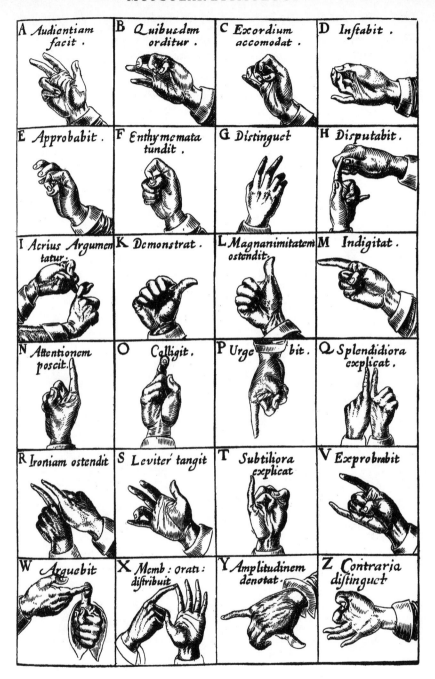

FIG 6. Artificial manual signs in John Bulwer's chirograms

dialect of the fingers, such as finger-in-mouth (deep meditation), thumb up (approval), and both thumbs up (transcendence of praise), Bulwer identified 64 elements in the natural dialect of the hands, from stretching them out in supplication to imposing them in blessing.[26] All these were listed in a comprehensive dictionary with a separate engraving or 'chirogram' to illustrate each one. (See Figure 7 below.)

But the hands were not the only amphitheatre of the human body, and after recording the natural 'Nationall Dialects' of fingers and

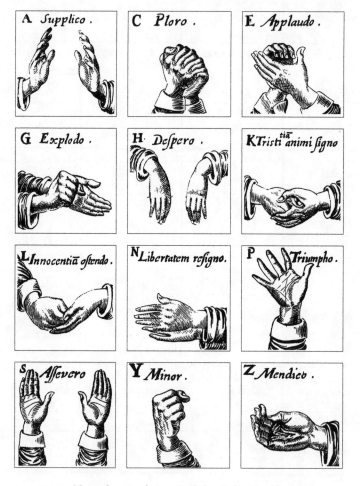

FIG 7. Natural manual signs in John Bulwer's chirograms

26 Bulwer, *Chirologia*, pp. 11–188.

hands, Bulwer extended his researches to 'the Naturall language of the Head'. The first principle of his *cephatologia* was that the head is like a clock, with the face as the 'Dyall of the Affections', and Bulwer offered a comprehensive description of the operation of the ten different 'significative muscles' which controlled its various expressive features – for example, the muscle which moves the whole head (nodding); those which govern the entire face (smiling and laughter); and others which regulate the forehead, eyelids, eyes and ears.[27]

Bulwer was especially fascinated by ears, and he steadfastly maintained that their expressiveness had never been properly appreciated, declaring that 'all Semeioticall philosophers are here lost'.[28] Conversely, he held that the significance of the tenth and last item in his inventory of the muscular clock-work of the head had always been grossly overestimated. Bulwer was referring to that proud but somewhat disgusting instrument, the tongue, which he described as the 'muscle of Discourse or Orall Reason' even though in his opinion it was neither particularly reasonable, nor even a muscle in the strict sense, being merely a cephatological equivalent of the turgid 'virile member'. But Bulwer was grudgingly impressed by its versatility: the tongue could move very rapidly and flexibly, after all, and if for some reason we found ourselves unable to communicate by ordinary chirological means, then it would usefully provide us with 'another way to expresse all the motions of the minde'.[29] As a final postscript, Bulwer reminded his readers that the tongue can also be used to articulate sounds, thus providing an audible supplement to visible gestures; and this byproduct – otherwise known as speech – might, he conceded, be of some occasional use to those unfortunates who, through blindness or paralysis, could not participate in normal gestural communication.

Trivial as they were in Bulwer's estimation, the audible sounds of language also had their own etymological roots, no less than the visible gestures of the hands and head. These elementary 'significant sounds' – 'the interjection of laughter, as ha, ha, he; of sorrow as ha; of weeping, as oh; of crying out for aide, as O' – gave direct expression to the 'passions of the minde'. They were the original letters of nature's vocal alphabet, derived from 'the instinct of nature', and they were

27 Bulwer, *Chirologia*, 'To the Reader'; *Pathomyotomia*, pp. 55, A2.
28 *Pathomyotomia*, p. 181.
29 *Pathomyotomia*, pp. 240, 234.

understood by all of us, including the dumb. But the simple origins of audible vocal gesture had been lost and buried by the artificial collections of sounds which constituted conventional languages.[30] Echoing Bacon, Bulwer recalled that human beings were not obliged to resort to the languages of the tongue for the purposes of communication:

> there's no native law, or absolute necessity, that those thoughts which arise in our pregnant minde, must by mediation of our Tongue flow out in a vocall streame of words . . . since whatsoever is perceptible unto sense, and capable of a due and fitting difference hath a naturall competency to expresse the motives and affections of the Minde.[31]

Spoken languages were essentially degenerate and confused, therefore: they were not a mark of human nobility but a solemn reminder of man's disobedience and fall. So we would do well to turn away from the sounds of speech, and rediscover the freedom of natural visible gestures: the only means of communication, as Bulwer said, which had 'had the happiness to escape the curse at the confusion of Babel'.[32]

---

30 Bulwer, *Philocophus*, pp. 126, 190, 156.
31 Bulwer, *Chirologia*, p. 4.
32 *Chirologia*, p. 7.

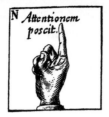

13

Time, syntax and the language of nature in a new academy for the deaf

Soon after its publication in 1644, a copy of Bulwer's *Chirologia* fell into the hands of two middle-aged sons of the gentry in the village of Willington in Bedfordshire. Both Sir Edward Gostwicke and his younger brother William were rather dull and slow; but to everyone's surprise they were moved and excited by Bulwer's 'chirograms' – his modest engravings depicting the 64 basic natural gestures of the hand. The two brothers were, if Bulwer's account is to be believed, 'not onely . . . affected but seemingly edified upon the sight of the alphabets of my *Chirologia*'. The drawings seemed to speak to them directly; and yet the unfortunate gentlemen were exceedingly backward – they could 'neither heare nor speake', in fact, for both of them were 'born deaf and dumb'.[1]

Sir Edward was something of a prodigy nevertheless. Despite his deafness, he had been allowed to succeed to his Baronetcy in 1630, and the Bishop of Lincoln noted him as 'a sweet creature', and 'of rare illumination from God'. He could not understand language, but his 'behaviour, Gestures, and zealous Signs' spoke quite as eloquently

---

1 John Bulwer, *Philocophus*, p. A3.

'as if his tongue could articulately deliver his mind'. He had therefore been admitted to the rites of the Church, and even into marriage with 'a Lady of a great and prudent family'.[2]

Bulwer's discovery about the effect of his chirograms on the Gostwicke brothers made him realize that his work in praise of gesture might also be of some practical help to the deaf, and his second book – *Philocophus: or the Deafe and Dumbe Mans Friend*, which came out in 1648 – was an attempt to defend and vindicate their condition. Bulwer admitted that if you were deaf, you might be cut off from all 'verball contrivances of man's invention'. But still, you would be blessed with a compensating fluency in visible natural gestures, and should therefore 'want nothing to be perfectly understood, your mother tongue administering sufficient utterance upon all occasions'. Being dumb did not really mean you could not speak: 'You want not *speech*,' Bulwer said, 'who have your *whole Body*, for a *Tongue*.'[3]

Bulwer then floated a proposal for an Academy dedicated to the needs of pupils 'originally deafe and dumb'. Thanks to Kenelm Digby's recently published account of Luis de Velasco, he already knew about the triumphs of Ponce de Leon and Bonet in teaching the deaf to talk. But Bulwer regarded their single-minded emphasis on speech as misplaced; and in any case he realized that their method required years of individual attention from a private tutor, which put it beyond the means of all but the very wealthy. At Bulwer's projected Academy for the Deaf, the emphasis would fall on signs rather than words, so that instruction could be delivered economically by a single schoolmaster acting and gesticulating before a whole class of pupils at the same time.

Bulwer envisaged that the scholars at his Academy would first be taught the arts of reading and writing, or '*visible* and *permanent speech*' as he called it, on the basis of gestural signs supplemented by a manual alphabet. But he assumed that once they could read a script, they would have no difficulty in learning 'Lip-Grammar', or the art of recognizing words by looking at a speaker's face as they were being

2 The future Archbishop of York's observations, made in 1634, are recorded in John Hacket, *Scrinia Reserata, a Memorial of John Williams*, London, 1692, Part 2, p. 61; see also William Page, ed., *Victoria History of the County of Bedford*, London, Constable, 1912, Vol. 3, pp. 203, 264.
3 *Philocophus*, pp. A3–4.

pronounced. According to Bulwer's reasoning, the movements of the speaking face – or 'the Characters of Nature's Alphabet' as he called them – should be as readily identifiable as the characters of the artificial alphabet when chalked up on a slate. Articulate speech could be '*seen* as well as *heard*', and did not require 'the audible sound of the voyce'. Bulwer concluded that his deaf scholars would soon be able to see the words people were uttering, just as readily as others could hear them. He also assured his readers that deaf children, having become adept in 'hearing with the eye', would automatically learn to 'speak with the tongue', without needing any further training.[4]

But these were the promises and predictions of a fantasist. Bulwer never put his project into practice, and it is unlikely that he ever worked with deaf children at all: if he had, he could hardly have retained his optimism about the ease and effectiveness of 'Ocular Audition', and he would certainly have realized that the deaf could never learn to speak merely by watching other people do it. (The difficulties ought to have been obvious anyway: if speech could really be recognized by sight as easily as by hearing, the deaf should never have had any difficulty in learning to understand languages in the first place; and if simply watching other people talk was going to enable deaf children to speak, they would not have been backward in their speech either.)

But Bulwer was not much interested in the practical problems facing an Academy for the Deaf. The real obstacles, he thought, were theoretical and philosophical – creatures of the stubborn traditional prejudice against every means of communication except speech. The idea of gesture as a self-sufficient medium was bound to be scorned, he thought, by all who were 'too superstitiously devoted to the received Phylosophy'.[5]

Bulwer was flattering himself, of course. Like many other thinkers who have imagined themselves to be heroically at odds with the Western philosophical tradition, he was actually reverting to a time-honoured theme – in this case, an argument proposed by Plato, recently revived by Montaigne, Bacon and many others.[6] But their idealized philosophical view of gestural communication as the true and

4 *Philocophus*, pp. A4–6, 49, 156, 190–1.
5 *Philocophus*, p. A5.
6 See above, pp. 119–20, 121–2.

natural pre-linguistic root of language was to become increasingly popular over the following century. It was taken up again in 1673, for example, when Isaac Vossius argued that eloquence in the ancient world depended on movements of the feet and hands as much as on the articulation of the voice by the tongue. Over the centuries, according to Vossius, classical rhetoric had declined into excessive intellectualism; it had lost its original force as a result of becoming separated from the muscular rhythms of the body. In fact humanity would do itself no harm if it turned its back on verbal language and 'interpretation' altogether, and returned to the simple and undeceptive medium of 'signs, nods, and actions' instead.[7]

Giambattista Vico, too, believed that there must have been a historical stage before the invention of vocal language, a period when humanity was 'mute' – a word which he (an incorrigible etymological dreamer) believed to be identical with the Greek *mythos*, or story. The 'first words of the earliest nations', he wrote in 1725, were 'mute'. Just like the deaf and dumb, our original ancestors expressed themselves by visible 'signs or actions' with a natural expressive relationship to their ideas, rather than through the artificial medium of audible words. Or, taking up Bacon's comparison, he argued that they 'originally spoke by writing' or in 'hieroglyphs'.[8]

In 1741, William Warburton, Bishop of Gloucester, put forward a similar speculation about the use of visible hieroglyphs and gestures in 'the first Ages of the World'. When language was in its infancy, he argued, and still 'extremely rude, narrow and equivocal', our early ancestors must have been driven to 'supplying the deficiencies of speech by apt and significant *signs*'. This gestural discourse corresponded exactly to the earliest forms of writing, which, having begun as 'mere picture' amongst the Mexicans, had been progressively improved and abbreviated by the Egyptians and then the Chinese, until eventually, 'by a gradual and easy descent' it arrived at the compendious perfection of the Greek and Roman alphabet, which represented the sounds of spoken language rather than the outward and

---

7 'Signis, nutibus, gestibusque': see Isaac Vossius, *De poematum cantu et viribus rythmi*, Oxford, 1673, pp. 65–6.
8 Giambattista Vico, *The New Science* (1744, first edition, 1725), translated by T. G. Bergin and M. H. Fish, Cornell University Press, 1948, §§225, 226, 401, 429, 431, 434; pp. 68, 114, 124, 125, 127.

visible appearances of things. 'Speaking by action', according to War-burton, was the exact equivalent of 'writing by picture'.[9]

Bishop Warburton's speculative history of gestures and hieroglyphs was promptly translated into French,[10] and in 1746 it was endorsed by Condillac, who reasoned that communication must logically have begun with signs – or 'the language of action' as he preferred to say – but that articulate sounds had gradually replaced them because they were more convenient. The language of action was originally indis-tinguishable from 'dancing' – both the 'dance of gestures' which expresses thoughts, and the 'dance of the feet' which communicates the various conditions of the soul. The movements of dance thus lay at the origin of all languages, as of every other technique for expressing ideas; and although they were somewhat irrational and disorderly, they could never be surpassed for vivacity and figurative fertility.[11]

The great advantage of the language of action, for Condillac, was its instantaneousness. In spoken language, you could not portray a moment of mingled feelings – say excitement tinged with hatred and fear – without separating them out and expressing them one by one in a temporal sequence of distinct words, even though the various ideas obviously do not 'come one after the other in our minds'. On the other hand, all sorts of different things could be visibly embodied in a single spatial array by means of a momentary expressive gesture, and actions therefore constituted the 'language of simultaneous ideas' – a language of nature, moreover, in which it was impossible to express anything that was not genuinely being felt at the actual moment of utterance.[12] Civilization, however, was bound up with the temporal or sequential character of spoken language, and human progress had therefore been bought at the expense of the immediacy and directness of gestural signs. By adopting the habit of communicating by sounds, we had broken the immediate link between expression and feeling, and fallen into a world of dissimulation and delay. Nevertheless our

9 William Warburton, *The Divine Legation of Moses*, Vol. 2, London, 1741, Book iv, section iv, pp. 81–3, 67, 87.
10 William Warburton, *Essai sur les hiéroglyphes des Egyptiens*, Paris, 1744.
11 Étienne Bonnot de Condillac, *Essai sur l'origine des connaissances humaines*, Amsterdam, 1746, Part 2, pp. 11, 15–16, 178, 222.
12 Étienne Bonnot de Condillac, *Cours d'instruction du Prince de Parme*, 16 Vols, Parma, 1775, Vol. 1, p. 13.

bodies still harboured many vestiges of natural actions and, to those who knew how to decipher them, these original signs continued to provide a reliable guide even to our most secret, mobile and complicated sentiments. But unfortunately the influence of spoken language was now spreading back into gesture itself: 'the language of action is not what it used to be,' as Condillac sadly observed.[13]

Condillac's unhappiness about the disparity between the simultaneities of experience and the temporal successiveness of spoken language was shared by Diderot, who may in fact have suggested it to him in the first place. Our soul, Diderot wrote in 1751, could experience vast swarms of impressions within an 'indivisible instant', thousands of different events happening 'as a whole and all at once'. But when we tried to give them vocal utterance, we collided with a very stubborn physical constraint, since each of us has only one mouth, which means we can only say one thing at a time.[14] (The idea of having several mouths will have reminded Diderot's readers of his scabrous novel, *Indiscreet Jewels*, in which fine ladies were conjured into talking through their vaginas, revealing aspects of their souls which would never have been voiced by the prim little mouths in their heads.)[15] According to Diderot, expressing one's mind in language was like the time-consuming art of landscape painting, in which 'the brush must execute at length what the painter's eye can take in all at once'. The sublime torrent of our soul was like a 'moving picture', but the only way we could talk about it was by cutting it up into separate details and expressing them in a pedestrian procession of words.[16]

Over the centuries, however, the labour of dividing the 'total impression' in our souls into the string of details required by language had become so habitual that we were scarcely aware of it any more. We had thus become susceptible to the illusion that our affections and sensations file through our soul one after the other, just like their expressions in spoken language. We failed to notice that the regimentation, clarity and explicitness of civilized human language was gradually squeezing out the hasty and negligent warmth of more natural

13 *Cours d'instruction du Prince de Parme*, Vol. 2, pp. 261–4.
14 Denis Diderot, *Lettre sur les sourds et muets à l'usage de ceux qui entendent et qui parlent* (1751), edited by Paul Hugo Meyer, *Diderot Studies* VII, 1965, pp. 64, 61.
15 Denis Diderot, *Les Bijoux Indiscrets*, Amsterdam/Paris, 1748.
16 Diderot, *Lettre sur les sourds et muets*, p. 64.

and primitive forms of expression. Increasingly, we were hanging up our souls in 'chains of syntax' – especially in French, a language which, Diderot thought, had gone further than any other in sacrificing rough ancient instantaneous beauty on the altar of plodding modern prose. It was as if our thoughts had grown ashamed of their natural nakedness, and would no longer allow us to draw near unless they were decorously covered by the conventional garments of spoken language. 'Ah, monsieur, how our understandings have been modified by signs!' he lamented. 'And – however lively our diction – how cold the copies we make of what is passing through our minds!'[17]

In order to investigate the effects of the temporal ordering that our early ancestors imposed on experience when they began to express it in vocal sound, Diderot sought out the testimony of those 'born deaf and dumb'. Their ignorance of language, he assumed, would have protected them from the corrupting prejudices of syntax, and indeed made them into a near-perfect replica of archaic humanity in its natural state. He referred in particular to a (nameless and probably fictional) 'deaf-and-dumb' friend, who – apart from being entranced by Louis Bertrand Castel's colour harpsichord and offering Diderot unwanted good advice on how to improve his game of chess – showed, Diderot said, a consistent syntactic pattern in his pantomimic gestures, always placing the 'principal idea' at the beginning of each phrase, so as to identify the topic to which his subsequent signs would refer. Diderot inferred that the same simple rule of precedence must have been used in the most primitive forms of spoken language, but that as speech began to develop (first Hebrew, then Greek and Latin), the restriction was gradually removed, until word order became entirely arbitrary. At first this made for loose, lively, and rapid forms of expression, and the ancient languages – especially Homeric Greek – were able to nurture complex works of poetic art unified by astonishingly original images, emblems, and nested hieroglyphs; but at length this youthful vitality was dissipated and language settled into the dull uniform trudge of modern science and philosophy, strung out along the predictable straight line of Syntax.[18]

The meditations of Condillac and Diderot on the primitive poetic

---

17 *Lettre sur les sourds et muets*, pp. 64, 87, 68, 46, 64.
18 *Lettre sur les sourds et muets*, pp. 47–51, 53, 77, 85, 70.

energy of visible gestures, and how it had been suppressed by the cold delaying calculations of modern spoken language, were one of the inspirations for the notorious *Discourse on the Origin of Inequality*, published in 1755 by their subtle but difficult friend Jean-Jacques Rousseau. The careless habit of invoking an age of natural gestural language prior to the institution of linguistic conventions struck Rousseau as question-begging, because it presupposed that society could have existed before the first invention of language. Rousseau glimpsed a frightening range of paradoxes here: for if language depends upon conventions, conventions also depend on language, and we could never have felt the need for language unless we had attained a level of social intercourse that already presupposed it: 'if humanity needed to speak in order to learn to think, still more did it need to think in order to discover the art of speech.' Thus the philosophical appeal to pre-linguistic gestures was of no theoretical use, according to Rousseau; and in any case gestures were intrinsically so coarse and ambiguous that they could never be more than a supplement to speech, used occasionally for pointing out obvious visible objects or actions.[19]

But then, in a timorous footnote, Rousseau quoted Vossius's praise of primitive gestures, and refused to reach any final opinion on the virtues of gestural signs and 'the advantages and disadvantages of the institution of spoken languages'.[20] And in the posthumous *Essay on the Origin of Languages* he elaborated a sustained and poignant ambivalence about the relation between gestures and speech. He accepted that our faculty for conventional language could operate with visible expressions as well as audible ones, and he agreed with Condillac and Diderot that gestures were 'more expressive', and able to 'say more in a shorter time'. But he went on to suggest that vocal languages are emotionally superior, for precisely the reasons that made Diderot and Condillac regard them as cold and calculating: temporal sequence allowed for artful exploitation of inversion and suspense, according to Rousseau, and therefore made speech more apt to move the heart and inflame the passions. He also accepted the view that the general quality

19 Jean-Jacques Rousseau, *Discours sur l'origine et les fondements de l'inégalité parmi les hommes* (1755), Part One, *Œuvres Complètes*, Vol. 3, edited by Bernard Gagnebin and Marcel Raymond, Paris, Pléiade, 1964, pp. 146–8.
20 See Rousseau, *Discours sur l'origine et les fondements de l'inégalité*, note 13, where Vossius is quoted (misquoted in fact – *motibus* for *nutibus* – see p. 132 n. 7, above) with approval: *Œuvres Complètes*, Vol. 3, pp. 148, 218.

of gestural communication had declined since the time of ancient Greece and Rome, and that the only remaining touchstone for investigating the natural language of action was the repertory of gestures used by the deaf. On the other hand, unlike his companions, he did not believe that gestural signs were particularly natural or primitive: sign language, in Rousseau's considered opinion, was 'no less complex' than speech itself.[21]

The French philosophical arguments over the vivacity, simultaneity and naturalness of the primitive hieroglyphical 'language of action' as compared with the slow successive artifices of speech were soon taken up again in Scotland. In *Of the Origin and Progress of Language*, which he began to publish in 1773, Lord Monboddo argued that the invention of speech marked the epoch at which humanity ceased to be a mere natural animal and became 'a new creature', no longer limited to sensual automatism, but capable of freely exploring an 'intellectual world' as well. Although speech was essential to civilization, it was not 'natural to man', as was proved by the existence of several groups of human beings who had yet to 'come the length of language'. For example there were the orang-utans, whom Monboddo (like Rousseau) considered to be fully 'of our species'; and then there were various kinds of wild children and 'solitary savages'. But the group that interested Monboddo most was the deaf, who were 'precisely in the condition in which we suppose men to have been in the natural state', and who still 'communicate their thoughts by looks and gestures, which we call *signs*'.[22]

Unlike earlier contributors to the philosophy of gesture, Monboddo was able to speak from real experience of the education of the deaf. For he had observed the work of a school in Edinburgh owned by one Thomas Braidwood, 'who professes a most curious art . . . the art of teaching the deaf to speak'.[23] Braidwood appears to have encountered his first deaf pupil in 1760, and though he probably knew nothing of John Bulwer's schemes, from 1764 onwards he gradually implemented

21 Jean-Jacques Rousseau, *Essai sur l'origine des langues* (1781, but written in the 1750s), edited by Charles Porset, Bordeaux, Ducros, 1970, pp. 29–37.
22 James Burnet, Lord Monboddo, *Of the Origin and Progress of Language*, Vol. I, Edinburgh, 1773, pp. 130, 174–6, 177–8.
23 *Of the Origin and Progress of Language*, Vol. I, pp. 131–2, 179.

a similar plan for an Academy for the Deaf and Dumb. He took on an assistant in 1770, and ten years later had up to twenty scholars regularly in residence, twenty being the most, he believed, that could be taught together in one class.[24]

The Edinburgh Academy took both boys and girls, aged between 5 and 20, and Braidwood soon noticed that on arrival they could be expected to have some fluency in a range of 'signs and gestures' which were immediately understood by the others, and possibly in quite general use amongst the deaf population of Scotland. He told the philosopher Dugald Stewart that 'his dumb pupils, from whatever part of the country they came, agreed, in most instances, in expressing asssent by holding up the thumb, and dissent by holding up the little finger' – a point which suggested to the philosopher that these must have been 'abbreviations of those signs by which assent and dissent are generally expressed in the language of nature'.[25]

Braidwood went to the trouble of learning the gestural language used by his pupils, so that he could use it for teaching them their first lessons. He claimed, however, that gestures were essentially a very limited medium, incapable of referring beyond the range of the five senses (though it is hard to see how he reconciled this opinion with the fact that they had signs for assent and dissent). But Braidwood considered that even if the stock of ideas available to his new deaf pupils was 'confined to visible objects, and to the passions or senses', nevertheless it was large enough to allow him to set to work immediately on their education. His first task was to get them to recognize written expressions corresponding to ideas they could already express in signs – a 'very hard task', he said, given that writing is 'purely arbitrary', whereas gestures are 'only hieroglyphical'. But, with the help of a manual alphabet, he managed to teach them such words as *high*, *low*, *hard*, *tender*, *clear*, and *cloudy*, at least in their literal application to ordinary physical things. Then he somehow cajoled them into understanding how this vocabulary could also – by a process of figurative or metaphorical extension – be 'applied to mind', so that eventually

24 Francis Green, '*Vox Oculis Subjecta*'; *A Dissertation on the Most Curious and Important Art of Imparting Speech and the Knowledge of Language to the naturally DEAF, and (consequently) DUMB*, London, 1783, pp. 139–41.
25 Dugald Stewart, *Philosophy of the Human Mind: Continuation of Part Second* (1826), in *Collected Works*, edited by Sir William Hamilton, Vol. IV, Edinburgh, 1854, p. 16.

they would be conducted, through written language, into the civilized spiritual world from which they had formerly been shut out.[26]

Having learned to read, the scholars at the Edinburgh Academy would be taught to write, and eventually – since 'spoken language hath so great and essential a tendency to confirm and enlarge ideas, above the power of written language' – they would be trained in speech as well. Braidwood proceeded by showing them how to make 'that concussion and tremulous motion of the windpipe which produces audible sounds', and then progressed to the far more difficult lesson in the pronunciation of the letters of the alphabet. He passed from one scholar to the next holding a specially made silver rod, flat at one end and with a ball at the other, which he would use to guide the movements of their tongues. After five or six years, they should be able to pronounce quite clearly – they could recite the Lord's prayer, for instance, better 'than many clergymen do in the desk', and even conduct conversations with strangers by following the movements of their lips.[27]

In 1780, a well-educated Bostonian called Francis Green, Sheriff of Halifax in Nova Scotia, despatched his beloved eight-year-old son Charles across the Atlantic to become a student at Braidwood's Academy in Edinburgh. The boy was totally deaf and, as his father wrote, he could not 'produce or distinguish vocal sounds, nor articulate at all, neither had he any idea of the meaning of words'. Green came to visit his son a year later, and was completely overwhelmed: 'it exceeds the power of words,' he said, when he tried to describe his delight as his son recognized him and 'eagerly advanced, and addressed me, with a distinct salutation of speech.' The young Charles could also repeat several set pieces, and read from any book, though he did not yet know what most of the words meant. He made further progress in the following year, and Green could scarcely contain his admiration for Braidwood and his Academy. One of the most monstrous misfortunes had been turned into 'little more than a disadvantage in conversing'. Children like his son Charles, he wrote, were being utterly

26 Hugo Arnot, *The History of Edinburgh*, Edinburgh, 1779, pp. 425–6.
27 This account of Braidwood's technique is drawn from Francis Green, *'Vox Oculis Subjecta'*, pp. 146–7, 157, and James Burnet, Lord Monboddo, *Of the Origin and Progress of Language*, Vol. I, pp. 180–1; see also Arnot, *The History of Edinburgh*, and John Herries, *The Elements of Speech*, London, 1773, p. 78.

transformed by the new Academy – so much so, that they could 'truly be said to be the offspring of these professors', who took on children with the behaviour of impassive idiots and transformed them into 'rational and conversible beings, capable of spiritual as well as temporal felicity'.[28] Having completed his extraordinary education, Charles Green returned to his devoted father in Nova Scotia, only to die there by drowning during a shooting expedition at the age of 15.[29]

When passing through Edinburgh in 1773, Samuel Johnson also paid a visit to Braidwood's Academy for the Deaf and Dumb, and he too was astonished:

> They not only speak, write, and understand what is written, but if he that speaks looks towards them, and modifies his organs by distinct and full utterance, they know so well what is spoken, that it is an expression scarcely figurative to say, they hear with the eye.[30]

The great lexicographer, as Boswell records with admiration, wanted to know if Braidwood's pupils could manage long words too, and therefore wrote down one of his *sesquipedalia verba*. Boswell could not recall the monstrous polysyllable, but he remembered that it was duly pronounced by Braidwood's brave scholars, leaving Dr Johnson very satisfied.[31] Johnson was delighted, too, to find that the children's spelling was almost perfect, no doubt because, being deaf, they were not misled 'by imperfect notions of the relation between letters and vocal utterance'. To crown it all, they could do arithmetical calculations as well. 'It was pleasing,' he said, 'to see one of the most desperate of human calamities capable of so much help.' The prospect was most edifying, for 'whatever enlarges hope, will exalt courage', and 'after having seen the deaf taught arithmetick,' Johnson asked, 'who would be afraid to cultivate the *Hebrides*?'[32]

28 Green, 'Vox Oculis Subjecta', pp. 148–50, 157–8.
29 Alexander Graham Bell, 'A Philanthropist of the last century identified as a Boston Man', from the *Proceedings of the American Antiquarian Society*, Worcester, Mass., 1900, p. 9.
30 Samuel Johnson, *A Journey to the Western Islands of Scotland*, edited by J. D. Fleeman, Oxford University Press, 1985, p. 136.
31 *Boswell's Life of Johnson*, edited by George Birkbeck Hill, revised by L. F. Powell, Oxford University Press, 1950, Vol. 5, p. 399.
32 Johnson, *A Journey to the Western Islands of Scotland*, pp. 136–7.

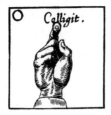

14

Methodical signs and spiritual salvation

In 1731, reports of miracles were hurtling round the streets of Paris. They concerned a tomb in the churchyard of Saint-Médard, on the Left Bank, where the remains of a Jansenist deacon called François de Pâris were buried. He had died in abject poverty four years before, relentlessly persecuted for the uncompromising purity of his faith; and thousands of unfortunates were now crowding round the church, hoping for miraculous cures. According to the atheistical Diderot, the mouldering remains of Deacon Pâris seemed to be performing more miracles every day than Jesus Christ had managed in his entire lifetime.[1] Even David Hume was impressed. 'There surely never was a greater number of miracles ascribed to one person,' he wrote, than to that 'famous Jansenist, with whose sanctity the people were so long deluded.'[2]

The miracles of Saint-Médard were such a threat to public order that the church was closed by royal decree in 1732. But there was already a large archive of signed depositions attesting to the astonishing number of invalids who had watched and fasted and prayed at the tomb of Deacon Pâris, and been cured. There were the lame, the

1 *Pensées Philosophiques* (1746), LIII, in Diderot, *Oeuvres Philosophiques*, pp. 42–3.
2 David Hume, 'Of Miracles', *An Inquiry concerning Human Understanding* (1748), Section 10, Edinburgh, John Brown, 1804, p. 131.

blind, the paralytics; but most remarkable of all, there were the deaf and dumb, especially the notorious Catherine Hogue-Bigot, 'the mute of Versailles', a girl in her early twenties who, after several days watching at the tomb, had suffered a fit of convulsions and recovered to find herself able to hear and, 'more or less', to speak as well.[3]

But the idea that speech could be given to the dumb by natural means as well as miraculous ones was by now beginning to gain ground in France. In 1745, Jacob Pereire, a young Spanish Jew who had recently moved to La Rochelle from Estramaduras to avoid persecution, claimed that he had invented an unprecedented new method for teaching speech to the deaf. To prove it, he mounted a public performance at which a deaf-and-dumb tailor's apprentice named Aaron de Beaumarin managed to pronounce most of the letters of the alphabet, and even a handful of words and phrases as well – *Madame, chapeau, vaisseau, que voulez-vous*. To all appearances, the boy could converse with his tutor too, if not with anyone else.[4]

Pereire's audience in La Rochelle arrived sceptical, but left impressed. His fame spread, and a year later he was entrusted with another young man, d'Azy d'Étavigny. His parents had been consulting doctors and surgeons throughout Italy and Germany as well as France, ever since they first realized that d'Azy was 'born deaf and dumb'. But medical science had not been able to help, and for seven or eight years the boy was left in the care of an elderly deaf man who, though well educated, could not get beyond teaching him to 'use signs to make requests for basic necessities'. Within a few days of transferring to Pereire, however, d'Étavigny was pronouncing his letters, and articulating a few simple words such as *pa-pa, ma-ma, Madame, châ-teau*. His tone was a little strange, and he isolated the syllables unnaturally, giving equal stress to them all. But after four months he could speak 1,300 words, and allegedly understand their meanings too. In November 1746 he was exhibited in Caen, where he was able to salute the Bishop of Bayeux with a recognizable *Monseig-neur, je vous sou-haite le bon-jour*.[5]

Three years later, Pereire set himself up as a trainer of the deaf and dumb in Paris, assisted by his brother and sister. He brought d'Azy

3 See Maryse Bézagu-Deluy, *L'abbé de L'Épee*, pp. 59–64, 276.
4 *Journal des Scavans*, Amsterdam, December 1747, pp. 513–20, p. 514.
5 *Journal des Scavans*, December 1747, pp. 515–17.

d'Étavigny along too, and displayed him to the Royal Academy of Sciences in 1749.[6] Buffon was convinced that Pereire had achieved what had always seemed impossible, communicating 'exact and precise notions of abstract general matters' to the deaf,[7] and in its report, the Academy declared that

> it would be impossible to give him too much encouragement in developing his art, which could deliver numerous subjects to society who would have been of no utility at all without this assistance; it is as if they had been transferred, by a happy metamorphosis, from the condition of mere animals, to become men.[8]

Pereire took his pupil to Versailles early in 1750. Louis XV, Mme de Pompadour and the young Princesses all marvelled at the spectacle of a deaf-and-dumb boy reciting the whole of the Pater Noster, and the King gave Pereire a pension of 800 livres for life, to help him continue his valuable work.[9]

Following this royal endorsement, Pereire received an inquiry from the Duc de Chaulnes, who happened to be godfather to a deaf-and-dumb child, an army officer's son called Saboureux de Fontenay. A few years earlier, at the age of about nine, the boy had been sent to stay with a gentleman in Montpellier, who communicated with him by pantomimic gestures and tried, without much success, to teach him writing and a two-handed manual alphabet. Saboureux was now thirteen, and had just been brought to Paris, where (as he recalled later) he was astonished by the spectacle of people constantly communicating by means of speech, and apparently understanding each other 'very perfectly'. He was then introduced to Pereire and d'Étavigny, who soon convinced him that he should learn their elegant one-handed Spanish manual alphabet and start studying language seriously, first reading and writing, and perhaps eventually speech.[10] Sabou-

6 Pereire's paper to the Academy was published with additions in *Mercure de France*, August 1749, pp. 141–51.
7 Buffon, *Histoire Naturelle*, Vol. 3. Paris 1749, pp. 348–9.
8 *Histoire de l'Académie Royale des Sciences de 1749*, p. 183; see also *Mercure de France*, August 1749, pp. 152–9.
9 See Édouard Séguin, *Jacob-Rodriques Pereire*, Paris, Baillère, 1847, p. 85.
10 'Lettre de M. Saboureux de Fontenay, sourd et muet de naissance, à Mlle ***, 26 Décembre 1764', in *Suite de la clef, ou Journal Historique sur les matières du temps* (*Journal de Verdun*), October 1765, pp. 284–98, and November 1765, pp. 361–72; see pp. 287–8, 292–4. Selections from this important document are translated in *The Deaf Experience*, edited by Harlan Lane, translated by Franklin Philip, Harvard University Press, 1984.

reux de Fontenay became Pereire's pupil in September 1750, and the following January he was examined by a distinguished committee of the Academy of Sciences, who certified that he could not only carry out all sorts of detailed instructions, transmitted either in finger-spelling or in writing, but also pronounce the letters of the alphabet and recite the Lord's prayer from beginning to end.[11]

Over the next thirty years, Pereire's home on the Left Bank provided lodging for three or four boys and girls at a time, while they followed their course of instruction in finger-spelling, written language, and articulation, which normally lasted several years.[12] Pereire became a philosophical celebrity too, supported and promoted by Buffon, Diderot, and Rousseau, and in 1759 he was also elected to the Royal Society in London.[13] He claimed that his method was quite distinct from the 'false' techniques of Wallis and Amman,[14] but never explained the difference, saying that his livelihood depended on the secret, which he planned to pass on as a legacy to his son. When he died in 1780, however, the son was still young, so Pereire took the mystery with him to his grave. It is probable, though, that he was a close follower of the Spanish tradition of Ponce de Leon and Bonet, and that his innovations amounted to no more than some enrichments of the Spanish manual alphabet and the use of gold and silver spatulas to guide his pupils' tongues when teaching articulation. Apart from this, the only invention which can be reliably attributed to Pereire is, it seems, a novel form of ear-trumpet.[15]

Pereire's position as a Jew who made a living as a tutor to young people was delicate, and as far as religious instruction was concerned he dared not go beyond reminding his pupils of their obligation to

---

11 Record of an examination conducted by de Mairan, Buffon and Ferrein on 13 January 1751, *Académie Royale des Sciences*, 27 January 1751, cited in Séguin, *Jacob-Rodrigues Pereire*, pp. 70–3.
12 See Renée Neher-Bernheim, 'Un pionnier dans l'art de faire parler les sourds-muets: Jacob Rodrigue Péreire', *Dix-huitième siècle*, 13, 1981, pp. 46–61.
13 See Rousseau, *Essai sur l'origine des langues*, p. 37; Buffon, *Histoire Naturelle*, Vol. 3, pp. 350–1; Diderot, 'Muet', in *Encyclopédie ou Dictionnaire Raisonné*, Vol. 10, 1765, p. 849, and Séguin, *Jacob-Rodrigues Pereire*, p. 100.
14 *Journal des Sçavans*, December 1747, p. 519.
15 The spatulas were 'a device to abuse the ignorant', according to his critics: see Charles-Michel de l'Épée, *La Véritable Manière d'instruire les sourds et muets, confirmée par une longue expérience*, Paris, Nyon, 1784, pp. 281–6. For the ear trumpet, see Maryse Bézagu-Deluy, *L'abbé de L'Épée*, p. 164.

worship the one God. They were sent out to other teachers for their lessons in Christianity, especially to a priest named Simon Vanin, who, as Saboureux de Fontenay recalled, would try to convey the essentials of Sacred History and Christian Doctrine by showing them prints of scenes from the Bible.[16] Vanin used the same method with several poor deaf children, whose parents could not afford Pereire's fees, and who lacked even the most rudimentary understanding of language.

Father Vanin died at the end of 1759, leaving his poor deaf pupils without a teacher. As it happened, though, two of them – twin sisters, deaf from birth – were discovered shortly afterwards by a prosperous and rather indolent middle-aged Abbé, who had known Vanin slightly. They were grieving for their lost teacher, and although the Abbé had no idea what could be done for them, he felt obliged to try and help. This is how he recalled the event some fifteen years later.

> Father Vanin . . . had begun the instruction of two twin sisters, deaf and dumb from birth, making use of prints (in itself a very weak and doubtful method). Now that the loving minister was dead, the two poor girls were utterly helpless: quite a long time had passed, and no one had come forward to continue his work or start it over again. Realizing therefore that these two children would live and die in ignorance of their religion if I did not try to find some way to teach it to them, I was filled with compassion. I said they could be brought round to me, and I would do what I could to help them.[17]

The author of the reminiscence is Charles-Michel, Abbé de l'Épée. He was born into a rich family in 1712, his father an architect to the King, and received an excellent education, being inspired first by Adrien Geffroy, a philosophy master at the Collège Mazarin in Paris who taught the Lockean doctrine that our minds are shaped entirely by experience, and then studying law at the University and qualifying in 1733 as an advocate.

But the Abbé de l'Épée was also susceptible to piety. As a young man he had been sympathetic to Jansenism, and an enthusiast for the

16 'Lettre de M. Saboureux de Fontenay, sourd et muet de naissance', pp. 366–7.
17 Charles-Michel de l'Épée, *Institution des Sourds et Muets par la voie des signes méthodiques, Ouvrage qui contient le projet d'une Langue Universelle, par l'entremise des Signes naturels assujettis à une Méthode*, Paris, Nyon, 1776, p. 8.

miracles of Deacon Pâris. In 1736 he had become a curate and then a minor priest (not competent to hear confessions, but entitled to the name of Abbé) in a country parish in the Champagne. After three years in the provinces he came back to Paris, to take up residence in a grand house, newly acquired by his father, at 14 Rue des Moulins in the parish of Saint-Roche on the Right Bank. He led, it seems, an undemanding life, though he accepted a chaplaincy in 1747, and continued to interest himself in miracles: he even took responsibility for validating a miraculous cure which took place in his local church in 1759, the year of the death of Vanin.[18]

It was probably in 1760 that the twin deaf girls first came to visit the Abbé de l'Épée in his spacious rooms on the first floor of his father's house, and set him the task of finding a means of communicating with them, in the hope of eventually teaching them the elements of Christianity. By his own admission, de l'Épée had no idea how to proceed. He knew about miraculous cures, such as the one granted to Catherine Hogue-Bigot through the intercession of Deacon Pâris, but he had never even heard of the educational methods advocated by Bonet, Wallis, or Amman. It seems certain, too, that he was unaware of the work that Pereire had been carrying out for more than ten years, just a few minutes' walk away from the Rue des Moulins, on the other side of the Seine.[19]

The Abbé de l'Épée was convinced from the outset that Vanin's use of pictures to teach Christianity could never succeed. The pupils might be able to pick up the literal physical meaning of the Bible by this method, but its deeper, spiritual significance – its relation to what Locke called 'abstract ideas', or to metaphysical matters inaccessible to the five senses – would always elude them unless they could somehow acquire a knowledge of language. Their deafness seemed to make this task impossible; but, as the practical and unpretentious Abbé put it to himself: 'if you cannot bring it through the door, you must try to get it through the window.'[20] Recalling the philosophy lessons at which he had learned that there is no natural or necessary connection between ideas and articulate sounds, de l'Épée decided to try to impart language to the girls through their eyes rather than their ears. He

18 Charles-Michel de l'Épée, *Relation de la maladie et de la guérison miraculeuse de Marie-Anne Pigalle*, Paris, 1759.
19 Charles-Michel de l'Épée, *La Véritable Manière*, pp. vi-vii.
20 *La Véritable Manière*, p. iv.

would teach them reading and writing by a direct visual method, simply pointing to objects with one hand, while writing their names on a slate with the other. Then he would guide the girls' hands as they learnt to write letters and words for themselves. And, reactivating another memory from his childhood, he also taught them the two-handed manual alphabet which he had used for communicating with friends in class without being detected by the master. Within a matter of days the two girls were able to read, write and finger-spell the names of dozens of familiar everyday things; and the Abbé was astonished and elated at the easy success of his humble scheme.

It was a gratifying start; but soon the progress of de l'Épée's pupils came to a dead halt. As he eventually realized, his method had run into a double barrier. First, the only words he could teach were ones which stood for obvious visible physical things that he could point to, and however long they pursued this path, the girls were never going to get any closer to an understanding of those spiritual matters, vital to their salvation, which 'cannot be perceived by the senses at all'.[21] Secondly, they were only learning isolated names, without any syntax to connect them up; and this was obviously no use for helping them 'think in an orderly manner and join their ideas together'.[22] He would never be able to lead the twins to reflect philosophically on spiritual matters until he had equipped them with a system of 'combined signs', grammatically interconnected so as to apply to 'things absent as well as present, whether dependent on the senses or not'.[23]

At first, the Abbé de l'Épée was completely baffled by the problem of teaching a system of 'combined signs' from scratch. But then he realized there might be no need: it was possible that his pupils already had a system of their own. He had observed that the twin girls, having grown up together all their lives, used fluent gestures to communicate with each other; and it occurred to him that this gestural language might already be equipped with syntax. Even the bands of wildly gesticulating deaf-and-dumb orphans who were to be seen wandering the streets of Paris might not be such idiots as he had always supposed: they too could conceivably be communicating in combined signs. And

21 de l'Épée, *Institution*, p. 9.
22 de l'Épée *La Véritable Manière*, p. ix.
23 de l'Épée *Institution*, p. 9.

so the Abbé jumped to the astonishing conclusion that 'every deaf and dumb child . . . is already fluent in a language' – not a spoken language, of course, but 'the language of signs'.[24]

Several previous pioneers, particularly John Wallis, had already recommended learning the gestures used by deaf children in order to initiate communication with them. And in Edinburgh, Braidwood was also beginning to pay attention to the signs used by his pupils, very possibly in exactly the same year as de l'Épée (1760 or 1761), though quite independently. But none of them ever put so much faith in 'sign language' as the Abbé de l'Épée. They regarded it as useful or even necessary for gaining the trust of their new pupils, and teaching them their first lessons; but they considered it unsuitable for prolonged use, since it could divert the child's energy from the learning of grammar, and from reading, writing and speech. As George Dalgarno had put it, you should teach your pupil the alphabet as soon as possible, and then 'you must keep him from any other way of signing, than by letters'.[25] Philosophers like Montaigne and Vico, Condillac, Diderot and Rousseau had all connected gestural communication with instantaneous animal instincts, primitive hieroglyphics and the earliest forms of human society, and whilst that might have been a partial recommendation from their point of view, it could hardly be so to the pious and conventional Abbé de l'Épée.

De l'Épée knew nothing of these earlier attempts to educate the deaf, however, nor did he care for arcane philosophical speculations about speech, time and the language of nature. He easily convinced himself that the gestural discourse of the deaf was a genuine 'combined' language: it comprised verbs, nouns, pronouns, prepositions, conjunctions and adjectives, he said, and implicitly made basic grammatical distinctions of person, number, tense, mood, case and gender.[26] Teachers of the deaf must become the pupils of their pupils, learning their signs so that they could then give them lessons 'in their own language'. Otherwise their efforts would be as fruitless as trying to get French children to learn German 'by giving them a German grammar written in German rather than French'.[27]

24 de l'Épée, *Institution*, pp. 36–7.
25 George Dalgarno, *Didascalocophus*, p. 47.
26 *Institution*, p. 38.
27 *Institution*, p. 36.

Despite his faith in the syntactic sophistication of sign language, however, the Abbé de l'Épée admitted that the progress of civilization had done so much to enrich the structures and vocabularies of spoken languages that they now far outstripped those of the language of signs. Sign language was still in a 'brute state', rough and irregular and incapable of expressing many of the fine distinctions enshrined in modern speech. So just as peasants had to cultivate and transform natural crops, teachers of the deaf must cultivate and transform natural sign language: they must 'perfect it', he said, 'by subjecting it to rules'.[28]

De l'Épée therefore set about constructing a range of 'methodical signs' based on materials he found in the gestural language already used by the deaf. Then, like a Platonic poet inventing new words from nothing, he created special signs to indicate pronouns, plurals, tenses and genders, and also signs for spiritual ideas. The idea that *I believe*, for instance – in the sense of having faith in the articles of revealed religion – was analysed by de l'Épée as *saying 'yes' with the mouth, the heart and the spirit, but at the same time seeing nothing with the eyes*, and he expressed it in signs accordingly.[29] This artificial sign, he argued, would give the deaf an excellent grasp of the idea of belief, and indeed they would surely understand it far better than ordinary children, who often learn to say things whose meanings they could never analyse even if they tried.[30]

The Abbé's ambition was to extend the native sign-language of the deaf with supplementary methodical signs until it became the intellectual equal of any spoken language, and capable of translating it exactly, sign for word. Since its essentials came naturally to the young, it could be taught to them without difficulty: they would take to it like a game. Indeed, if the rulers of each state would take care to ensure that all children were taught methodical signs at an early age, it could become

---

28 *Institution*, p. 135.
29 'I first make the sign of the first person singular by pointing to myself with the index finger of my right hand . . . Then I place my finger on my forehead, on the concave part which is supposed to contain my spirit or faculty of thinking, and then I make the sign for "yes". Then I repeat the sign, while placing my finger on that part of myself which is ordinarily regarded as the seat of what we call the heart . . . I then make the same sign on my mouth, whilst moving my lips. Finally, I put my hand to my eyes, and by making the sign for "not" I show that I cannot see. It only remains to make the sign for the present tense, and to write out the words *je crois*. It goes without saying that all these signs are executed in an instant.' See *Institution*, p. 9.
30 de l'Épée, *La Véritable Manière*, p. 128.

a meeting-place for the whole of humanity – the 'universal language' of which Renaissance metaphysicians and grammarians had always dreamed, and the perfect medium for 'people of all nations' to 'make themselves understood to each other'.[31]

But the Abbé de l'Épée was more interested in remedying the spiritual plight of the children in his care than in speculating about the future of humanity. By 1763 several more deaf children had joined the twin girls to benefit from lessons given in 'their own language' – the language of natural signs, 'subjected to a method' by the Abbé.[32] He established a routine which he kept to till his death many years later, giving two lessons a week, every Tuesday and Friday afternoon, four hours in winter, five in summer, eventually to as many as sixty children at a time. He called himself an *instituteur* – a schoolmaster, that is to say, who taught an open, public class at his own premises, as opposed to a private tutor employed by a wealthy household. His principle was to turn no one away, and to accept no payment; he also paid, from his own pocket, for a number of respectable women in the neighbourhood to take in his pupils as lodgers.

The Abbé's most notorious pupil was a boy who had been found – unconscious, filthy, starving and half-naked – on a roadside in Picardy in 1773. He was about eleven years old, apparently an idiot, and incapable of any kind of communication. But in 1776 he was brought to the Abbé de l'Épée in the Rue des Moulins. He was not idiotic, it turned out, but deaf, and the Abbé allowed him to explain himself, at last, in his native language, the language of signs. Was he French? He did not know. But he was certain he came from a prosperous family, comprising his mother and three sisters, with a large house, and a garden full of flowers, and trees bearing fruits that could be eaten in winter. And then one terrible day he had been put on a horse, blindfolded, taken on a long journey, and abandoned to the mercies of an uncomprehending world.

Information about the Abbé de l'Épée's foundling was printed up and sent round to state marshals throughout France, and within a few weeks he received a response stating that the boy, whom he called

31 *Institution*, pp. 135–7.
32 Proof that his lessons began in 1763 at the latest is given in Maryse Bézagu-Deluy, *L'abbé de L'Épée*, pp. 146–7.

Joseph, must be the son of the late Comte de Solar of Clermont-en-Beauvaisis in the Oise. There was no doubt that there had been a deaf child in the family, who had probably been beaten and locked in a cellar, but the Dame de Solar claimed that her poor son had died of smallpox in 1774, so de l'Épée's Joseph must be an impostor. There were uncanny correspondences, though – a birthmark, a wild tooth – so, despite some strange discrepancies (the sister of the missing boy did not recognize Joseph, nor did he recognize her) the Abbé was convinced that his dumb boy must be the true Comte de Solar.

In 1778, a young man who had been mysteriously intimate with the Solar family was arrested in connection with the alleged abduction, and in 1781 he was brought to trial. The verdict was a triumph for de l'Épée: although the accused was acquitted, Joseph's claim to the title and dwindling estates of the Comte de Solar was upheld. For the first time, charges had been brought in a French court by an accuser who was deaf and dumb, and who could communicate only by means of gestures. (He was allowed an interpreter, trained by the Abbé de l'Épée.)[33]

Public agitation about the case brought to light dozens of other deaf and dumb children, abused, exposed, or confined, or exploited as meek and unprotesting chimney-sweeps, and the Abbé found himself converted into a public symbol of enlightened good works: the genial champion of poor little voiceless children, heralding an epoch where they would at last be able to enjoy their natural birthright. The work of the Abbé de l'Épée was proof, as the great philosopher Condorcet said in 1779, 'that it is not only in the field of books that this has been the century of reason and humanity'.[34]

The Abbé de l'Épée himself saw it slightly differently, however: 'my element is theology', as he said.[35] The purpose of his methodized sign language was to teach his pupils the truths of religion, so that they could become members of the Church. It was not human judges, after all, who were going to decide their ultimate fate. The right to use sign

33 The finding was overthrown by another court in 1792, however. A full but excessively imaginative account of the case is to be found in G. Lenôtre, *L'impénétrable secret du sourd-muet mort et vivant*, Paris, Perrin, 1929; a shorter but sharper description is given in Maryse Bézagu-Deluy, *L'abbé de l'Épée*, pp. 189–201.
34 Marie-Jean-Antoine-Nicolas Caritat de Condorcet, cited in an article on Pierre Desloges, *Mercure de France*, 18 December 1779, p. 142.
35 Charles-Michel de l'Épée, *Institution*, p. 57.

language in a court of law was one thing; but it was far more important to use it to teach 'the mysteries of religion and the sacraments – if not completely, then at least sufficiently to ensure that, should they be called away from this life, the spiritual aids which Christ has provided for our salvation can save them, redeem them, and admit them to eternal bliss at last'.[36] The Abbé also arranged for them to use sign language in the confessional, with him as their interpreter. 'They declare their sins to me, gazing into my eyes,' he said; then he translated for the confessor, who 'could but weep and offer absolution'. Eventually he restored confidentiality by assuming (rather irregularly) the right to hear confessions himself.[37] The language of methodical signs might not be perfect, he admitted; but he could not be altogether displeased with his work, if it 'led the deaf and dumb to salvation'.[38]

36 de l'Épée, *La Véritable Manière*, p. iv, second letter to Heinicke, pp. 244–76.
37 Letter of 1779, cited in Maryse Bézagu-Deluy, *L'abbé de L'Épée*, p. 228. It was as a result of these letters that de l'Épée obtained tacit permission to hear confessions on his own.
38 de l'Épée, *Institution*, p. 57.

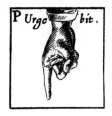

15

Reactions against signs:
sight, sound and the taste
of language

By 1764, the Abbé de l'Épee had about a dozen children attending his lessons in the Rue des Moulins every Tuesday and Friday afternoon. New pupils would be given a month or two of private tuition before being admitted to the class, so that the Abbé could establish a relationship with them based on their own natural signs, introduce them to the elements of Christianity, and – perhaps most important of all – prepare them for the revelation that any ideas they were able to express in signs could also be represented by alphabetic characters, either written or manually spelt.[1]

On their first day in the class, new pupils would be given chalk and a slate by the older ones, and assisted in tracing out the letters of the alphabet. Then they would play some classroom games, using cards with names of parts of the body written on them, or a kind of printer's case containing the letters of the alphabet written on slips of paper. By the end of the first lesson they would be expected to know the meanings of about twenty everyday words of written French. In their second lesson, the Abbé himself would teach them the infinitive form

---

1 Charles-Michel de l'Épée, *La Véritable Manière*, second letter to Heinicke, pp. 244–76.

of some obvious French verbs, writing them on the board, spelling them in his manual alphabet, and explaining their significance by performing actions like carrying a book or beating on the table. Later, he would teach the personal pronouns and their corresponding verb endings – *je porte, tu portes, nous portons*, for example – by getting some of the senior students to join in a pantomime of carrying a book. After a few lessons, the pupils would have no difficulty matching a basic vocabulary of written French to a range of gestural signs which they already understood. Having started on the familiar territory of their own language of signs, they would be 'very delighted to realize how ours [French] corresponds to it'.[2]

But the main business of each session was the Abbé's lecture on a passage from the Bible, delivered entirely in methodical signs, except for supplementary finger-spelling of names and unfamiliar words. All but the most junior pupils would be expected to write down the lesson while it was being dictated, translating the Abbé's signs back into French, and the more advanced ones would have their slates held up as an example for the others to imitate. They could also copy out their dictations in notebooks, so that over the years they would accumulate a collection of transcripts of all the Abbé's explanations of the New and the Old Testament.[3]

The Abbé de l'Épee may have been indifferent to personal fame, but he made every effort to advertise his ministry to the deaf and dumb, always encouraging members of the public to observe his lessons, and inviting them to suggest improvements to his technique, or even learn it for themselves so that they could carry on his work around the world. This openness was of course an implicit reproach to the crabbed secrecy of other educators of the deaf. Braidwood of Edinburgh, for example, was determined to maintain a family monopoly in Scotland, and when in 1783 he moved his Academy to Hackney, then on the outskirts of London, he placed his new assistants under a bond to keep his method secret. This attitude so disgusted Francis Green, the lawyer from Nova Scotia whose short-lived son had owed everything to Braidwood, that he withdrew his support and transferred it to the frank Abbé in Paris instead.[4]

2 Charles-Michel de l'Épée, *Institution des Sourds et Muets*, pp. 45–6.
3 *Institution*, pp. 111–15.
4 See Alexander Graham Bell, 'A Philanthropist of the last century', pp. 9–10. Green visited Paris in 1790 and 1791, and later translated some of de l'Épée's works into English.

The Abbé's generosity was also a threat to the livelihood of others, especially Pereire, still labouring away at training deaf pupils in writing, finger-spelling and articulation on the other bank of the Seine, with no family wealth to support him. On several occasions thereafter, the public at de l'Épée's lessons included Saboureux de Fontenay, the well-connected pupil of Pereire whose ability not only to read and write but to speak as well had so impressed the Academy of Sciences in 1751, when he was just thirteen. He had gone on to spend five more years with Pereire, and although he had now given up trying to communicate by speech, he read widely and wrote excellent French, and was able to finger-spell with astonishing speed and dexterity.

The gratitude that Saboureux de Fontenay felt towards Pereire led him to loathe his master's prosperous and easy-going rival in the Rue des Moulins. One afternoon, for example – probably in 1764 – he rudely disrupted the Abbé's lesson, to ridicule his use of the French two-handed manual alphabet. But when de Fontenay showed off the one-handed Spanish system he had learned from Pereire, the Abbé's cheerful receptiveness quite disarmed him: he acknowledged the advantages of the new method, and within fifteen minutes (or so he claims, no doubt with some exaggeration) he and his pupils had switched over to it, never to go back to the cumbersome French system again.[5]

Then in 1765, Saboureux de Fontenay published a long autobio-graphical article in the *Journal de Verdun* explaining how, despite the efforts of various teachers before Pereire, he had reached the age of twelve without understanding anything about language: the problem was, he observed, that most words do not correspond to visible objects, and this made them 'extremely difficult' to explain to the deaf. But then Pereire took charge of his education, and he was soon learning French almost as naturally as an ordinary hearing child. The key had been simply to 'substitute eyes for ears, and replace sounds and writing with the signs of the Manual Alphabet'. As de Fontenay explained, Pereire had developed an improved 'dactylology' comprising more than eighty handshapes, representing not only the vowels and conson-ants, but also numerals, punctuation points, and accents, not to men-tion 'large and small letters, and standard abbreviations, and . . . the

5 *Institution*, p. 102.

long, medium or short rests which are to be observed in pronun-ciation'.[6]

Once you had got into the habit of using Pereire's dactylology, de Fontenay continued, you would be able to write French in the air as fast as anyone could speak it: your hand would act 'like a pen', and you would be relishing a fluent experience of language which, prejudice apart, was equal to that enjoyed by those who could speak and hear. You could even develop a fondness for particular forms and styles of manual spelling, just as others may take delight in 'the sounds of speech and *viva voce* conversations'. Citing the philosophical common-place that 'there is nothing in this world except pure convention', de Fontenay claimed that Pereire's dactylology would allow the deaf to become 'as knowledgeable, as cultivated, and as capable of reasoning and proper reflection, as anyone else'.[7]

But, de Fontenay went on, Pereire's method depended on a strict rule forbidding the use of gestures. This forced his pupils to explain themselves 'in French, without using signs', and placed them 'under the happy necessity of attending meticulously to the meanings of nouns, verbs and particles', and so impelled them to make their belated journey into the world of 'intellectual, abstract and general ideas'. For it was impossible to teach spiritual matters, particularly religion, through gestural signs. In the first place, it would mean burdening the memory with tens of thousands of separate elements, one for each word, plus others for all their inflections; and for all its difficult complexity, such instruction was purely 'mechanical, and very similar to the training of animals'. In any case it would never lead pupils beyond the immediate world of the senses. De Fontenay recalled the shameful results of his brief period as a student of the late Simon Vanin, friend and precursor of de l'Épée: 'I then believed,' he wrote, 'that God the father was a venerable old man who lived in the sky, that the Holy Spirit was a dove surrounded by light, and the devil a hideous monster dwelling in the bowels of the earth.' The experiments to which he had been subjected before being sent to Pereire proved, in short, that pictures and signs reinforced the 'sensory, material or mechanical' ideas of the deaf: the only way to impart abstract ideas to

6 'Lettre de M. Saboureux de Fontenay, sourd et muet de naissance', pp. 361, 286, 369–70.
7 'Lettre de M. Saboureux de Fontenay', pp. 369–70, 297, 371, 295.

them and hence to save their souls was by finger-spelling or dactylology.[8]

Yet the Abbé de l'Épée persisted in dictating his lessons in 'methodical signs', apparently unperturbed by de Fontenay's attack. Pereire himself did not believe that the technique could ever succeed, and in 1772 he turned up in person at one of the Abbé's classes, bringing a letter with him and challenging the Abbé to dictate it to one of his pupils without using a manual alphabet. De l'Épée left his own description of the encounter with his rival. 'He sat down opposite me,' he recalled:

> There was a table between us, and a young girl, deaf and dumb, sat beside him on his left. The young lady followed my signs and wrote out the first five or six lines of the letter he had given me. At that point, he made me stop, saying, 'Enough of that, sir, enough. I would never have believed it: and you have as many signs as the Chinese have characters.'[9]

De l'Épée was obviously gratified by this little victory over Pereire, and he stirred himself at last to write a reply to the criticisms that had been published by Saboureux de Fontenay seven years before. His book on *The Education of the Deaf and Dumb by means of Methodical Signs*, which eventually appeared in 1776, showed him still smarting at allegations that gestural communication, with all its wagging of heads and waving of arms, was ugly and uncivilized, fit only for vulgar pantomimes or the guards of the seraglio of the Grand Turk. The Abbé professed himself astonished that Saboureux de Fontenay, who had often visited his rooms in the Rue des Moulins and seen him conversing with his pupils in signs, could think it anything but beautiful and dignified. Surely it was the use of manual alphabets, whether one-handed or two-handed ('dactylolias' and 'chirolalias' as the Abbé sarcastically called them) that was really barbaric and unsightly. Of course he himself had to resort to them on occasion – with new pupils, or when explaining how to spell unusual words and proper names. But apart from these special cases, it was absurdly cumbersome and time-wasting to have to spell out every letter, accent, and punctuation

8 'Lettre de M. Saboureux de Fontenay', pp. 367–8.
9 *Institution*, Part Two (Letter Two, 1772), p. 34; see also the re-telling of the story in the second letter to Heinicke, *La Véritable Manière*, pp. 244–76.

point with a separate handshape, when his own methodical signs seldom required more than one or two gestures for each word.[10]

The Abbé then took on the main argument of the dactylologists and turned it against them: it was finger-spelling, he said, not sign language, that was the uncultivated and unintelligent means of communication. Although it was useful as a method for specifying how words should be written, it gave absolutely no indication or analysis of what they meant. In fact it could just as well be used for dictating passages in a language which none of the participants could understand. Teachers who explained themselves in signs, however – especially if their pupils were making a simultaneous transcription in French – could be sure that all the ideas associated with each word were being taken up and analysed, one by one. *Messieurs les Dactylologistes*, on the other hand, were only giving their pupils a mechanical skill, reducing them to 'the same class as parrots'. The effect was all too evident, said the Abbé, in the scowling countenance of the dactylological Saboureux de Fontenay, which contrasted so starkly with the exuberant gaiety of his own signing pupils in the Rue des Moulins.[11]

Meanwhile a second attack on the methods of the Abbé de l'Épée was being prepared. Whereas Saboureux de Fontenay had chosen to fight him on a matter which struck most outsiders as specialized and abstruse – the relative merits of finger-spelling and gestural signs – the issue this time would be the far more inflammatory question of speech.[12] The author of the new assault was Claude François Deschamps, a priest who had been offering free instruction to deaf children in Orléans since 1776.[13] Despite several visits from the Abbé de l'Épée, Deschamps refused to be won over. Uncompromisingly, he argued that a choice had to be made between 'the two systems', which he defined as that of signs on one side, and that of speech on the other. According to Deschamps, it was of the most urgent spiritual importance that deaf children should be taught reading, writing and speech, because these provided the only means of equipping the human soul with the abstract ideas that are essential to religion and morality. De l'Épée's method

10 *Institution*, pp. 119, 26–7.
11 *Institution*, pp. 29, 151, 109.
12 See *Journal Encyclopédique*, 1 March 1776, p. 262.
13 See *Journal Encyclopédique*, 1 August 1777, p. 533.

of signs, he argued, confined the deaf to a purely sensory and physical experience of the world, and its use should therefore be severely discouraged.[14]

Of course, de l'Épée entirely accepted the importance of teaching the deaf to read and write: indeed he favoured sign language partly because he thought it the best means to this end. But then, according to Deschamps, he shied away from the supreme task: the teaching of speech itself. The problem was, presumably, that the simple Abbé lacked a philosophical grasp of the true relation between speaking and writing. Acknowledging the lead given by Pereire, and more remotely by Amman and Helmont, Deschamps pointed out that when people speak, the movements of their lips are a visible trace of their spoken words. But if – as was agreed on all sides – writing is essentially speech made visible, then it would be illogical not to regard the changing shape of the lips as a variety of writing. From a philosophical point of view, according to Deschamps, lip shapes are exactly like written characters, only fluent and fugitive rather than frozen and permanent. Speech, in its visible aspect, should be regarded as 'writing on the part of the speaker' and 'reading from the point of view of the listener'. Since everyone agreed that the deaf and dumb could be taught to read permanent written characters, it was absurd not to encourage them to hold conversations with hearing people by a process of 'continuous reading and writing', or 'mutual writing composed of characters imprinted on the organs of speech'. Provided they were relieved of the time-wasting task of learning sign language, the deaf could be taught to speak and hear as well as anyone else – writing out their thoughts on their own lips, and also, as Deschamps put it, 'reading from the lips' of others.[15]

Deschamps's attack on the Abbé de l'Épée and his use of sign language drew another participant into the debate. Pierre Desloges was a master bookbinder who had contracted smallpox as a child of seven and then, as he put it, 'become deaf and dumb'. Luckily, Desloges had learned to read and write before his illness, and for the next fifteen years, including the period when he served out his apprenticeship, reading and writing were his only means of communi-

---

14 Claude François, Abbé Deschamps, *Cours Élémentaire d'éducation des sourds et muets*, Paris, 1779, pp. 59–67.
15 *Cours Élémentaire*, pp. 210, xxii, 49, 22, 40, xxviii.

cation. Around 1770 he left his provincial home near Tours and came to work in Paris. And in 1774, when he was 27, he made the acquaintance of an Italian servant, deaf and dumb from birth, who at last initiated him into the riches of the Parisian 'language of signs'. (Desloges explained that, having passed his youth in provincial isolation, he had never had the chance to learn any but the most rudimentary signs; but it was very different to be deaf in a great city like Paris, 'the epitome of the wonders of the universe'.) Within six weeks he was fluent in Parisian signs, and by now, after several years of practice, he could express all kinds of thoughts in his second language – 'even those which are most independent of the senses' – and with as much order and precision as could be desired.

Naturally, he was angered by Deschamps's attack on signs: it made him feel, he said, as his compatriots would if they heard an ignorant German ridiculing the French language. Desloges therefore considered himself 'obliged to avenge my language, and so justify the method of the Abbé de l'Épée, which is based entirely in the language of signs'.[16]

Desloges continued his riposte to Abbé Deschamps by describing a whole network of poor deaf-and-dumb working people in Paris. They had never had any education apart from 'common sense and the company of their fellows', and most of them could neither read nor write.[17] But they all shared the language of signs, and it served their needs very well: 'there are no events, whether in Paris, or France, or at the four corners of the world, which lie beyond the range of our conversations,' he said. And the poor signing deaf of Paris were well instructed in religion too: well enough, at any rate, to be admitted to the sacraments, 'even the Eucharist and marriage' in one enlightened parish.[18] As for the estimable Abbé de l'Épée: he was not the inventor of sign language, nor had he ever claimed to be. He had merely picked it up from the deaf, extended its vocabulary, and regularized its grammar. As far as Desloges was concerned, then, Deschamps's

16 Pierre Desloges, *Observations d'un sourd et muet sur un cours élémentaire d'éducation des sourds et muets*, Paris, 1779, pp. 14, 13, 3. The text is translated in Harlan Lane, ed., *The Deaf Experience*, pp. 30–48.

17 Desloges, *Observations d'un sourd et muet*, p. 3.

18 See *Observations d'un sourd et muet*, pp. 13–15 (the parish in question was St Étienne du Mont). See also the review in *Journal Encyclopédique*, 1 February 1780, pp. 446–65, and the 'Lettre de M. Bellisle' (presumably by Desloges), *Journal Encyclopédique*, 15 August 1780, pp. 125–32.

criticisms of de l'Épée were really an attack not only on an excellent and well-established means of communication, but also on the humanity of all those poor creatures who had to depend upon it.[19]

The Abbé Deschamps responded to the artisan Desloges in a brief pamphlet, heavy with languid disdain. He was amused by the thought of this self-educated deaf bookbinder promoting himself as the champion of illiterate deaf-and-dumb paupers with their strange and primitive substitute for a language. If signs were really so wonderful, he asked, why did Desloges still read and write in French? If sign language was natural, why did he have to come to Paris to learn it? And if it was perfect, why had de l'Épée been obliged to improve it and subject it to a method? Why should the deaf have any need for teachers, indeed, when they knew everything already? If the deaf were so blessed, why should they deserve any sympathy and consideration at all?[20]

Of course Desloges might have expected special weight to be given to his opinion, as a member of the class about which he spoke; but Deschamps neutralized this advantage by reproducing a testimonial from the sophisticated Saboureux de Fontenay, who had even more authority than Desloges, since he was born deaf, whereas the little gesticulating bookbinder admitted that he had not lost his hearing till he reached the age of seven. In his letter, de Fontenay also pointed out that the glory of being the first deaf-and-dumb writer to appear in print belonged to himself, with the article in praise of dactylology that he had published in the *Journal de Verdun* in 1765, rather than to Desloges with his pamphlet defending de l'Épée of 1779. What is more, in the battle of the two systems, it was himself, Saboureux de Fontenay, the most learned of the educated deaf and dumb, who had the honour of being the first to denounce 'the habit of conversing by means of gestural signs', and the courage to 'declare war' on sign language, in the name of the deaf.[21]

Despite all the controversies raging around him, the serene Abbé de l'Épée got on with teaching his pupils in the Rue des Moulins – and

19 'Lettre de M. Desloges', *Mercure de France*, 18 December 1779, pp. 147–8.
20 See Claude François, Abbé Deschamps, *Lettre à Mr de Bellisle pour servir de réponse aux observations d'un sourd et muet sur un cours*, Paris, 1780, pp. 8, 12, 26.
21 'Lettre de M. Saboureux de Fontenay à M. Desloges', appended to Deschamps, *Lettre à Mr de Bellisle*, pp. 35–6.

by 1780 he had nearly seventy attending each lesson. He also had the satisfaction of training sign-language teachers to extend and carry on his work. One of the first was a young priest called Friedrich Storck, who was sponsored by the Empress Maria Theresia and then entrusted with the direction of an Academy for the Deaf in Vienna, which she set up in 1779. Within a few months the pupils of de l'Épée's disciple were giving acclaimed performances before an illustrious public in the imperial city.[22]

But the success of Friedrich Storck in Vienna was to provoke yet another scornful attack on de l'Épée and the language of signs. It was launched by a teacher and inventor called Samuel Heinicke, who had been working with the deaf since about 1765, first in Dresden, then in Hamburg, and had recently opened a School for the Deaf in Leipzig under the patronage of the Elector of Saxony.[23] All his efforts were concentrated on articulation, since, as he saw it, the deaf would never be able to understand the spiritual truths of religion until they had learned to express 'abstract and general ideas' in speech. Heinicke recognized several precursors in this vocation – Bonet, Wallis, Amman and Pereire amongst others – but he considered that they had all committed the same basic mistake as the egregious Abbé de l'Épée: they wanted to 'substitute the sense of sight for the missing sense of hearing', and thus increased their pupils' dependence on the 'visible world' when they should have been doing exactly the opposite, and trying to wean them away from it.[24]

In his *Observations on the Dumb*, published in 1778, Heinicke argued that the intellectual life of those who can hear depends to a large degree on the use of sounds as names: all of us make use of vocal patterns in order to fix and recall our ideas, he said – not just musicians, but everyone else too, 'from the cook to the algebrist'. Echoing Herder, Heinicke affirmed that 'we think by means of sounds', and

---

22 See *Journal Encyclopédique*, 1 April 1780, pp. 133–4.
23 On Heinicke, claimed as founder of the 'German school' of deaf education, see Eduard Walther, *Geschichte des Taubstummen-Bildungswesens*, Bielefeld and Leipzig, Velhagen and Klasing, 1882, pp. 105–23; but Walther's claim that Heinicke opened a school in 1754–5, at least six years before de l'Épée, is unpersuasive given that in 1784 Heinicke said he had been combating prejudice against the dumb for 'nearly twenty years': see Samuel Heinicke, *Wichtige Entdeckungen und Beyträge zur Seelenlehre und zur menschlichen Sprache*, Leipzig, 1784, p. 4.
24 Samuel Heinicke, *Beobachtungen über Stumme, und über die menschliche Sprache*, Hamburg, 1778, pp. 26, 18, 28.

that our thoughts 'resonate within us through the sounds of their names'.[25] The problem facing the uneducated deaf was that – being cut off from the world of sound – they had no 'names' either for things or for concepts, which meant that they lived like infants or animals, their various 'impressions and representations' passing straight through them in uncontrollable confusion, leaving no mental trace behind them.[26]

Of course it was perfectly possible to teach the deaf to write – to use 'visible names', that is, instead of audible ones. But Heinicke considered this recourse to vision to be wasted effort. In the first place, it overlooked the fact that the sense of sight is 'mostly deceptive and always cold'. For another, it violated the 'fundamental law, that two different impressions can never be distinctly experienced at the same time'. It forgot, therefore, that 'written thoughts go far less quickly' for the deaf than 'thoughts in sound' do for the rest of us: visible names file slowly through our imaginations, one letter after another, whereas spoken ones course through the soul 'with the greatest clarity and rapidity', letting us think our thoughts 'like lightning'. For this reason, if the deaf could not be taught the language of sound, they might as well be left to their subhuman 'mother tongue', the gestural pantomine championed by the Abbé de l'Épée of Paris and his deluded disciples.[27]

Even if Heinicke's readers accepted his opinion about the rapidity of spoken signs compared with visible ones (a view which was exactly opposed, as they may have noted, to that of Condillac, Rousseau and Diderot), they must have been puzzled as to how he would dispense with vision in the training of his deaf pupils. Part of the answer, he revealed, was his *Sprachmaschine* or Language Machine – an exact replica of the throat and the tongue, which enabled him to show how all kinds of vocal sounds are produced, and exhibit the mechanism to the sense of touch as well as to the eye. But the cornerstone of Heinicke's non-visual technique was rather more special and unexpected. It was a new invention, based on the clearest 'psychological results', and, according to Heinicke, 'very simple, yet also certain'. It involved

25 'Sie sind durch ihre tönenden Benennungen in uns tonhaft', *Beobachtungen über Stumme*, p. 33.
26 *Beobachtungen über Stumme*, p. 36.
27 *Beobachtungen über Stumme*, pp. 94–5, 40, 32, 41, 55.

connecting vowel sounds to another sensory faculty – a faculty which, though generally despised, is actually capable of 'the most manifold and extensive' sensations. Heinicke would lead the deaf into the realm of speech and abstract general ideas, that is to say, by way of the sense of taste.[28]

Heinicke was not prepared to divulge the details of his invention beyond stating that he had devised 'a special scale' relating the experience of speech to a table of flavours.[29] This scale – the 'supreme article of our art' – was described only in a handwritten *Arkanum* which Heinicke bequeathed to his son-in-law Ernst Adolf Eschke (who went on to open the Royal Institute for the Deaf and Dumb in Berlin, but seems not to have exploited the family secret). The document was saved for posterity, however, and the secret turns out to consist in associating each vowel with a different flavour, using a feather to apply appropriate liquids to the tongue: the scale ran from sharp vinegar (corresponding to I), through extract of wormwood (E), pure water (A), and sugar-water (O), down to olive oil (U), with mixtures for diphthongs.[30] Once they had learned the taste of their vowels, Heinicke's pupils became so accustomed to naming their concepts with sounds, and so delighted with the rapidity and convenience of the practice, that they stopped using gestures altogether and paid the ultimate tribute to his method, by talking in their sleep.[31]

On more than one occasion, Heinicke was visited at his school in Leipzig by de l'Épée's pupil and follower, the Abbé Storck of Vienna; but the proud inventor refused to consider parting with his secret for less than 10,000 thalers.[32] He also composed a polemical book, contrasting his own 'de-dumbed' or 'demutized' students (*entstummte*, as he called them) with the unfortunate products of the sign-language method of de l'Épée and Storck. Speech, according to Heinicke, was not an ordinary mechanical skill, but an 'incomparable means of thinking', and his own students, thanks to his Language

28 *Beobachtungen über Stumme*, pp. 99–100, 61–2, 59.
29 *Beobachtungen über Stumme*, p. 62.
30 The manuscript explaining these flavour-vowel correlations (dated 1772) was eventually published in Heinrich Stötzner, *Samuel Heinicke. Sein Leben und Wirken*, Leipzig, 1870, pp. 53–4; and the hagiographer permits himself to comment that 'experience has sufficiently shown, how far Heinicke erred at this point.'
31 *Beobachtumgen über Stumme*, pp. 109, 105.
32 See Eduard Walther, *Geschichte des Taubstummen-Bildungswesens*, p. 113, where Heinicke's *Geheimnisthuerei* is described as 'einen unverzeihlichen Humbug'.

Machine and the secret 'special scale' of sounds and tastes, had direct contact with words and their associated concepts: they knew language intimately and 'through consciousness' (*Bewusstseyn*), rather than through the mere 'inner representation of absent, written names'.[33]

In 1782, the Abbé de l'Épée himself took responsibility for the argument with Heinicke, in an exchange of mutually uncomprehending letters. As far as de l'Épée was concerned, Heinicke's argument was the same as that of his old opponents Pereire, Deschamps and de Fontenay: he seemed to be calling for the suppression of sign language on the ground that 'the deaf and dumb must learn to speak before they can understand the meaning of words or of things'. Heinicke replied that de l'Épée was missing the essential point: that he was able to teach speech directly, without reference to signs or writing, simply by making 'taste supply any defect of hearing'. De l'Épée would have to come to Leipzig for at least six months to study the new method if he wanted to appreciate its power; but even then, Heinicke warned, de l'Épée would not be let into the secret of the flavour-vowel correspondences.[34]

Instead of undertaking a long journey and abandoning his beloved pupils, the 70-year-old Abbé de l'Épée sent a copy of the whole correspondence to a neutral body – the Council of the Zurich Academy – asking them to deliberate on the merits of 'the two methods, that of Paris and that of Leipzig'. Once again de l'Épée was rewarded with a gratifying verdict: in February 1783, two years after the Solar case, the Zurich jury concluded that whilst Heinicke's Language Machine was ingenious, his taste-sound scale was of doubtful utility. The Abbé de l'Épée's use of gestural signs to convey meanings, however, promised to be a great blessing to humanity: 'our frank sentiment,' they said, 'is that the utility of your method is so astonishing that it seems to us it would be salutary if all those deaf pupils trained by the oral method could be sent to you so that they could gain a proper understanding of the meanings of the words they have already learned.'[35] The elderly Abbé appeared to have finally won his battle.

---

33 Hanicke, *Wichtige Entdeckungen und Beyträge*, pp. 5, 58, 25–7.
34 The correspondence was published in Latin in 1784 as an appendix to de l'Épée *La Véritable Manière*; see pp. xvi, 276, 277, 280. A French translation appeared in *Corpus*, 2, January 1986, pp. 87–115; see pp. 96, 101, 102.
35 See *La Véritable Manière*, p. 286, *Corpus*, p. 108.

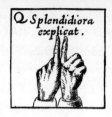

16

Sign language and
the philosophers

During the 1770s, more and more deaf people were to be observed on the streets of Paris, conversing fluently in gestures or 'the language of signs'. The reason was not that more children were being born deaf, according to the Abbé de l'Épée, but simply that they were no longer being concealed or removed from society. Certainly they were not killed off as they used to be. Customs had changed, the Abbé said, and 'today, such cruelty would make us shudder'. The sighs and moans of families with deaf children had given way to tears of tenderness and joy. Parents who would once have regarded deaf children as monsters and sent them away to 'the secrecy of a cloister, or the obscurity of unknown lodgings' now showed them off with pride, and expected them to bring their family great honour and fame.[1]

The Abbé's regular lessons in his rooms in the Rue des Moulins were exciting so much public interest that, starting in 1771, he also mounted annual public exercises, to let a larger audience admire the accomplishments of his pupils. In one celebrated routine, he would deliver an improvised discourse in methodical signs, and different pupils would write it down in different languages – some in French, others in Italian, Spanish or Latin. This was taken by certain observers

---

1 Charles-Michel de l'Épée, *Institution des Sourds et Muets*, pp. 1–5.

– a little hastily no doubt – as positive proof of the universality of sign language, confirmation that it was untouched by the arbitrariness and multiplicity of speech; but the real motive for the performance, as far as the practical Abbé was concerned, was the hope of getting foreigners to realize that his methods could be brought back and used in their own countries as well.[2]

Even the regular lessons in the Rue des Moulins took on an aspect of public exercises, and the Abbé and his pupils grew accustomed to welcoming all sorts of visitors there, especially 'persons of the highest quality', who might with luck be inspired to found new academies of 'methodical signs' and pay for the training of staff to run them. De l'Épée received guests from Spain, Italy, Germany, Ireland and Scotland, and on one occasion in 1777 he broke with tradition and held a class on a Thursday for the benefit of a great visitor travelling incognito who turned out to be the Emperor Joseph II. On another occasion there was a special audience for the Papal Nuncio, Prince Doria Pamphili.[3] As a result of visits like these, de l'Épée was eventually to train a total of twenty teachers, half of them foreigners who went back to implement his methods at home – Storck to Vienna, others to Rome and Zurich and various cities in Spain, Ireland and the Netherlands.[4] In 1778, Louis XVI himself decided to take the Abbé de l'Épée under his protection, and promised to endow an establishment in Paris to carry on his work in perpetuity.[5] (The promise was not kept.)

Scientists and philosophers were also drawn to the lessons and exercises, perhaps excited by the publicity given to them by the ubiquitous Baron Grimm, who in 1773 described de l'Épée as 'a credit to philosophy and to humanity'.[6] Lord Monboddo came from Edinburgh on several occasions, to be charmed by the civility of the Abbé, and he took away particularly pleasing memories of one of the female students.[7] The Viennese gentleman-scientist Wolfgang von Kempelen also visited, in 1783. (Kempelen was fascinated by the human voice, and had invented

2 *Institution*, Part Two, First Letter, p. 12.
3 See Charles-Michel de l'Épée, *La Véritable Manière*, p. 100; also Maryse Bézagu-Deluy, *L'abbé de L'Épée*, pp. 206–7.
4 See Bézagu-Deluy, *l'abbé de l'Épée*, p. 216; *La Véritable Manière*, p. 159.
5 See Bézagu-Deluy, *l'abbé de l'Épée*, p. 209.
6 Friedrich Melchior von Grimm, Letter for September 1773, *Correspondance Littéraire*, edited by Maurice Tourneaux, Vol. 10, Paris, Garnier, 1879, pp. 295–6.
7 James Burnet, Lord Monboddo, *Of the Origin and Progress of Language*, Vol. 1, 1773, pp. 178–9.

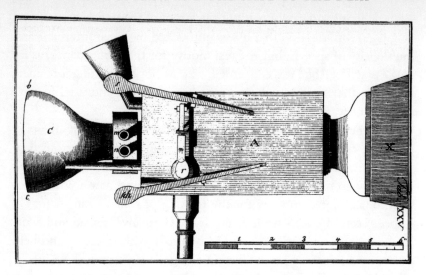

FIG 8. Wolfgang von Kempelen's 'Speaking machine' (1791)
(Air is pumped into the voice box (A), and can be released noiselessly through the
vent (X) or resonantly through the horn (C). The heel of the right hand rests on
X to control the release of air, whilst the fingers cover the nostril-holes (m,n) and
throat-aperture levers. The left hand, placed firmly over the opening of the horn,
is moved in imitation of the motions of the lips.)

an ingenious apparatus, composed of bellows, a modified oboe-reed,
and a box containing movable parts corresponding to lips, palate,
tongue and nostrils, with which he could synthesize all the ordinary
vowel sounds and most of the consonants: a true *machine parlante* or
speaking machine, as he rightly boasted, with which he managed to
cause great consternation to his family and servants. See Figure 8.)
Despite his immoderate affection for the human voice, de Kempelen
acknowledged that the Abbé's 'methodical signs' were capable of the
same perfection as any spoken language; and he too was singularly
moved by a 'pretty girl, twenty years of age', who turned out to be
deaf and dumb, though he did not realize it at first.[8]

Another visitor at de l'Épée's classes was Alexis Copineau, a theological
grammarian and linguistic reformer who published a judicious account
of the origins of language in 1774, much influenced by what he saw
at the Rue des Moulins. Summarizing the arguments over visible signs

8 Wolfgang von Kempelen, *Le mécanisme de la parole, suivi de la description d'une
machine parlante*, Vienna, 1791, p. 18.

and hieroglyphs, audible words and temporal succession developed by philosophers like Warburton, Diderot, Condillac, Rousseau, and Herder, Copineau proposed that spoken language should be seen as a natural development of a general human instinct for forming vocal sounds. It had progressed through the successive stages of mimicry, expression, and imitation until at last, through the gradual accretion of analogies, it embraced even the most abstract, refined and universal ideas, organizing them so far as possible in accordance with the rational principles of grammatical logic.

But there was one form of language which was unmarked by the progress of civilization and uncontaminated by social convention. The language of visible gestures avoided the arbitrariness of speech by functioning like 'a kind of painting' and 'placing objects themselves, so to speak, before our eyes'. Copineau observed that gestural language was not only 'very normal in infancy', but also 'the only language that the dumb can use amongst themselves'.[9] And for anyone who doubted its power, Copineau recommended a visit to the Rue des Moulins, to see the Abbé de l'Épée silently addressing his students and observe how, starting with signs 'taken from nature', the Abbé had raised sign language 'to such a degree of perfection that every idea has a sign of its own'. The result was like a system of fleeting hieroglyphs, where 'what the Egyptians used to draw with lines is painted in gestures instead'. Nothing could be more touching, Copineau explained, than the sight of the good citizen de l'Épée delivering edifying silent lessons to the poor dumb students who thronged gratefully around his desk.[10]

A year or two later, Copineau befriended the deaf bookbinder Pierre Desloges, and encouraged him in the composition of his indignant reply to the Abbé Deschamps's attack on sign language. Copineau not only corrected Desloges's spelling and grammar, but added notes of his own explaining the different philosophical principles underlying gestural and spoken language. Signs, he maintained, were intrinsically more exact than words because they 'depict ideas immediately', without getting sidetracked by 'the intermediary of sounds'. Copineau went on to declare himself 'so convinced of the advantages of the

9 (Alexis Copineau), *Essai synthétique sur l'origine et la formation des langues*, Paris, Ruault, 1774, pp. 21–2.
10 *Essai synthétique sur l'origine et la formation des langues*, fn. pp. 22–3.

language of signs, that if I were responsible for the education of an ordinary child, I would make frequent use of it ... so as to be sure that I was not simply training a parrot'.[11]

Once Desloges had published his book, he was taken up by the illustrious Condorcet, who was fascinated to observe the bookbinder's mastery of a means of communication which, though a little primitive (simpler and less regular than de l'Épée's, for example), was almost entirely 'natural, and independent of arbitrary conventions', and yet perfectly adequate to the necessities of a complex working life.[12] And then an even more eminent philosopher came forward to give his theoretical endorsement to de l'Épée, Desloges and their language of signs. This was Étienne Bonnot de Condillac, who, thirty years before, had followed Vico and Warburton in praising the naturalness, honesty and simplicity of gestures, or what he preferred to call the 'language of action'.[13] A little later, in the course of arguing (in agreement with Montaigne and in opposition to Descartes and Buffon) that animals can think and have feelings just like humans, Condillac had claimed that animals too made use of the language of action: their 'physical actions are signs of their thoughts,' he said, and anyone who was familiar with the way domestic animals could be trained to respond to vocal commands would know that animal signs could also be used as a foundation for teaching the language of articulate sounds.[14]

Towards the end of the 1770s, Condillac attended several lessons and exercises at the Rue des Moulins and cross-examined the Abbé de l'Épée about his methods, but without revealing his identity. To his delight, his old speculative theories about the language of action seemed to be thoroughly corroborated by de l'Épée's practical work with the deaf. As Condillac saw it, the generous Abbé had first observed the language of action in a more or less pristine state, as used amongst his fellow citizens, the Parisian deaf and dumb. Realizing that it remained 'of necessity very limited', he had ingeniously extended it by means of 'analogies' until it became capable of 'rendering all the conceptions of the human spirit', so that he could now use it to convey

11 (Alexis Copineau), in Pierre Desloges, *Observations d'un sourd et muet*, pp. 16–18.
12 Jean-Antoine-Nicolas Caritat, Marquis de Condorcet, *Mercure de France*, 18 December 1779, pp. 142–6.
13 See above, pp. 133–4.
14 Étienne Bonnot de Condillac, *Traité des Sensations* (1755), Part 2, Chapter 4, Paris, Fayard, 1984, pp. 371–2.

'all kinds of ideas to his pupils'. According to Condillac, indeed, de l'Épée's signs were distinctly superior to any other form of language, because they left no room for ambiguity or vagueness. The basic signs, after all, were pantomimic: they imitated simple actions like eating, beating or caressing – actions which were, so to speak, signs of themselves, and left no room for misunderstanding. Since the Abbé had to explain the meaning of every other sign in terms of these basic ones, patiently constructing abstract ideas out of their simple sensory components, it was logically impossible to utter inane and meaningless discourse when using his methodical signs. The Abbé's teaching, as Condillac interpreted it, consisted essentially in 'analysing ideas, and getting his pupils to analyse them with him'. The language of action was a philosophical education in itself; it was not only the intellectual equal of speech, but distinctly superior to it.[15]

The Abbé de l'Épée enjoyed being the hobby-horse of the philosophers, often quoting their enthusiastic endorsements of his methods. He himself warmed to the idea that 'the language of signs' might be the currency 'of nature herself, and common to all humanity'.[16] At any rate, he was certain that it was the most expressive of all means of communication, since the gestures of which it was ultimately composed – unlike the words of speech, or the characters of Chinese script for that matter – had a rational connection with the ideas they denoted: *breadth* being represented by a broad gesture, for example, and *sadness* by a sad one.[17]

In practice, however, the Abbé never approached sign language in the same spirit as his philosophical sponsors. For him, it was not so much a self-sufficient form of communication, as a means for enabling his pupils to understand enough French (or on occasion Spanish, Latin or Italian) to be able to grasp the elements of Christian belief. Furthermore, his supplementary artificial signs were explicitly modelled on French. Having observed, for instance, that the uneducated deaf of Paris gestured over their shoulder with their right hand to indicate the past, or extended it in front of them to indicate the future, he decided to modify this practice in order to bring it into harmony with part of

15 Condillac, *Cours d'Instruction du Prince de Parme*, Vol. 1, pp. 11–12, fn.
16 de lo'Épée, *Institution*, p. 36.
17 *Institution*, p. 120.

the tense system in French, using one throw over the shoulder to indicate the imperfect tense, two the perfect, and three the pluperfect. Or again, finding no equivalent for particles in the natural language of signs, he noted that the definite articles *le* and *la* served as link-words, which might be compared in function with the joints of the fingers. So he made up a 'rational sign' for them, by crooking his right forefinger, and moving it to his head, where a man's hat would be, for the masculine *le*, or to the ear, where a woman's hair would end, for the feminine *la*. By devices like these, he built up a way of signalling all the words of everyday French, so that his pupils could easily make exact, one for one, word-for-sign transcriptions of his gestural lessons. 'The great utility of methodical signs,' he wrote, 'is for dictating every-thing that we want our deaf and dumb pupils to write down.'[18] He conceived his lessons in French, that is, and then dictated them in signs, intending his pupils to transcribe them in exactly the same French words he originally had in mind.

Thus the Abbé's practice with his pupils did not quite correspond with the theories about the origins of language that the philosophers projected onto it. He never seriously supposed that the language of signs, either in its wild natural state or subjected to his methodical rules, could be an adequate substitute for civilized languages based in speech. His paradigmatic language was always French, as seen through the Latinizing eyes of the grammarians, rather than natural signs, as glimpsed in the etymological utopias of the philosophers. In reality, his methodical signs were just an abbreviated way of identifying French words, or their equivalents in any other language with similar tenses particles, and syntactic rules. From this point of view, there was not such a huge gulf between de l'Épée's signs and the 'dactylography' or finger-spelling of his rival Pereire: it was not much greater, in fact, than the difference between writing in shorthand and writing in full.

Nor did the Abbé de l'Épée conform to the precepts of his philo-sophical sponsors on the most divisive of all the great issues in the education of the deaf. When he began his work in the early 1760s, he assumed that only a miracle could restore speech to the dumb, and his mission was simply to use methodical signs as a means of teaching the written form of French or some other ordinary language, in which

18 *Institution*, pp. 48–50, 60, 72.

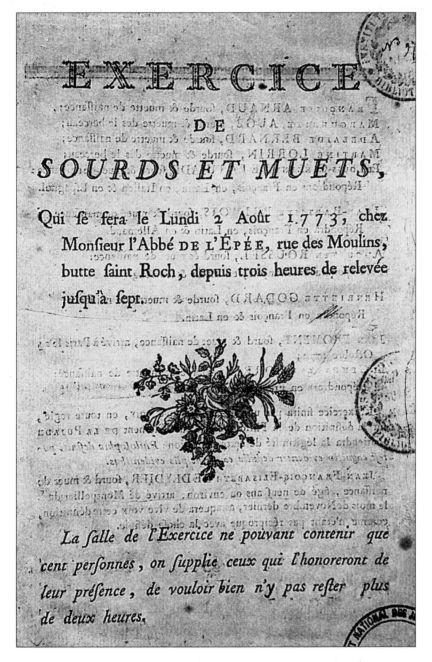

EXERCICE

DE

SOURDS ET MUETS,

Qui se fera le Lundi 2 Août 1773, chez Monsieur l'Abbé DE L'ÉPÉE, rue des Moulins, butte saint Roch, depuis trois heures de relevée jusqu'à sept.

La salle de l'Exercice ne pouvant contenir que cent personnes, on supplie ceux qui l'honoreront de leur présence, de vouloir bien n'y pas rester plus de deux heures.

FIGS 9 and 10. Notice for a public demonstration of speech by de l'Épée's deaf pupils in 1773, featuring a disputation on the definition of philosophy

Françoise ARNAUD, sourde & muette de naissance;
Marguerite AUGÉ, sourde & muette dès le berceau;
Adelaide BERNARD, sourde & muette de naissance;
Martine LORRIN, sourde & muette dès le berceau;
Et Louis-Clément DE LA PUJADE, sourd & muet de naissance:
Répondront en François, en Latin, en Italien & en Espagnol.

Jean-Baptiste PRIMOIS, sourd & muet de naissance :
Répondra en François, en Latin & en Allemand.

Augustin ROUSSEL, sourd & muet de naissance:
Répondra en François, en Latin & en Anglois.

Henriette GODARD, sourde & muette de naissance:
Répondra en François & en Latin.

Jean FROMENT, sourd & muet de naissance, arrivé à Paris le 24
Octobre 1772;
Et Genevieve LORRIN, sourde & muette de naissance:
Répondront en François seulement.

L'Exercice finira par une dispute de vive voix, en toute reglé,
sur la définition de la Philosophie. Louis-Clément DE LA PUJADE
soutiendra la légitimité de cette définition : *Philosophia definiri po-
test cognitio evidenter deducta ex principiis evidentibus.*

Jean-François-Elisabeth DE DEYDIER, sourd & muet de
naissance, âgé de neuf ans ou environ, arrivé de Montpellier dans
le mois de Novembre dernier, attaquera de vive voix cette définition,
comme n'étant pas réciproque avec la chose définie.

they could then receive their religious indoctrination. But in 1764 or thereabouts, he changed his mind. According to his own account, a stranger came to observe one of his early lessons and suggested that he could go further, and teach his pupils to speak. This 'unknown man' presented de l'Épée with a copy of Bonet's book on the *Simplification of the Letters of the Alphabet,* and he set about learning Spanish in order to read it.[19] Soon he discovered the works of Amman too, and then began his own experiments in teaching speech to his pupils. He would make them wash carefully, and then let them explore the inside of his mouth with the fingers of their left hand whilst feeling his throat with their right; then he would spell out the letters of the alphabet, vowels first, then consonants, simultaneously writing them down on a slate. Afterwards they would be expected to imitate him by feeling their own throats and the insides of their mouths whilst trying to pronounce the alphabet for themselves. By following this procedure, de l'Épée said, his pupils soon learned to replicate all the elementary actions of speech, and thus start making articulate vocal utterances just like anyone else.[20] After only four lessons, he would have 'opened their mouth, and unshackled their tongue', a task he had originally assumed to be impossible.[21] It turned out not to be difficult at all, he said, in fact it was so 'purely mechanical' that it required no great talent or intelligence, merely patience. The sole difficulty was that it was expensive and time-consuming, because lessons had to be given individually, not in class, so he recommended leaving them to junior assistants who could keep up a course of regular daily training until full vocal fluency was achieved.[22]

Having adopted Bonet's solution to the problem of speech, de l'Épée decided that the manual alphabet was also strictly superfluous, and could be replaced by the 'labial alphabet' – what Deschamps had called 'reading from the lips'. It was considerably harder to teach, but it was more effective too, and of course entirely natural: the match between lip-shapes and sounds was absolutely universal and common to every country and every people.[23] De l'Épée claimed that by opening

19 de l'Épée, *La Véritable Manière*, p. 159.
20 *La Véritable Manière*, p. 170.
21 de l'Épée, *Institution*, pp. 191–4, 220.
22 *Institution*, pp. 220–3.
23 de l'Épée, *La Véritable Manière*, p. 209.

his own mouth no more than a finger's breadth, he could show his deaf pupils various different positions of his vocal organs, one for each letter, and that they could then write them in the ordinary alphabet just as he pronounced them. No doubt he began by spelling out each letter separately, but before long, he claimed, the children were able follow his normal speech, and take it down letter by letter, even correcting for any faults, slurs and idiosyncrasies in his pronunciation. He boasted that there was nothing, absolutely nothing, that his advanced scholars could not write from his spoken dictation, and without any prompting from either finger-spelling or signs.[24]

At the first public exercise in the Rue des Moulins, in 1771, de l'Épée's scholars gave spoken answers to his questions, and delivered prepared speeches in Latin or French, so rapidly but so well that some of the ladies laughed out loud, suspecting a trick. At another exercise a couple of years later, two of his students sustained a formal disputation *viva voce*, albeit only a brief one, concerning the proper definition of philosophy. (See Figures 9 and 10 pp. 173–4.) In addition, the Abbé gave a dictation by the lips alone, without using any gestures at all, or even making a sound; but, as he put it, the children 'heard me through their eyes, and either wrote down what I said, or repeated it out loud'.[25] Kempelen, too, observed a deaf boy taking dictations from the Abbé's lips,[26] and Monboddo recalled a girl 'who spoke so pleasantly that I should not have known her to be deaf'.[27] Only the dullest of the Abbé's pupils were left to make do with sign language, therefore; for all its philosophical notoriety, and the antagonism it aroused in critics like Deschamps, the language of signs played a strictly limited role in the work of the Abbé de l'Épée. His main aim was simply to 'deliver the deaf and dumb completely to society', and – like his critics but unlike his philosophical admirers – he thought that meant teaching his pupils to progress beyond sign language and 'hear with their eyes and express themselves with their voice'.[28]

24 de l'Épée, *Institution*, pp. 107–8, 155–6.
25 *Institution*, Part Two, First Letter, p. 15, Third Letter, pp. 56–7.
26 de Kempelen, *Le mécanisme de la parole*, p. 23.
27 James Burnet, *Of the Origin and Progress of Language*, Vol. 1, p. 179.
28 *Institution*, p. 155.

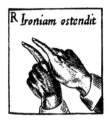

17

Signs and the French Revolution

The systematic philosophers who came to praise the Abbé de l'Épée for vindicating the natural truthfulness of gesture against the artificial conventions of speech may have misunderstood him, but he accepted their compliments all the same. Perhaps he felt they made up for the equally uncomprehending hostility shown by rival teachers of the deaf, like Deschamps and Heinicke. In any case, he was happy to let the two parties exhaust themselves in theoretical disputes over the merits of natural and methodical signs as compared with spoken and written language, while he persevered with his eclectic and empirical collection of educational techniques regardless. He was, after all, a rich amateur, living off rents and inherited wealth. The support promised by the King in 1778 had never materialized,[1] but his private income allowed him to continue giving free lessons in his rooms in the family home, as well as maintaining four boarding houses for his poorer pupils – three for girls and one for boys – on the Rue d'Argenteuil, and keeping himself in solid bourgeois comfort.[2] The Abbé de l'Épée had no need for patrons; he was responsible only to his own conscience.

The confusion surrounding the nature of his work was compounded by a certain obtuseness in the Abbé himself. By 1779, under the

---

1 See Maryse Bézagu-Deluy, *L'abbé de l'Épée*, pp. 222–3.
2 See Ferdinand Berthier, *L'Abbé de l'Épée*, Paris, Michel Levy, 1852, p. 82.

pressure of public curiosity about his methods, as well as his own concern for the needs of future teachers of the deaf, he decided to write a 'dictionary' of signs, and even sought a grant from the state to support its publication. He had little enthusiasm for the project however: gestures would lose their special virtue, he thought, as soon as they were put down on paper. The experience of reading a cold record of signs in black and white could never rival the joy of seeing them performed in real life; '*signes lus*', as he put it, would never replace '*signes vus*'.[3] But he undertook the duty anyway, and since he did not propose to include the methodical signs – which represented elements of French grammar – he expected it to be quite easy to write.

The more he worked at the dictionary, however, the more difficult the task became. The problem was not that he had too much to say, however. Most everyday objects could either be pointed at, or else their shape could be sketched out in gestures: no definitions were required. And you could indicate physical actions simply by carrying them out in pantomime. If you already understood a spoken language, then you would know the meanings of such verbs as HURRY, WONDER, SHELTER, LOOK or SEE, and you would not need to be told what actions they represented. On the whole then, it was superfluous to describe the gestures themselves. So some typical entries in the Abbé's diction-ary ran like this:

> HURRY: to make haste, come forward promptly; *natural sign*.
> WONDER: to look with astonishment; *natural sign*.
> SHELTER: to keep sheltered from rain and sunshine; *natural sign*.
> LOOK: to fix the eyes on something.
> SEE: *natural sign*; not to be confused with LOOK.

Even WINE and ACCIDENT were presented as *signes naturels*, and all de l'Épée said about VOWEL was: 'sign known to everyone'. Of course the Abbé was able to include the analysis of BELIEF on which he had always prided himself ('say yes with the spirit, yes with the heart, yes with the mouth; yet the eyes do not see'), and a few definitions which were neither grammatical nor analytical at all, such as 'BRUTALIZE: wine

---

3 See Copineau's note in Pierre Desloges, *Observations d'un sourd et muet*, pp. 19–20.

brutalizes those who drink too much too often.' But the dictionary was becoming little more than an alphabetical list of a few hundred French words, with occasional comments and elucidations. For example:

ABASEMENT: figuratively, taken as humiliation.
ABBEY: religious establishment: *give examples.*
ABBREVIATE: hold your thumb and index-finger apart, then bring them closer together.
ADOLESCENCE: the age between 14 and 25 years.
ANCHOR: iron instrument thrown to the bottom of the water to halt a vessel: *make a drawing.*
AFTER: what follows: 'after the rain we get fine weather.'[4]

The Abbé worked desultorily on the project for several years, and then in 1786, with some bitterness but, it seems, more relief, he gave it up. After all, his own pupils had always been perfectly good at writing what was dictated to them in signs, without ever being put to the trouble of 'leafing through dictionaries'. It was his personal responsibility as their teacher to ensure that their minds were stocked with 'the words they ought to choose as well as the ideas that they signify', and whenever this failed, he would always explain unfamiliar words or ideas as he went along. 'If anyone asked me whether I had also written a dictionary, I could answer that my deaf and dumb children have no need for a written or printed one, because I myself am their living dictionary in all my lessons.'[5]

Before long the Abbé de l'Épée knew that death was approaching: more and more ailments were adding themselves to his chronic gout, and he died at last on 23 December 1789, at the age of 77. His servants were grief-stricken, and so of course were his pupils, or his 'children', as he liked to call them. But when his will was read out, there was consternation too: he left all his worldly goods to the elder brother with whom he shared the house in the Rue des Moulins, and made no provision at all for the continuation of his school, or the financial needs of his pupils.[6]

4 De l'Épée's dictionary was eventually published as *Dictionnaire des sourds-muets,* edited by J.A.A. Rattel, Paris, J.-B. Baillière, 1896.
5 de l'Épée, *La Véritable Manière,* pp. 145–7.
6 See Bézagu-Deluy, *L'abbé de L'Épée,* p. 232.

Though the Abbé did not care for such matters, these were, as it happens, days of political turmoil too: the Bastille had fallen less than six months before, and an enlightened new political order was currently under construction. At the memorial service two months after his death, the congregation mourned the Abbé de l'Épée not only as a philanthropist, but as a hero of the revolution – a 'wise friend of Liberty', and an uncompromising defender of 'the rights of Man and of the Citizen'. The oration was given by Claude Fauchet – 'christian democrat', eloquent hero of the storming of the Bastille on 14 July, and, some said, the most handsome of all the revolutionaries. De l'Épée's methodical signs were the language of the angels, Fauchet proclaimed: 'their precision is incredible, and their rapidity seems supernatural.' While the rest of us were left to 'fumble with our words', the Abbé's pupils could present dozens of ideas simultaneously, 'taking wing with their signs'. De l'Épée was more than a priest: he was a citizen, who had raised his deaf fellow-citizens from their half-bestial condition, up into the same sphere as the celestial spirits; he was a benefactor of the nation, who had 'presented the State with a whole new class of useful Citizens'.[7]

The Commune of Paris expressed its grief within hours of the Abbé's death, and a few days later resolved that the needs of his pupils should be met from public funds. In the early months of 1790, it recommended that a national public institution be created in Paris to perpetuate the Abbé's work. The Constituent Assembly endorsed the plan, entrusting the task of choosing a 'head teacher' (*premier instituteur*) to a committee which included that old philosophical partisan of sign language, Condorcet. After a bitter competition, the post was awarded to the energetic and ambitious Roche-Ambroise Sicard, an Abbé who had already spent a year training with de l'Épée in 1785 before returning to run a school for the deaf in Bordeaux.[8]

Sicard was much closer to the philosophers' ideal of an educator of the deaf than de l'Épée had ever been. In fact he accused his late master of misunderstanding the entire nature of sign language, and drastically underestimating its power. De l'Épée had succeeded in exciting vulgar curiosity by teaching articulation and lip-reading, but

7 Claude, Abbé Fauchet, *Oraison Funèbre de Charles-Michel de l'Épée*, Paris, 1790, pp. 14, 32–4, 30.
8 See Ferdinand Berthier, *L'Abbé Sicard, Célèbre Instituteur des Sourds-Muets*, pp. 5–6.

these activities, according to Sicard, were perfectly meaningless from the point of view of the deaf themselves, and should have no place in their education. Sicard preferred not to treat his pupils as monsters, giving sign-language performances for the diversion of the public; instead he would address them directly as his brothers and sisters. With the spread of the sacred names of *Liberty* and *Equality*, he wrote, such unfortunates need suffer oppression no more; deaf citizens must lay claim to their human rights, confident that in the new age that is dawning they can no longer be ignored.[9]

In the same democratic spirit, Sicard brought his favourite deaf pupil with him from Bordeaux, and appointed him his assistant. Jean Massieu, who was just twenty, had already made legal history two years earlier by appearing before a judge in Bordeaux and using pen and paper to make accusations against a man who had tried to rob him, and he now became the first deaf person ever to be given a post as an educator of the deaf.[10] As a further symbol of his commitment to the dignity of the educated deaf, Sicard carried out a small but significant linguistic reform. Henceforth those he sought to serve should be referred to as *sourds-muets* rather than *sourds et muets* (*deaf-mutes* as opposed to *deaf and dumb*, in the translation which entered English some forty years later): this was in order to prevent the damaging imputation that, apart from their defective hearing, the deaf had something inherently wrong with their vocal and mental capacities as well.[11]

After a delay of more than a year, the Constituent Assembly voted that what it called 'the Institution of the Abbé de l'Épée' should henceforth be maintained at the State's expense, 'as a monument worthy of the French nation'.[12] So the Institution Nationale des Sourds-Muets finally opened in September 1791, sharing the old Célestins priory with a school for the blind, before moving, in 1794, to a large seventeenth-century building in the Rue St Jacques, a former Oratorian seminary which has remained the headquarters of deaf education in France ever since.

9 Roche-Ambroise Sicard, *Cours d'instruction d'un sourd-muet de naissance*, Paris, 1800, pp. xxv-xxvi.
10 Sicard, *Cours d'instruction*, pp. 573–4; on Massieu, see his own account of his early life in Berthier, *L'Abbé Sicard*, pp. 141–57.
11 See Berthier, *L'Abbé de l'Épée*, p. 357; Bézagu-Deluy, *L'abbé de L'Épée*, pp. 252–3.
12 See Bézagu-Deluy, *L'abbé de L'Épée*, pp. 252–3.

Unfortunately, the head teacher of the new Institution Nationale was destined for political trouble. In August 1792, Sicard was arrested and imprisoned for sheltering 'refractory priests'. His deaf-mute assistant Jean Massieu led a delegation of deaf pupils to plead for his release, and Sicard defended himself by arguing that since deaf-mutes were more numerous amongst the poor than the rich, his mission to them automatically made him a friend of the disinherited people. Sicard escaped the guillotine, but he was suspended from his post on the grounds that, as an aristocrat, he might corrupt 'the sublime method invented by the immortal de l'Épée'. He returned to his responsibilities in 1796, but the following year he was driven from his post again, this time for being implicated in the dissemination of illegal religious tracts.[13]

At the end of 1799, just five weeks after Napoleon's seizure of power, the fashionable dramatist Jean-Nicolas Bouilly presented a new play called *L'Abbé de l'Épée* at the Théâtre de la République. It told an idealized version of the case of the Comte de Solar, with the silent role of the Count taken by a young actress who had been painstakingly coached in sign language by Massieu himself. In the play, the poor and saintly Abbé befriends a deaf boy in the streets of Paris, and after conversing with him in signs 'at the speed of thought', he discovers that the child has been deprived of his wealth and title by a scheming guardian. The Abbé bravely denounces the conspiracy, and there is an affecting scene of clemency and reconciliation at the family château in the fifth act. At the second performance (attended by Josephine Bonaparte, according to some accounts), the play was interrupted just before the end. At the moment when the Abbé de l'Épée announces that he must leave the reinstated Count and hurry back to his needy pupils in Paris, a whole section of the audience rose, shouting that Sicard should be allowed to return to his needy pupils too; and following another campaign led by Massieu, Napoleon granted Sicard an amnesty at the beginning of 1800.[14] Bouilly himself was a guest at the ceremony marking Sicard's triumphant return after 28 months'

13 See Berthier, *L'Abbé Sicard*, pp. 8–42, and Harlan Lane, *When the Mind Hears*, pp. 24–9.
14 Berthier, *L'Abbé Sicard*, p. 44; Jean-Nicolas Bouilly, *L'Abbé de l'Épée, Comédie Historique en Cinq Actes* (1799), London, Dulau, 1877. English versions were produced throughout the nineteenth century, starting in 1801 in a translation by Thomas Holcroft, with Charles Kemble as de l'Épée; a German translation was made by Kotzebue.

enforced absence: Massieu kissing him passionately on the mouth as he mounted the tribune, the boys swarming over their master till he was completely hidden from view, and the girls at last shyly crowning him with a wreath of poppies and dried flowers, symbols of their grief in his absence, and of the immortality he had earned by his patience and good works.[15]

The Abbé Sicard used his periods of enforced leisure to perfect a method of deaf education that would conform with the latest developments in philosophical theory. He was an associate member of the Institut National des Sciences et Arts, which was created in 1795 to take responsibility for reforming all branches of learning. Specifically, Sicard was associated with the section concerned with 'analysis of sensations and ideas', which began its proceedings by instituting a competition for the best work on one of the great theoretical questions of the day: the 'influence of signs upon the formation of ideas'.[16]

The ensuing discussions ranged widely; but everyone who contributed seems to have accepted that all but the most rudimentary mental functions depended on language: it was only thanks to words, that is, that we could fix our attention on simple ideas, analyse complex ones, or form any comparative or abstract conceptions at all. There was Destutt de Tracy for example, who gave a sequence of lectures to the Institute between 1795 and 1797 arguing for a systematic science of ideas – a bold young science, for which he invented a brave new name: *Idéologie*. The general principle of Ideology was that all ideas could be traced to experience of the real world, and one of its main arguments was that it is impossible to think – that is to say, to manipulate, combine, and refine ideas – without recourse to linguistic signs, whether written or spoken. Sign language, however, or the 'language of action', was regarded by de Tracy as an extremely ineffectual means of thinking; hence, he thought, the pitiful intellectual limitations of those deaf-mutes who are obliged to rely upon it. In addition, spoken and written languages also served to 'transmit to the individual all the

---

15 J.-N. Bouilly, *Rentrée du Cn. Sicard à l'Institution Nationale des Sourds-Muets*, Paris, Dupont de Nemours, 1800, pp. 11–15.
16 *Mémoires de l'Institut National des Sciences et Arts. Sciences Morales et Politiques*, Vol. 1, Paris, 1798, pp. i-iii.

ideas accumulated by the human race', and de Tracy concluded that uneducated deaf-mutes were deprived not only of the means of thinking, but also of access to the human intellectual heritage.[17]

The Institute's prize for the best discussion of the relation between signs and ideas was awarded early in 1799 to a young man called Joseph-Marie de Gérando. Six years before, at the age of 21, he had been condemned to death for fighting on the royalist site at Lyon, but he escaped, and eventually joined the French army, while beginning to immerse himself in the study of philosophy, including the latest fashions from Germany. He was impressed by the new Kantian theory of experience, but not persuaded by it: all the problems of philosophy had already been solved in principle, he thought, when Locke rebutted the theory of 'innate ideas' and showed how there is nothing in the mind except what enters it from experience.[18]

In his prize-winning essay on *Signs and the Art of Thinking* – a vast work in four large volumes – de Gérando argued, like Destutt de Tracy, that it is language that turns us into intellectual and social beings. Learning a language not only enables us to think, but also introduces us to a vast store of human experience. To lack a language, in other words, is to be isolated from 'a system of signs created long, long ago, and perfected by the simultaneous contributions of thousands of individuals, and the successive labours of numerous generations'.[19]

But this was precisely the fate of the deaf: cut off from language, they found themselves intellectually imprisoned, 'confined to a very narrow circle of ideas'. Their inability to cross the boundary which separates 'the material and sensible world from the philosophical world' was yet another refutation, if any were needed, of the doctrine of innate ideas. Anyone who knew a language was automatically 'reaping the fruits of a labour to which society as a whole has contributed', whereas an uneducated deaf-mute, being cut off from language, was 'reduced to his own individual resources', much like our ancestors in the first ages of history. Compare two uneducated children, one with

17 Destutt de Tracy, 'Mémoire sur la faculté de penser', *Mémoires de l'Institut National*, Vol. 1, pp. 286, 324, 418, 406–9.
18 Joseph-Marie de Gérando, *Des Signes et de l'Art de Penser considérés dans leurs rapports mutuels*, 4 Vols, Paris, 1800, Vol. 1, p. xxxvii.
19 *Des Signes*, Vol. 4, pp. 454–5.

normal hearing and the other born deaf, de Gérando said: 'The two may be contemporaries, but their minds are separated from each other by many centuries.'[20]

On the other hand, de Gérando also admired the 'language of action', and praised the ingenuity that the deaf had shown in trying to raise it from its primitive natural state to a 'high degree of perfection'. Compared with the other two forms of language – speech and writing – it was, he conceded, uniquely favourable to the development of the visual imagination. Because of the 'material nature of the signs it uses' – visible gestures made by several parts of the body at the same time – it occupied the mind with a simultaneous profusion of vivid spatial ideas, as simple as they are natural. But, de Gérando went on, the efficiency and rapidity of sign language meant that it was 'far more favourable to the development of the imagination than to the progress of the meditative faculties'. It could never foster a capacity for steady deliberation, and it did not embody any of those artificial or 'arbitrary' ideas which are essential to the formation of intellectual judgement. It was not till the Abbé de l'Épée ('whose very name inspires recognition and respect') had shown how to teach the deaf to read and write, that they were released from the mental isolation imposed on them by sign language.[21]

But if the deaf were denied access to the riches of tradition by their exclusion from language, they were also, for the same reason, protected from time-hallowed prejudice and confusion. Louis-François-Joseph Alhoy, a pupil of de l'Épée who acted as head teacher at the Institution Nationale during the period when Sicard was banned, used the principles of the 'science of ideology' to argue that whilst hearing children receive their intellectual ideas ready made, as part of a language that they absorb without effort or reflection, deaf-mutes are forced to construct their own out of natural materials, by laborious processes of comparison and generalization. In an opening address to the Institution in 1799, just three days before Napoleon's seizure of power, Citizen Alhoy explained that those who are blessed with hearing are like 'children born to opulence' – incapable, that is, of appreciating the unearned riches that are showered negligently upon them. The

20 *Des Signes*, Vol. 1, p. xxiv; Vol. 4, pp. 459, 455.
21 *Des Signes*, Vol. 1, pp. 128–9; Vol. 2, pp. 325–44; Vol. 4, pp. 467–8.

deaf, on the other hand, provided they were guided by an instructor with a gift for philosophical analysis, would acquire language without the risks of luxury: 'their progress may be slower,' he wrote, 'but it is also more certain: for the deaf-mute never takes a step without first testing the firmness of the ground.'[22]

Sicard went along with the basic claims of Ideology, as far as his belief in the revealed truths of Christianity allowed. His fundamental principle, constantly reiterated, was that 'speech is an art'. It was neither natural nor mysterious: it was just an artificial collection of human techniques for organizing thought, a set of tools which each generation inherits from its predecessor, and passes on, hopefully a little improved, to the next. Originally, speech must have comprised only a few instinctive sounds, barely sufficient to give expression to our simplest feelings. Then it had developed into a 'nomenclature', a collection of names for simple objects and perhaps a few basic actions as well. Finally it had been transformed with the invention of 'the art of combining these sounds, and multiplying them'. Speakers acquired the habit of linking words together, that is to say, and connecting them into syntactically organized sequences. These linguistic constructs – sentences or propositions – allowed us to anatomize our thoughts into their constituent ideas, and fit them together again to create new ways of thinking. Without the aid of verbal propositions, Sicard argued, our intellectual capacities would never have exceeded those of animals.[23]

The progress of both the individual and the race depended therefore on the cultivation of the art of speech. In Europe it had reached several historic peaks of perfection – the Greek of ancient Athens, the Latin of ancient Rome, and the French of the age of Louis XIV. There were some unfortunate nations who had never mastered it properly – the Chinese, for example, whose language consisted of words rather than propositions, and who could 'scarcely combine their ideas at all'.[24] But of course the most calamitous case of linguistic inanition was that of

22 Louis-François-Joseph Alhoy, *De l'éducation des sourds-muets de naissance, considérée dans ses rapports avec l'Idéologie et la Grammaire, prononcée à la rentrée de l'École Nationale des Sourds-Muets,* 15 Brumaire A, VIII, Paris, 1799, pp. 13, 18–21, 24, 28.
23 Roche-Ambroise Sicard, *Élémens de grammaire générale* (1799), second edition, Paris, Imprimerie des Sourds-Muets, 1801, vol. 1, pp. xv-xix, vi-viii, 12.
24 Sicard, *Élémens de grammaire générale,* p. xv.

the deaf-mutes. Even in Europe, the deaf lacked any settled conventional signs with which to fix and retain ideas in their minds, or reflect and make comparisons, or accomplish even the most elementary tasks of reasoning. Without language, they could make no sense of morality itself, as they had no way of entering into the feelings of others: they lived lives of the most terrible solitude, surrounded by unimaginable depths of silence.[25]

But the only reason for the idiocy of the deaf, Sicard argued, was that they lacked an adequate set of signs for organizing their thoughts. They would be as intelligent as anyone else, if only they could be provided with a language adapted to their special needs; and, contrary to the opinion of philosophers like Destutt de Tracy, there was no reason why a 'language of action' should not be devised which would be the intellectual peer of any spoken one. If the deaf themselves had never developed gestural language beyond a few rudimentary natural signs, it was only because they had always lived in isolation, and therefore 'never had the chance to perfect the language of action through habitual communication'.[26] Sicard even permitted himself to imagine – rather as Leibniz had at the beginning of the century – 'an entire nation of deaf-mutes in some corner of the world'. They would undoubtedly develop a rich and sophisticated system of signs, he thought, a language both clear and sincere, and then there was no limit to the heights of civilization that such a people might attain.[27]

In fact even the most isolated and uneducated of deaf-mutes already possessed a rudimentary innate language of grimaces and gestures, according to Sicard: 'their eyes can blaze with indignation, their brow furrow in sadness, or a smile play on their lips.' And what eloquence they displayed in their natural language! 'Who could fail to recognize their signs of love, hate, hope and desire, fear and terror?' But the basic language of signs was desperately impoverished, however vivid it might be: it contained very few 'words', and possessed none of the syntactic structure necessary for the development of analytical thinking. The minds of the deaf remained virgin territory, a vast emptiness in

25 Sicard, *Cours d'instruction*, pp. viii-xii.
26 Sicard, *Théorie des signes*, Vol. 1, p. 2.
27 '*Tout un peuple de sourds-muets*', see Sicard, *Cours d'instruction*, p. xxiii. On Leibniz, see above, pp. 116–7.

which 'everything has yet to be created, or at least remade'. Deaf-mutes were like brutes who must be softened, savages to be humanized; they were automatons, and it was the mission of their teachers to give them 'a new being', and even to endow them with 'a soul'.[28]

Sicard held that the only practical way of reclaiming the deaf for society was by constructing an artificial sign language for them, or rather helping them to do so for themselves. He acknowledged that de l'Épée had embarked on the task back in the 1760s; but by some astonishing oversight the good Abbé had failed to make any record of either the signs or the syntax of his language. 'Was it reasonable, was it wise, to entrust it to a kind of oral tradition?' Sicard asked.

He knew it was not for want of trying: in the 1780s de l'Épée had discussed his projected dictionary with Sicard, eventually handing over all his papers and entreating him to complete the task.[29] But Sicard considered de l'Épée's conception of the dictionary so fundamentally mistaken that a completely new start was required. Sicard's dictionary, unlike de l'Épée's, would specify the precise sequence of gestures which constituted each sign, so that readers could learn to make them for themselves. And it would be thorough – covering 3,000 separate manual signs corresponding to 3,000 elementary French words. Definitions would be given for all of them, and verified by a congenital deaf-mute, Sicard's indispensable assistant Jean Massieu.[30]

Sicard also considered that most of the signs used by de l'Épée were so faulty, idiomatic, and illogical that they were not worthy of being recorded in a dictionary anyway. The philosophers who praised de l'Épée for constructing signs based on clear analyses of ideas had been more kind than rigorous, according to Sicard. For instance, de l'Épée had simply made a gesture towards his coat as the sign for *black*, or touched his lower lip as the sign for *red*. He had also been so bewitched by his own native language that he assumed that sign language needed to supply a distinct equivalent for every separate word of French – even when the words were synonyms, or embodied unfounded analogies or

---

28 Sicard, *Théorie des signes*, pp. 9–10, 1–2; *Élémens de grammaire générale*, p. xxiii; *Cours d'instruction*, pp. xiv, lvi.
29 Sicard, *Théorie des signes*, pp. xxxix-xv.
30 Sicard, *Cours d'instruction*, p. 437; *Théorie des signes*, Vol. 1, pp. xl, 2–4.

pointless distinctions. Furthermore, he had often allowed himself to be misled by superficial verbal forms and false etymologies: for example, he arrived at his gestural translation for *intelligence* by dividing it into the Latin *intus* ('inside', *signe naturel*) and *legere* ('to read', also *signe naturel*). This analysis, as Sicard observed, is not only historically false (the correct derivation would have traced the word back to *inter* and *legere*, meaning *to choose between*, not *to read inside*) but also a thoroughly baffling and misleading explanation of the idea attached to the word *intelligence* in modern languages. Even those celebrated exercises where de l'Épée's scholars transcribed his signed dictations had been absurd: the unfortunate children were matching words to signs, and signs to words, without having to consider or even conceive the corresponding ideas.

> He [de l'Épée] imagined that he had given them the meaning of words, when he had only given them the signs. He did not see that nothing was easier than to make them write words for signs; and that as they knew as little of the latter as of the former, he did but lead them from the *unknown* to the *unknown*.[31]

The Abbé de l'Épée had drilled his scholars to take dictations, but never encouraged them to compose discourses of their own, either in French or in signs. In the ardour of his benevolence, the inventor of methodical signs 'never even suspected that he was not being understood'.[32]

De l'Épée's great theoretical failing, according to Sicard, was that he did not appreciate the vast historical gulf between the natural language of signs – which encompassed very few ideas, had no tradition, and lacked syntax – and spoken languages like French, which had been 'perfected through the experience of many centuries'. Because he ignored the first obligation on hearing teachers of the deaf – to 'mistrust their own facility in speaking and understanding' and endeavour to think in the gestural language of their pupils – de l'Épée had never been able to grasp the magnitude of his task.[33]

31 Sicard, *Cours d'instruction*, pp. xxxvii-xxxviii; *Théorie des signes*, Vol. 1, p. xxxvi; J. H. Sievrac, ed., *Recueil des Définitions et Réponses les plus remarquables de Massieu et Clerc, Sourds-Muets, à Londres*, London, Cox and Baylis, 1815, p. xiii.
32 Sicard, *Cours d'instruction*, pp. xli-xliii.
33 Sicard, *Théorie des signes*, Vol. 1, pp. 15–16; *Cours d'instruction*, p. xix.

The correct method, Sicard went on, was to set aside all one's knowledge of spoken languages, and then try to identify the small stock of genuinely simple ideas, expressed by natural signs, which are available to the uneducated deaf. 'The best way to find the most appropriate signs for indicating different objects is to show each object, demonstrate how it is used or worked with, or in the case of food, how it is prepared and how eaten.' The most suitable sign for BREAD for instance would be discovered by pretending to mix flour with water, putting it in the oven, then taking it out again, and cutting and eating it. The deaf pupils should then be allowed to take up the gestural description in their own way, abbreviating and stylizing it to their taste and convenience, 'and in this way the sign of the object becomes fixed, communicated first by the pupil, and adopted by the master.'[34]

The teacher would then construct artificial signs from these simple roots, in such a way that their meaning and structural complexity would be obvious from their form. (Sicard's model of a well-made language was the chemical nomenclature introduced by Lavoisier in 1787, where terms like *sulphuric acid* or *carbonic acid* gave a direct representation of the real constitution of the compounds they referred to.)[35] In Sicard's monumental dictionary, then – eventually published in 1808 – the specification of each sign would automatically bring with it a genuine analytical knowledge of its meaning. For instance:

> AFFIRMATION: (1) represent two persons, one reporting an extraordinary event to the other; (2) the action of the latter who refuses to believe it; (3) the action of the former who, with head and gestures, affirms it; (4) noun sign.
> EFFECT: (1) suppose some active cause, such as fire; (2) represent fire burning wood; (3) display the ashes.
> BLACK: (1) sign for an opaque and porous body which absorbs light; (2) sign for darkness; (3) adjective sign.
> RED: (1) sign for blood; (2) sign for only looking; (3) adjective sign.[36]

---

34 Sicard, *Théorie des signes*, Vol. 1, pp. 27–9.
35 See Antoine Lavoisier, *Méthode de nomenclature chimique*, Paris, 1787, p. 12.
36 Sicard, *Théorie des signes*, Vol. 2, pp. 22, 141; Vol. 1, pp. 367–8.

Geographical and cosmological terms were based on sketching maps in the air:

> IRISHMAN: (1) indicate the map of Europe; (2) point to England, then Ireland to the west of it; (3) add the sign for male inhabitant.
> YEAR: (1) indicate the sun, with your left hand held still; (2) indicate the earth making a full circle round it.
> DAY: (1) indicate the sun, with your left hand held still; (2) turn your right hand on itself in front of the left.[37]

Sicard admitted that it cost his pupils much study to learn sign language on these principles, especially compared to the carefree way in which hearing children learn their mother tongue. But hard work is never a misfortune, and in this case it meant that the deaf acquired their intelligence by analysis, not routine. In contrast with those who could hear, they would never be tempted to use expressions they did not understand. They were like simple working folk, who knew the value of their possessions, because they had slowly acquired each one of them by their own honest toil, unlike the idle rich who derived neither profit nor happiness from their wasteful luxury. The language Sicard taught at the National Institution, in short, was so simple and pure that his pupils were happier, kinder, and more intelligent than they would have been if they were so unfortunate as to be able to hear.[38]

In the fifteen years following the amnesty granted him by Napoleon, Sicard built up the school in the Rue St Jacques – the Institution Impériale des Sourds-Muets, as it was now called – until it had about a hundred residential pupils. They attended his three weekly lessons in sign language (Tuesdays, Thursdays and Saturdays at noon) and spent the rest of the time learning a trade under one of ten masters in the Institution's workshops – cutting precious stones, engraving copperplate, drawing, wood-turning, mosaic-making, shoe-making, cabinet-making, gardening, and (largest by far) printing. These classes laid the basis for some astonishingly successful careers, creating in particular a remarkable tradition of deaf painters and sculptors in

---

37 *Théorie des signes*, Vol. 1, pp. 275, 291.
38 Sicard, *Cours d'instruction*, pp. xiv, xx-xxii.

France;[39] and all Sicard's own books were printed, exceptionally beautifully, on the presses of the Sourds-Muets.

In 1805, the Pope himself visited the Institution. (See Figure 11.)
He picked an a paragraph from a book at random, and got Massieu
to dictate it in signs to a young man called Laurent Clerc, now in his
eighth year as a pupil at the Institution, and so fluent in sign language
that he was already beginning to outstrip his teachers. The Pope was
very satisfied with the version that Clerc returned to him in written
French, and stayed for more than two hours before blessing them all
and taking his leave.[40]

Sicard also revived de l'Épée's old practice of getting his pupils to
perform regular public exercises. There were to be no vulgar displays
of mechanical skills like speech or lip-reading, however, nor signed
dictations taken down by groups of pupils in several languages. The
purpose of the performances was simply to demonstrate the intellectual
virtues of sign language by exhibiting the personal culture of the
Institution's individual pupils, especially their deftness with artificial
and abstract ideas. (See Figure 12.) The audience would test them by
asking questions, to which they would reply by writing on a board.

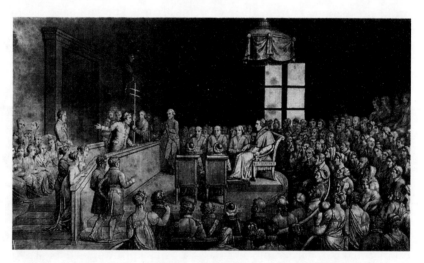

FIG 11. Sign language demonstrated to Pope Pius VII at the Institution
Nationale, 1805

39 Nicholas Mirzoeff has identified more than 100 deaf artists emerging from the
Institution during the nineteenth century: see his *Silent Poetry*, p. 3.
40 Berthier, *L'Abbé Sicard*, pp. 71–2.

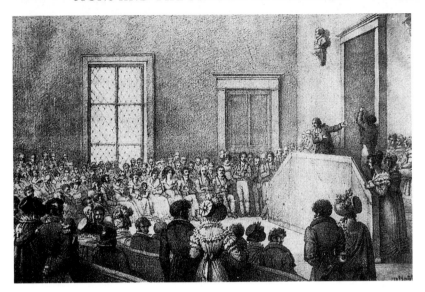

FIG 12. A public exercise at the Institution Nationale, *c.* 1810, with Sicard
addressing the audience and Massieu at the board, chalk in hand

'What is hearing?' 'Auricular vision' was Massieu's well-received
reply. And gratitude? 'The remembrance of the heart.' Sense? 'An idea-
carrier (*une porte-idée*).' Hope? 'It is the flower of happiness,' he replied
in a flash. And eternity? 'A day without either a yesterday or a
tomorrow.'[41]

Massieu – 'the amazing Massieu', as one regular visitor put it, 'the
coryphée of the deaf-mutes' – composed a touching autobiographical
sketch, extracts of which were read out at the Institutional exercises.[42] In
it, he evoked his childhood as one of six deaf children of poor peasants
in the Gironde, and his desperate attempts to get himself an education:
how after repeated refusals from his stubborn father he ran away to
implore help from the village schoolmaster, only to be 'harshly refused
and driven away again'. At the age of 13, he still had no language except
the signs he had improvised with his brothers and sisters; but then a
gentleman passing through the village took pity on the tearful boy, and
eventually placed him with Sicard, who had just opened his school in
nearby Bordeaux. It was thanks to Sicard, of course, that his yearning

41 Sicard, *Théorie des signes*, Vol. 2, pp. 646–7.
42 See U.R.T. le Bouvier Desmortiers, *Mémoire ou Considérations sur les sourds-muets de
naissance*, Paris 1800, pp. 252–4.

for education, not to mention love, was gratified at last.[43] For as Massieu's personal history showed, Sicard's deaf-mutes could think for themselves, and understand and analyse their ideas. Where de l'Épée had produced deaf-and-dumb speakers and scriveners, Sicard had formed self-conscious citizens, all with their own story to tell.

43 The public reading of Massieu's autobiographical sketch is mentioned by le Bouvier Desmortiers (p. 252) and a version is printed in an appendix to Sicard's *Théorie des Signes*, Vol. 2, pp. 623–49, from which these passages are taken. See also Berthier, *L'Abbé Sicard*, pp. 146–56, and Lane, *When the Mind Hears*, p. 418.

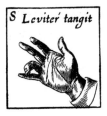

S *Leviter tangit*

18

The deaf nation
and its language

In the summer of 1815 the Abbé Sicard paid a visit to London, accompanied by his two most accomplished pupils: the faithful Jean Massieu and the brilliant Laurent Clerc. Clerc was now employed as an assistant teacher at the Institution, and unlike Massieu he was worldly, fashionable, and elegant, far surpassing him both in the verve of his sign language and in his popularity with pupils.[1] During the trip to London, Clerc made a strong impression on his English hosts, with whom he exchanged written notes in French, though he was beginning to learn English as well. 'You seem frank,' said one young lady, at a reception in a private house off Cavendish Square, after he had made a remark about English ladies being prettier than French, but not so well dressed; and she treasured his suave and ironic riposte: 'It is the privilege of the man of nature.'[2]

There was a series of public presentations in London throughout June and July, at which Sicard gave an opening lecture, and then Massieu and Clerc stood at a blackboard, responding in writing to

1 See Harlan Lane, *The Wild Boy of Aveyron* (1976), London, Granada, 1978, p. 211. An imaginative first-person account of Clerc's career is to be found in Lane's *When the Mind Hears.*
2 J. H. Sievrac, *Recueil des Définitions et Réponses les plus remarquables de Massieu et Clerc*, pp. 11–13.

questions and requests from the audience. On one occasion the Duke of Kent handed a French book to Massieu, who rendered a passage in signs, which Clerc then translated back into written French. But most of the time, they simply had to satisfy the public's curiosity as to whether they could really understand abstract or artificial terms, words whose meanings were linguistic rather than sensory. 'What is an admiral?' for example, or 'What is the difference between love and friendship? . . . between simplicity and ingenuousness? . . . mind and matter? . . . mind and intellect . . . authority and power?' They were constantly asked their opinion of Napoleon, too: a brilliant soldier but a terrible statesman, was their considered opinion, and they gracefully thanked the British for defeating him at the battle of Waterloo, which had taken place in the middle of June. Altogether, Massieu and Clerc convinced fashionable London that, despite being deaf and unable to speak, they had 'a perfect acquaintance with abstract and purely intellectual ideas'.[3]

But the visit to London was not such an unqualified pleasure for Sicard as for his deaf-mute assistants. He had perhaps been unaware that London already had an institution rivalling his own in Paris – the Asylum for the Deaf and Dumb, the first charitable school for the deaf in England, founded in Bermondsey in 1792 with half a dozen pupils and now taking nearly two hundred at its premises in the Old Kent Road. It was run by Thomas Watson, a nephew of Thomas Braidwood, and it followed the same educational principles as Braidwood's academies in Edinburgh and Hackney: manual signs were used in the first stages, but then actively discouraged as the emphasis shifted to written language and then lip-reading and speech.

Sicard imagined that the old dispute between the 'French' and 'German' systems – between de l'Épée's use of signs and Heinicke's 'oral' method – had been satisfactorily settled thirty years before, with victory going to sign language and to France. But when he visited the Asylum in the Old Kent Road, accompanied by an old patron of his, Laffon de Ladébat, he had to admit that the oral education it offered was 'excellent', and that the pupils could speak effectively, with voices 'not disagreeable'. And when Dr Watson defended his method by pointing out that 'artificial speech', as he called it, was 'peculiarly useful for the

3 Sievrac, *Recueil des Définitions et Réponses*, pp. 120, 5, 7, 15, 145, Advertisement.

deaf and dumb among the poor, because children of this description are placed out in manufactories, and they are thus enabled to communicate more easily with their masters,' Sicard had to concede that, at least from the point of view of 'convenience and charity', Dr Watson had a point.[4]

There was another blemish on Sicard's success in London. At their public performances, both Massieu and Clerc were asked to clarify the distinction between natural and artificial languages. Massieu explained how the greater part of written and spoken language was not natural but 'conventional', having been 'invented by the union of several persons, which is called *society*'. Clerc agreed, arguing that ordinary languages, whether written or spoken, were of their nature 'imitated, borrowed, and conventional'. In these answers, of course, the pupils were supporting the notions of their master. They were also in agreement with him when they praised the clarity and universality of the spontaneous natural cries and gestures used by those with no knowledge of conventional languages. But when they went on to argue that their own sign language was itself 'as simple as nature', and that spoken and written languages should be regarded as so many artificial translations of its universal natural gestural code, they were beginning to show more intellectual independence than Sicard can have liked.[5]

Sicard had never doubted that a complex gestural language such as the one he taught in the Institution must be just as conventional as ordinary speech and writing. Furthermore, he thought that the signs used by Massieu and Clerc were essentially his own personal inventions, though he paid tribute to Massieu and other pupils for helping him perfect them. To Sicard, like de l'Épée before him, signs were little more than an educational method, a classroom technique for explaining the meanings of written words to deaf children. Sign language might have its roots in pantomimic actions and instinctive gestures, but, as Sicard conceived it, it was broadly comparable to modern Latin: a scholastic or academic language, known only to those who had learned it from a teacher in a school; in fact it was even more academic than Latin, since it had never enjoyed the unruly autonomy of a popular living language, and had no literature and no past.

4 *Recueil des Définitions et Réponses*, p. 169.
5 *Recueil des Définitions et Réponses*, pp. 137–9.

Laurent Clerc, however, had always been noted for the vigour and originality of his signs: he regarded them as his first language, his mother tongue. And when he paid a visit to the pupils at the London Asylum, accompanied by Laffon de Ladébat, his experience confirmed him in his unorthodoxy. This is how de Ladébat recalled the occasion, in a letter to Sicard:

> It was at the moment when one hundred and fifty pupils, assembled in the eating-room, were all sitting at table. As soon as Clerc beheld this sight, his face became animated; he was as agitated as a traveller of sensibility would be, on meeting all on a sudden, in distant regions, a colony of his countrymen . . . On their side, the one hundred and fifty deaf and dumb fixed all their looks on your pupil, and recognized him as one of themselves. He made signs and they answered him by signs. This unexpected communication caused a most delicious sensation in them [*une jouissance délicieuse*].[6]

Here was a phenomenon that Sicard could never account for. The London deaf were officially discouraged from making any signs at all, and Clerc was using a system of gestures which was supposed to be a recent invention of his master in Paris, and yet they were conducting an animated conversation with each other, as if they were natives of the same country. Even if their sign system was artificial and academic in origin, it had now escaped from the classroom and was spreading amongst the deaf beyond the control and even the knowledge of those who could hear. The pupils at the new schools for the deaf seemed to know far more than they had ever been taught.

During the visit to London, Laurent Clerc also attracted the attention of a pious young American called Thomas Gallaudet, who – moved by the predicament of a deaf girl back in New England – had come to Europe in 1815 to investigate methods for instructing the deaf. Gallaudet began by approaching Braidwood's heirs and successors in Edinburgh and Hackney and the Old Kent Road, but they all refused to divulge their special techniques. Then he attended Sicard's exercises in London with Massieu and Clerc, and the intellectual results of the

6 *Recueil des Définitions et Réponses*, pp. 171–3.

French sign-language method made a deep impression on him. So did Sicard's generosity, when he offered him free training if he followed them back to France.

Once in Paris, however, Gallaudet chose to associate not with Sicard but with Laurent Clerc. Clerc, who was now thirty years old, had acquired a taste for travel and adventure, and readily accepted the proposition Gallaudet put to him: that he should separate himself from his master, renounce the sophisticated pleasures of Paris, and cross the Atlantic with Gallaudet to start a sign-language institution for the deaf in the wilds of North America.[7]

The Connecticut Asylum for the Education and Instruction of the Deaf and Dumb opened in Hartford in 1817, as a residential school for boys and girls, modelled on Sicard's Institution in the Rue St Jacques. The medium of instruction would be the sign language brought over from France by Laurent Clerc, supplemented by manual spelling. The pupils would be taught written English too, but not articulation and lip-reading: Gallaudet and Clerc stated that they were not willing to 'waste their labour and that of their pupils upon that comparatively useless branch of education'. Following a grant of land from Congress, the school changed its name in 1819 to become the American Asylum, and Clerc, having married one of its first students, presided expertly over the school for a further forty years, seeing its enrolment rise from 20 pupils to over 200, mostly aged between twelve and eighteen. He also had the satisfaction of training teachers who went on to staff more than twenty other 'manual' schools for the deaf.[8] By the time he died in 1869, aged 83, the gestural language he had imported from Paris was being propagated amongst 2,000 deaf pupils throughout North America.[9]

But Parisian sign language was altering as it spread. At the American Asylum it was regarded as the pupils' first language, and just like hearing children, they were expected to learn their first language for themselves, without much formal instruction. Even hearing children were observed to acquire signs as a first language if they were exposed

7 See Harlan Lane, *When the Mind Hears*, pp. 155–205, which includes transcripts of Thomas Gallaudet's letters about his visit to Europe.
8 See Gardiner Hubbard, *The Story of the Rise of the Oral Method in America, as told in the writings of the late Hon. Gardiner G. Hubbard*, Washington D.C., 1898, pp. 17–18.
9 See Harlan Lane, *The Wild Boy of Aveyron*, pp. 211–18.

to them in infancy: Thomas Gallaudet, like Clerc, had married a deaf woman, one of the first pupils at the Hartford School, and it was noted that their son Edward was fluent in sign language well before he learned to speak.[10]

The Abbé Sicard had once mused about how sign language might have developed in an 'entire nation of deaf-mutes', where it would be spared any competition from speech.[11] ('Oh happy nation!' as one of his philosophical supporters exclaimed: 'how sweet it would be to lose hearing and speech and be enfolded in its embrace!')[12] In America, this hypothetical Utopia soon became a real aspiration, and in 1831 a group of thirteen graduates from the American Asylum came together to try and purchase some land 'out west' where they might form themselves into 'a nucleus around and within which others of our class might, in process of time, gather'.[13] It came to nothing, but twenty-five years later a plan for a complete commonwealth of the deaf was being canvassed by a deaf property owner in Georgia called John James Flournoy. The deaf commonwealth would have 'political indepen-dence' and 'state sovereignty', Flournoy suggested, and would thus be able to provide for 'our peculiar necessities', without detraction from uncomprehending users of speech. 'We are not beasts, for all our deafness. We are MEN! The era of de l'Épée has been the epoch of our birth of mind.' For Flournoy, in other words, the deaf needed to assert not only their individual rights as human beings, but also their collective rights as a nation. Flournoy was dismissed by many leading American deaf-mutes as having an 'unbalanced mind', and his cam-paign for a deaf homeland came to nothing; but it gave notice that,

---

10 'My mother was a mute,' Edward Miner Gallaudet wrote, 'who never heard and who never spoke . . . I communicated freely [with her] by signs from the earliest days of my infancy; and I learnt to communicate [with her] before I learnt the use of my voice.' See Edward Miner Gallaudet and Alexander Graham Bell, *Education of Deaf Children: Evidence Presented to the Royal Commission of the United Kingdom (1886–8)*, edited by Joseph C. Gordon, Volta Bureau, Washington, 1892, p. 10.
11 Roche-Ambroise Sicard, *Cours d'instruction d'un sourd-muet de naissance*, p. xxiii.
12 U. R. T. le Bouvier Desmortiers, *Mémoire ou Considérations sur les Sourds-Muets de Naissance*, p. xxiv.
13 Edmund Booth, 'Mr Flournoy's Project', *American Annals of the Deaf and Dumb*, 10, 1858, pp. 72–3; cited in Carol Padden and Tom Humphries, *Deaf in America: Voices from a Culture*, Cambridge, Harvard University Press, 1989, pp. 112–13. See also Lane, *When the Mind Hears*, pp. 274–5, which mentions a similar proposal made in France by C. J. Richardin in 1834.

in an age of burgeoning nationalist aspirations, the deaf could also regard themselves as a specific 'variety of the Human Race', united not only by shared physical characteristics but also by a distinctive common language – in their case, the language of signs.[14]

But as well as provoking utopian dreams, the propagation of Parisian sign language in North America revealed some unexpected realities. In 1818, a year after the American Asylum opened, Laurent Clerc noticed that it was drawing a large proportion of its pupils from Martha's Vineyard, a small island about a hundred miles to the east, where as much as a quarter of the population were born deaf. There had never been any special school there, but when children from Martha's Vineyard arrived at the Asylum in Hartford, they turned out to be already fluent in a sign language of their own. Moreover, Clerc found that their gestures – like those he had discovered in the eating-room at the London Asylum three years before – had enough overlap with his own to enable him to converse with them immediately.

The population of Martha's Vineyard referred to their sign language as 'Deaf and Dumb', and they learned it automatically in infancy even if they were not deaf. All the inhabitants of the island could therefore converse in signs, though of course the hearing majority spoke English too. 'The community has adjusted itself to the situation so perfectly,' as one nineteenth-century observer put it, that its hearing members were as ready with signs as with words, and would 'pass from one to the other, or use both at once, almost unconsciously'; and as a result, the deaf-mutes of Martha's Vineyard were 'not uncomfortable in their deprivation'.[15] The nature of gestural communication might remain a mystery, and the philosophers could still debate whether it was essentially natural or not; but no one could ever again suppose that sign language was merely an educational device: indeed it was beginning

14 John James Flournoy, 'Mr Flournoy to Mr Turner' and 'Reply to Objections', *American Annals of the Deaf and Dumb*, 8, 1856, p. 142; and 10, 1858, pp. 149–50. See Padden and Humphries, *Deaf in America*, pp. 31, 112–13.
15 *Boston Sunday Herald*, 20 January 1895. The passage is quoted in Nora Ellen Groce, *Everyone Here Spoke Sign Language: Hereditary Deafness on Martha's Vineyard*, Cambridge, Harvard University Press, 1985, p. 53. All the rest of the information in this paragraph is also due to this excellent study: see pp. 73, 14, 23–35, 54. The sign language tradition on the island began to decay after the death of the last deaf inhabitant in 1952: see Oliver Sacks, *Seeing Voices: A Journey into the World of the Deaf*, Berkeley, University of California Press, 1989, pp. 35–6.

to look more and more like an ordinary language whose medium happened to consist of visible gestures rather than audible sounds.

When he left Paris in 1816 to sample life in a new country, Laurent Clerc could not have imagined how fruitful his work in North America would prove. On the other hand, he must have realized that his prospects would not be very bright if he stayed on at the school in the Rue St Jacques. The 'Royal Institution', as it was now called, was obviously in decline. Sicard was becoming senile and incompetent, but he refused to retire, choosing instead to preside over darkening chaos until his death in 1822, at the age of 80. His habits of praising his own sagacity and coveting academic titles were now openly ridiculed.[16] Even his sweet philosophical mascot Jean Massieu was becoming a figure of fun, the derisive young pupils finding his sign language quaint and his behaviour absurd. (One of them was to remember Massieu as a doddery eccentric who 'had a childish passion for collecting watches, seals and gold keys, and liked to walk around with as many as four different timepieces about his person'.)[17]

But Clerc's departure for America left the Paris Institution with at least one teacher who was highly competent in sign language, and who commanded the respect of most of the pupils. Roche-Ambroise Bébian was a native of Guadeloupe who had come to Paris in the early years of the century to acquire an education. He was a godson to the Abbé Sicard, and though not deaf he had stayed with him in the Rue St Jacques, soon acquiring fluency in sign language. ('It takes scarcely more than a few days to learn gestures,' he claimed.)[18] Like Clerc, Bébian despised the slow, old-fashioned, stiffly regimented signs used by Sicard and Massieu, and when Clerc left for America, he took over his job at the Institution.

Bébian now began to advocate the virtues of sign language with the feverish enthusiasm of a convert. The natural gestures of the deaf were honest, brave, simple, pure and strong, and de l'Épée and Sicard had

16 See Gabriel Michaud, ed., *Biographie Universelle*, 1843, s.v. Sicard.
17 Berthier, *L'Abbé Sicard*, pp. 119, 161.
18 Roche-Ambroise Bébian, *Essai sur les sourds-muets et sur le langage naturel, ou introduction à une classification naturelle des idées avec leurs signes propres*, Paris, Dentu, 1817, pp. 76–7. Parts of this essay are translated in Harlan Lane, ed., *The Deaf Experience*, but without the passages where Bébian expresses his belief in signs as the perfect and universal language of nature.

been profoundly wrong to try and alter and extend them and force them to conform to the artificial grammatical principles and arbitrary muddled vocabularies of Latin and French. 'Nowadays we admire the expressive gestures of the deaf-mute,' he wrote, 'in the same way that a fine Chinese lady, tottering on her tiny delicate feet, admires the peasant woman who can walk upright and straight.'[19] Reviving some old philosophical speculations on gesture and the origins of language, Bébian went back to Rousseau's paradox ('speech is not natural to man, but man cannot have invented it, because speech itself would be necessary for the invention of speech,' as he summarized it) and claimed that it could be resolved by reference to the language of signs.[20] Gestures were 'the natural language common to all mankind', a universal means of communication, 'a language which preceded all others in the first age of human society, just as it precedes all others in the first age of man'. It was the natural language not only of human infants but of wild animals as well:

> This is the language of the child before it can lisp a single word, smiling at the sight of its mother, and already holding out its little caressing arms to declare its love . . . Behold this terrified woman, as she sinks to her knees before a ferocious lion, stretching out her hands in supplication. She begs it to release the little child gripped between its jaws. The animal pauses, and gently lays the object of her tenderness and alarm beside the trembling mother.

And natural gestural language, being free of all the figurativeness and circumlocution of conventional speech, was not only a vivid way of expressing emotions; it was also the perfect means of communicating intellectual ideas.[21] More Rousseauist than Rousseau himself, Bébian argued that natural gestures constituted 'a language for all places and all times, everywhere uniform because it expresses our unchanging organic constitution; a language which preceded all spoken languages, and which presided over their formation'. Gesture was 'the language of those who have no language'. It was 'the language of deaf-mutes;

19 Roche-Ambroise Bébian, *Mimographie ou Essai d'écriture mimique propre à régulariser le langage des sourds-muets*, Paris, Colas, 1825, p. 2.
20 On Rousseau, see above, p. 136.
21 Bébian, *Essai sur les sourds-muets et sur le langage naturel*, pp. 80, 77, 97–8.

or rather, the true language [*le langage propre*] of the human race'. Thanks to the language of signs, according to Bébian, 'man is never a stranger to man'.[22] Questions that had always led to interminable wrangling in spoken language would be settled at once if translated into the language of signs – 'the language that cannot deceive, since it is the voice of nature itself.'[23]

Bébian's enthusiasm for the essential purity of sign language brought him into direct conflict with his godfather, the Abbé Sicard, as well as his own colleagues in the Paris Institution. In Bébian's opinion they were all guilty of 'corrupting' the natural language of man, under the guise of improving, enriching and regularizing it. They were adulterating it with 'the forms and vices of our languages', and it was now in imminent danger of losing 'the inestimable advantage of transmitting thought directly'. By 1821, Bébian's relations with Sicard's administration had become so hostile that he had to leave the Institution altogether, spending the remainder of his life drifting between various schemes for promoting interests of the deaf and their glorious language. None of them prospered, however, and he returned to Guadeloupe to die there in 1839, aged fifty.[24]

But Bébian had made a lasting impression on some of his pupils during his brief and unsuccessful career at the Institution – especially Ferdinand Berthier, who became his assistant, and stayed on as a senior teacher for a further forty years. Berthier was himself deaf, and a skilful writer and campaigner in the cause of *le peuple sourd-muet*.[25] He not only created such institutions as the Société Centrale des Sourds-Muets de Paris (the first ever autonomous organization for the deaf, founded in 1838), but also supplied them with a kind of national myth, based on pride in sign language and reverence for the Abbé de l'Épée. In Berthier's version of history, Sicard was an arrogant and evil tyrant who had insulted the deaf by slighting the expressive richness of their natural language, and trying to saddle it with the alien and pedantic rules of a foreign, verbal grammar. He had even presumed that the deaf could never be better than imbeciles and 'social non-entities' without the gracious help of his absurd artificial system of 'methodical

22 Bébian, *Mimographie*, pp. 1–2.
23 Bébian, *Essai sur les sourds-muets et sur le langage naturel*, p. 53.
24 See Bézagu-Deluy, *L'abbé de L'Épée*, pp. 267, 280–1.
25 Berthier, *L'Abbé de l'Épée*, p. 173.

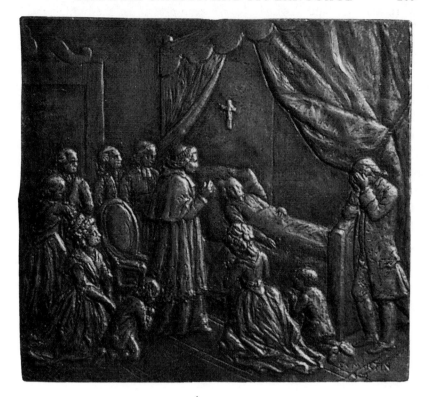

FIG 13. The death of the Abbé de l'Épée, from a memorial in the Rue St Jacques
by the deaf artist Félix Martin, 1909

signs'. Nor could Berthier forgive Sicard for the humiliating 'theatrical presentations' at which he paraded Massieu and other pupils before gaping crowds of tourists – performances in which the young Berthier had himself unwillingly taken part. Worst of all, this arch-enemy of the deaf had somehow managed to pass himself off as their friend.[26]

Fortunately, however – according to Berthier – the cruel Abbé Sicard had been opposed by the 'judicious and far-seeing' Bébian, worthy disciple of the virtuous tradition that had been usurped by Sicard – the tradition founded by the Abbé de l'Épée, 'spiritual father of the poor deaf-mutes'. The good Abbé de l'Épée was a 'quasi-divinity', the first man to look into the eyes of the deaf and offer them this prophetic assurance: 'and you too,' he said with his eloquent gaze, 'you too shall be men.' Berthier and other patriots of the deaf nation glossed over

26 Berthier, *L'Abbé Sicard*, pp. 65, 55–6.

the fact that all the criticisms they made of the Abbé Sicard were in fact far more pertinent to the Abbé de l'Épée (the public exercises, the use of methodical signs, and especially the preoccupation with lip-reading and speech). As befitted his posthumous role, they presented the Abbé de l'Épée dying a pauper's death, shivering in his humble unheated room, having spent all his wealth on founding the National Institution and providing for his adoptive deaf children. 'After a long night of wandering, our planet has at length attained an orbit round a central luminary,' as the American utopian Flournoy expressed it.[27] The Abbé de l'Épée was the sun of the nation of the deaf, the saviour or even the creator of their language, and his birthday – 24 November – would be honoured for ever as the principal date in the deaf national calendar.[28]

27 John James Flournoy, 'Reply to Objections', *American Annals of the Deaf and Dumb*, 10, 1858, pp. 149–50. See Padden and Humphries, *Deaf in America*, p. 31.
28 Berthier, *L'Abbé de l'Épée*, pp. 2, 243, 10, 173–5.

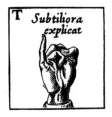

19

Tradition and the power of speech

Like other nationalists, the new patriots of the deaf people were unified by a sense of collective insecurity: their sign-language tradition might be sanctified by nature and seasoned by time, but at the present moment it was, they thought, in mortal danger – and not only from arrogant outsiders, but also from enemies within. By a terrible irony, as Berthier saw it, the work of the Abbé de l'Épée was being subverted from inside the Institution in the Rue St Jacques, direct successor to the great school founded by de l'Épée in the Rue des Moulins. Even the angelic deaf teacher Massieu was in the habit of telling his students to curtail their intellectual ambitions, warning them for example that Voltaire was 'so difficult that no deaf-mutes, however talented, could ever aspire to understand him'.[1] Added to this, there had been thirty years of duplicity on the part of Sicard, who, as leader of the hearing teachers of the deaf, would have liked to force deaf children to speak and lip-read, even if he did little enough about it in practice.[2]

But the most sinister traitor of all, from the point of view of the deaf nationalists, was Jean-Marc-Gaspard Itard, who had become medical supervisor at the Institution in 1800, and achieved great celebrity the following year through his work with a child he called Victor, the 'wild

1 Ferdinand Berthier, *L'Abbé Sicard*, p. 158.
2 Berthier, *L'Abbé Sicard*, p. 63.

boy of Aveyron', who had apparently been raised by animals in a forest, and lacked any understanding of language.[3] Despite his long career in the Rue St Jacques, Itard was never an advocate of sign language. Indeed he held that it was 'inherently defective and abbreviated', and persistently tried to wean the pupils away from it and offer them a training in vocal articulation instead. When he died in 1838 he left a handsome legacy to the Institution to fund a special class in spoken French, where the use of signs would be completely prohibited.[4] It was only thanks to the tenacious opposition of deaf members of the teaching staff, led by Berthier, that the implementation of Itard's will was prevented.[5]

Itard's hostility to sign language drew some sustenance from the work of his friend Joseph-Marie de Gérando, author of the essay on the 'influence of signs on the formation of ideas' which had won the gold medal of the Institut National des Sciences et Arts back in 1799.[6] In that treatise, de Gérando extolled the imaginative power of gestural languages, speculating inconclusively on whether, under favourable conditions, they might become intellectually equal to spoken ones. He also praised de l'Épee and Sicard for their use of signs in the education of the deaf, and criticized de l'Épee's rival Pereire for his efforts to get the deaf to speak. Pereire was guilty of treating his pupils like 'speaking machines', de Gérando said, and his assumption that the production of sounds was necessary for the proper expression of thought was nothing but a 'vulgar prejudice'.[7]

But de Gérando's own attitude to speech and signs was to grow increasingly complex. After the publication of his early essay, he had been released from military service so that he could apply himself to political work in Paris. Later he was appointed an administrator under Napoleon, who made him a Baron of the Empire, and after the restoration he became a valued servant of Louis XVIII. But throughout this flexible and influential political career, de Gérando maintained a primary commitment to philosophy – not only pure philosophy (he

3 E. M. Itard, De l'éducation d'un homme sauvage, Paris, 1801.
4 See Harlan Lane, The Wild Boy of Aveyron, pp. 52, 185, 250.
5 See Jean-René Presneau, 'Oralisme ou langue des gestes: la formation des sourds au XIXe siècle', in Jean Borreil, ed., Les Sauvages dans la Cité, Paris, Champ Vallon, 1985, p. 146.
6 See above, p. 184.
7 Joseph-Marie de Gérando, Des Signes et de l'Art de Penser, Vol. IV, pp. 467–8.

wrote lucid books on the History of Philosophy and the origin of knowledge)[8] but also philosophy as applied to practical problems, especially the education of the deaf. And he frequently participated in the daily work of the Institution in the Rue St Jacques, often deputizing for Sicard, and also developing a personal and intellectual friendship with Itard.

After Sicard's death, de Gérando was appointed to the Administrative Council of the Institution, and in 1827 he wrote a characteristically polished, vast, well-informed and clearly-argued report surveying and comparing all the rival approaches to the education of the deaf. Once again, he praised the 'mimic signs' employed by the deaf ('rich, expressive, even eloquent, and extremely picturesque'), but he judged them to be intellectually crude. On the other hand, their shortcomings were only contingent – a consequence of the fact that in the past most deaf-mutes had lived their lives in isolation, with no opportunity to associate together and create a continuing linguistic culture that would be passed on and enriched from one generation to the next. 'Whereas we receive our languages ready made from the society into which we are born,' de Gérando wrote, the deaf were obliged to create theirs 'entirely for themselves'. In ideal conditions, though – that is, 'if there were a nation of deaf-mutes somewhere' – gestural systems would, he had no doubt, develop 'all the characteristics of our languages'.[9]

Baron de Gérando was a pioneer of anthropological inquiry, and as a founder-member of the Société des Observateurs de l'Homme he urged explorers to learn for themselves the languages of any primitive peoples they might encounter, using Sicard's rational sign language as their starting point.[10] It was in this spirit of anthropological science that he made a study of the pupils at the Institution in the Rue St Jacques and compiled the first systematic descriptive record of gestural signs as actually used by the deaf amongst themselves.[11] (The diction-

8 See for example *De la génération des connoissances humaines*, Berlin, 1802; and *Histoire Comparée des Systèmes de Philosophie*, 3 Vols, Paris, 1804.

9 Joseph-Marie de Gérando, *De l'éducation des sourds-muets de naissance*, 2 Vols, Paris, 1827, Vol. 1, pp. 80, 240–1.

10 See Harlan Lane, *When the Mind Hears*, pp. 434–5, n. 82.

11 De Gérando refers to Justus Arnemann and Ernst Adolf Eschke, *Kleine Beobachtungen über Taubstumme*, Berlin, 1799 as an earlier attempt, and to Ferdinand Neumann's *Die Taubstummenanstalt zu Paris im Jahre 1822*, Königsberg, 1827, which includes comparative tables of signs used in Paris, Caen, Bordeaux etc.

aries of de l'Épée and Sicard, in contrast, had prescribed what signs ought to be used by teachers in the classroom, and gave little indication of their physical form.)

First of all, de Gérando noted the privately improvised 'mimic' gestures which uneducated deaf-mutes could be expected to know even before they arrived at the Institution. For example:

> BABY: Most of them make the sign for *little* accompanied by that for *to nurse*; some, that for *to cradle*; and others do an imitation of carrying a baby in their arms.
>
> BREAD: Some represent the various processes by which corn is transformed into bread; others make the sign for *to be hungry*, with that for *to cut*, and carrying to the mouth.
>
> NIGHT, DAY: They cross their hands and pass them in front of their eyes which they shut at the same time.
>
> WATER: By showing a little saliva; or imitating the action of rowing; mimicking a water-carrier; or representing a person working a pump. To these pantomimes, they always add the sign for *to drink*.[12]

He also noted certain systematic differences between the mimic signs used by boys and girls:

> AFFIRMATION (girls): bending the head forward and immediately bringing it back to its initial position.
>
> AFFIRMATION (boys): Some give a piercing glance and a toss of the head; others move the right hand forward with an air of assurance, as if they were hitting an object a little distance away at stomach-height.
>
> DOG (girls): designated sometimes by its height, its form, or its habit of barking . . . sometimes by the faithful way it follows its master, or beckoning to it to come nearer, or by extending a hand as if offering something to eat.
>
> DOG (boys): by the movement of its head when barking, or by pretending to call one.
>
> HORSE (girls): represented, by some, by indicating its noble form and its mane; by others, by harnessing it and showing it pulling a heavy cart.

12 De Gérando, *De l'éducation des sourds-muets de naissance*, Vol. 1, pp. 100–1.

HORSE (boys): Some like to characterize it by the mobility of its ears, some by putting the index and middle finger of the right hand astride the index of the left, and a few by putting a finger in their mouth to represent a bit . . .[13]

But when they started their new life in the Institution, de Gérando continued, deaf children would quickly discard these simple mimic signs in favour of the conventionalized signs in use amongst their fellows. For it was clear to him that the Paris Institution had, over the thirty-five years of its existence, unwittingly fostered what amounted to a miniature deaf nation amongst its inmates. There was now 'a tradition of signs which is the invention of the deaf-mutes', a heritage which they were continuously expanding by 'inventing more and more signs every day'. These signs 'owed nothing to the lessons of their masters', and each of them was of daunting complexity, depending on the movements and positions of hands, arms, and other parts of the body simultaneously, and on facial expressions too. Conventional signs such as these would normally be executed at such speed that it was impossible for the outsider to see exactly what was taking place, let alone describe it in words, so de Gérando confined himself to very simple examples:

EQUAL: the two index fingers are placed one against the other.
DIFFERENT: the two index fingers, placed against one another, are rapidly separated.

But many of the conventional signs were – like words of well-developed spoken languages – too nuanced to permit of exact translation:

When one pupil is being punished or suffers some other harm, and another rejoices at it, he will imitate the action of playing a violin: this action corresponds approximately to our expression: *c'est bien fait* [*a good thing too*].

When one deaf mute is tormenting another, and dead set against him, the latter will . . . always make the following sign: he will point at whoever he is accusing, and then rapidly put his hand to his chest, several times; this sign corresponds,

13 De Gérando, *De l'éducation des sourds-muets de naissance*, Vol. 1, pp. 100–3, 109–10.

roughly, to these words: *He won't leave me alone, he's torment-ing me, he won't leave me be.*[14]

In this way the children arriving at the Institution would discard their private mimic signs, and replace them with a system which, through the elaboration of analogies over many years, had become 'almost entirely conventional and arbitrary', and thus constituted 'a systematic and artificial language', broadly comparable to any other. Like a spoken language, it took a long time to learn; and although the pupils con-versed in it continuously, it was largely unintelligible to their hearing teachers, who were often 'unable to fathom the subject of their conver-sations'.[15]

The gestural language which was used as 'the essential means of instruction and translation' by the masters at the Institution consti-tuted a third system, alongside the private mimic signs of isolated deaf-mutes, and the artificial conventional system developed by the pupils collectively. It consisted of what de Gérando called 'reduced signs' – the simplified and stylized gestures devised by de l'Épée and Sicard for explaining the meanings of French words:

GOODNESS: The hand is raised to the lips, which kiss it; the face expresses sensibility.

CAUSE: Movement of closed hand, with thumb raised, moving from a lower to a higher position, as if imitating production.

EFFECT: The index and thumb of the right hand appear to detach something suspended between the index and thumb of the left.

COFFEE: Mimic the action of grinding it, imitating the mill with one fist, and the movement with the other.

DAILY: The thumb of the right hand is raised, with the other fingers closed, and after brushing the cheek while moving up from a low position to a high one, and from a position behind to one in front, it makes a vertical circle from left to right; then it executes a series of movements from a position behind to a position in front, while gradually moving horizontally towards the right.

BREAD: The outer edge of the right hand is dropped trans-

14 De Gérando, *De l'éducation des sourds-muets de naissance*, Vol. 1, pp. 116, 99, 116–25.
15 *De l'éducation des sourds-muets de naissance*, Vol. 1, pp. 125, 87.

versely to the back of the left hand, which is half closed.[16]

After presenting his sketch of the three kinds of gestural languages in use in Paris in the 1820s – the 'mimic', the 'traditional', and the 'reduced', which today might be distinguished as 'Home Sign', 'Paris Sign Language' and 'Paris Signed French' – de Gérando set about describing the two other great forms which language can take, namely writing and speech. Both of them, he believed, had been systematically misunderstood in European philosophy, because of its irrational metaphysical presumption in favour of speech. 'It has been supposed,' he wrote,

> that speech, and the sounds of the human voice, are invested with a kind of mysterious virtue, which makes them the natural and living expression of thought and feeling; appeal has been made to a few vague notions of Plato's about the relation between language and ideas; and the old metaphor, or rather equivocation, which enabled the word *logos* to have the dual function of referring both to *speech* and to *reason*, has been treated as if it embodied some profound truth.

Prejudices on behalf of speech, de Gérando continued, had in their turn been buttressed by a long-standing misconception about the nature of writing, through which non-European writing-systems – symbolic, ideographic or hieroglyphic – were systematically denigrated in comparison to alphabetic script.

> The practice which, amongst us, has reduced the function of writing to that of representing speech . . . has allowed speech to be accorded the exclusive privilege of representing thought; so much so, that the very name we apply to our idioms – the word *language*, or *tongue* – is borrowed from speech, from the organ which functions as its instrument.

Superstitions concerning speech and alphabetic writing, apart from being indefensible in theory, had in practice presented a terrible barrier to the progress of the deaf people of Europe. The philosophers' deluded idea that articulate sounds possessed a 'mysterious special power' repressed the fact that, given a chance, groups of deaf-mutes

16 *De l'éducation des sourds-muets de naissance*, Vol. 1, pp. 555, 579–92.

would always be able to institute for themselves a 'genuine conventional language' composed of gestural signs. Because of metaphysical prejudice, deaf-mutes had either been regarded as ineducable, or forced to learn speech like parrots, without understanding what it meant; or they had not been taught written language at all, on the specious grounds that it could not be meaningful to those who were unable to understand spoken words. And de Gérando was certain that deaf-mutes in countries with non-alphabetic writing systems, such as ancient Egypt and Mexico, and of course China, would be taught writing as a matter of course, 'and no one is surprised in the least'.[17]

It might seem that de Gérando was displaying a remarkably sympathetic and intelligent understanding of sign language and the injustices suffered by the deaf. But the deaf patriots did not see it that way. For them, de Gérando was a traitor like Itard, a reactionary ally of the 'method of speech' once espoused by Jacob Pereire, the deadly rival of de l'Épée. They accused him of deliberately confounding the authentic language of signs with gestural systems that had been corrupted and defiled by the alien conventions of speech. They could not accept de Gérando's suggestion that the sign language of the deaf was conventional, and that 'each community has its own dialect'.[18] True gestures, they believed, were pure 'mimicry', and intrinsically superior to speech. They were, as Bébian had argued, the only 'universal language', and Berthier insisted that they were innate rather than learned, 'sublime and universal, based on nature and on reason'.[19]

When de Gérando came to make his recommendations on the future linguistic and educational policies of the Institution in the Rue St Jacques in 1827, his treachery seemed to Berthier gross and unforgivable. De Gérando might point to the contradictory history of the Institution's attitudes to speech, explaining how the Abbé de l'Épée had criticized rivals like Heinicke for being obsessed with articulation and lip-reading, when it was also the chief goal of his own lessons. Or he might show how Sicard, 'having solemnly declared that artificial articulation was the necessary complement of the education of deaf-

17 *De l'éducation des sourds-muets de naissance*, Vol. 1, pp. 16–19, 13.
18 *De l'éducation des sourds-muets de naissance*, Vol. 2, pp. 452, 460.
19 Roche-Ambroise Bébian, *Essai sur les sourds-muets et sur le langage naturel*, p. 114;
Berthier, *L'Abbé de l'Épée*, pp. 39, 50.

mutes, neverthless abandoned it entirely in practice'. But de Gérando's own proposals struck his deaf critics as no less contradictory: after praising sign language for its intellectual potential, he went on to argue that its use should be severely discouraged. Of course he conceded that teachers of the deaf must start off by using the sign language of their pupils, but he urged that the children's signs should then be 'corrected' and 'rectified', and finally replaced by written words. Written language would be to their signs what paper money is to gold coins, he said: it would circulate in their place, and eventually make them unnecessary. Deaf children should be forced to give up gestures as soon as written words had been 'monetized' for them by the 'bold imprint of signs' – otherwise they would never learn to trust in written languages, or become fully integrated into the intellectual traditions of humanity as a whole.

To substantiate his case, de Gérando conducted an experiment in which one of the deaf teachers at the Institution dictated a simple story from a French book to six of his most able pupils. The dictation was given in signs, and the pupils took it down in French. When the six versions were inspected, however, they all turned out to be different, and none of them tallied exactly with the original text.[20] Of course a defender of sign language could point out that this is a quite normal result of translating from one language to another and back again: there would have been similar problems if English or German had been the intermediate language, rather than gestural signs. But de Gérando thought the experiment proved that the use of signs interfered with the pupils' direct understanding of French, and concluded that, having learned to read and write, the deaf should be given intensive instruction both in 'the labial alphabet, or the art of reading from the lips' and in 'the oral alphabet, or artificial pronunciation'. For only speech would allow the deaf to become citizens of the world, and once a deaf child had acquired speech, its need for signs would wither away.[21]

The year after the publication of de Gérando's report, an articulation class was started at the Institution. But the pupils refused to attend.

20 De Gérando, *De l'éducation des sourds-muets de naissance*, Vol. 1, p. 578; Vol. 2, pp. 463, 466, 495.
21 *De l'éducation des sourds-muets de naissance*, Vol. 1, p. 284; Vol. 2, pp. 398, 645.

Under government pressure, the class was restored, but the instructor, Léon Vaïsse, still found it impossible to get his students to substitute lip-reading for signs, as desired by the authorities.[22] The Director of the Institution, Jean-Jacques Valade-Gabel, who supported a new government policy of integrating deaf children into ordinary primary schools, tried to dispense with signs completely. He did not think it feasible for deaf children in school to be taught speech and lip-reading, but argued that they could easily be taught to read and write, using the 'direct' method, which meant 'introducing through the eyes, by means of writing, what the mother would have introduced through the ears, by means of speech'. In this way, he imagined, it should be possible to 'associate ideas with written words without any intermediary', and the 'jargon' of gesture (he considered it unworthy to be called a language) could be completely eliminated, even from the early stages of a deaf child's education.[23]

But the pupils still showed no inclination to stop using signs. After 1858 the French government began to despair of the Institution in the Rue St Jacques, and started encouraging a new kind of deaf school, where signs would be absolutely prohibited, and apprenticeship to a useful trade would be completely set aside to allow pupils to devote all their time to classes in 'demutization'.[24]

In this atmosphere, even the name of the Abbé de l'Épée was ceasing to command respect. By 1847, Itard's pupil Édouard Séguin was denouncing the pious Abbé as an atheistical disciple of Condillac, 'the high-priest of sensualism', and a collaborator of the Ideologists, for whom 'the language of natural signs was an excellent critique of the Revealed Word'. The only safe and godly means of educating the deaf was Pereire's method of articulation and lip-reading, but it had been cynically attacked by the wealthy Abbé de l'Épée, whilst the true friend of the deaf – the poor but selfless Pereire – had been libelled, spurned, and then forgotten.[25] Séguin's campaign was backed by Per-

22 See Presneau, 'Oralisme ou langue des gestes', p. 146, and Lane, *The Wild Boy of Aveyron*, pp. 237, 244, 247–9.

23 J.-J. Valade-Gabel, *Méthode à la portée des instituteurs primaires pour enseigner aux sourds-muets la langue française sans l'intermédiaire des signes*, Paris, 1857, cited in Presneau, 'Oralisme ou langue des gestes', p. 146.

24 The term *démutisation* appears to have been introduced by the deaf-educator Fourcade: see Presneau, 'Oralisme ou langue des gestes', p. 147, and Lane, *The Wild Boy of Aveyron*, p. 248.

25 Édouard Séguin, *Jacob-Rodrigues Pereire*, Paris, Baillière, 1847, p. 151.

eire's descendants, now a prosperous banking family, who endowed the Fondation Pereire both to celebrate the memory of their grandfather, and to support a new crusade against the insidious spread of signs.

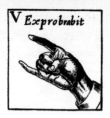

20

The gift of speech and
the care of the soul

In Boston in 1837, a young man called Samuel Gridley Howe agreed to undertake the education of Laura Bridgman, an eight-year-old girl who was not only deaf but also blind. He noted that she could already express herself in a spontaneous 'language of signs', a system which he took to be similar to that used in Laurent Clerc's American Asylum for the Deaf in Connecticut. But Howe convinced himself that Laura should be forced to stop using the 'natural language' of gestures. By providing 'a sign for every individual thing', he thought, it was holding up her intellectual and spiritual development, which required a grasp of the abstractions and generalities that were available only through 'the purely arbitrary language in common use'.

Howe began by making some cards with words printed on them in raised letters so that Laura could recognize them with her fingertips. Then he taught her to match familiar objects to the cards bearing their names. And before long he observed that 'her intellect began to work . . . her countenance lighted up with a human expression; it was no longer a dog, or parrot: it was an immortal spirit, eagerly seizing upon a new link of union with other spirits.' Howe next devised metal types for the letters of the alphabet, which his pupil could arrange in a frame to spell out words for herself, and he also taught her 'the manual alphabet, as used by deaf-mutes', which she could follow by lightly touching the hand of her teacher. Finally, she also learned to write with a pen for herself, in clear square letters.[1]

In 1841, Howe took his little pupil on a trip to Connecticut to visit the American Asylum and meet another deaf-blind child, Julia Brace. Although the girls disliked each other cordially, Howe was gratified by the meeting. 'What a difference between the two!' he said. Julia Brace was still communicating in sign language, and, just as Howe predicted, she seemed to be 'exercising only the lower propensities', little better than a domestic animal. The contrast with the 'moral and social nature' which the English language had awakened in Laura Bridgman was evident to all.[2] A year later Howe introduced his pupil to Charles Dickens, who gave a touching description of 'this gentle, tender, guileless, grateful-hearted being . . . built up, as it were, in a marble cell, impervious to any ray of light, or particle of sound'. She was completely at home in her 'finger language', however, and Dickens watched her spelling out English sentences with fluency and confidence. Even in sleep, when the rest of us might 'dream in words', she could be observed enacting many-sided conversations, entirely in the manual alphabet that Howe had taught her.[3]

Howe's opposition to sign language was reinforced the following year, when he accompanied Horace Mann, Secretary to the Board of Education of Massachusetts, on a tour of educational institutions for the deaf in Europe. Mann's report gave prominence to the oralist techniques used in Germany, which were 'decidedly superior' to the Parisian sign-language method still favoured in America. German teachers, Mann said, 'prohibit, as far as possible, all intercourse by the artificial language of signs,' and hence – 'incredible as it may seem' – the German deaf had all taken to spoken communication. In Germany, according to Horace Mann, it was 'almost absurd to speak of the dumb'.[4]

1 Samuel Gridley Howe's description of the education of Laura Bridgman is quoted extensively in Charles Dickens, *American Notes for General Circulation* (1842), Oxford, Oxford University Press, 1957, pp. 34–5.
2 This account of the meeting appeared in the *New York Commercial Advertiser* in November 1841, and is cited in F. B. Sanborn, *Dr S. G. Howe, the Philanthropist*, New York, Funk and Wagnalls, 1891, p. 162.
3 Dickens, *American Notes*, pp. 32, 41.
4 Horace Mann, *Seventh Annual Report of the Secretary of the Board of Education* (1843), reprinted in his *Annual Reports on Education*, pp. 230–418, pp. 253, 244.

Laura Bridgman never learned to speak, though, and twenty years passed before another campaign was launched in America to replace French methods with German ones. It began in 1862, when a four-year-old girl from Cambridge lost her hearing. She was Mabel Hubbard, and her father – a prosperous lawyer called Gardiner Hubbard – was told that he must wait till she was ten years old and then send her away to learn sign language at the American Asylum. This prospect filled him with despair, especially as Mabel had already begun to speak before she went deaf. But his despondency turned to anger when he took Mabel to see Thomas Gallaudet junior, a son of the creator of the American Asylum. Having heard Mabel speak, Gallaudet sighed with regret (according to Gardiner Hubbard's account) and said: 'But she will lose the beautiful language of signs.' In any case, he advised Hubbard that nothing could be done to save his daughter's speech: within three months she would be as dumb as she was deaf.[5]

Mabel's mother and father were determined that she should grow up as an ordinary American, speaking the language of Americans, rather than being consigned to 'a distinct race' with 'a language of their own', like those unfortunates at the Asylum who were permitted or even encouraged to use signs. Mabel apparently shared their revulsion. In middle age, she looked back to her childhood and recalled 'my own feelings of awe, not unmixed with horror, when I first saw some of these strange people'. They were 'truly dumb – extraordinary beings whose sometimes graceful, more often uncouth gestures and facial contortions made them in public places objects of curiosity, sometimes of pity, at others of ridicule; always things strange and apart.'[6]

At last, Mabel's parents turned to Samuel Gridley Howe, the teacher of Laura Bridgman, who assured them that Mabel's speech could be saved after all. She should always be spoken to very distinctly and directly, and everyone must insist that she 'read' their faces, and express herself only in clearly enunciated speech. Above all, they must take care 'not to allow any signs, and never to understand them'. Hubbard hired a governess to carry out this plan for him, and Mabel took swiftly to reading and writing, though her speech remained hard for strangers to follow. Meantime Hubbard began to campaign for the creation

5 Gardiner G. Hubbard, *The Story of the Rise of the Oral Method in America*, edited by Mabel Gardiner Bell, pp. 21–2.
6 Hubbard, *The Story of the Rise of the Oral Method in America*, pp. 18–19, 4–5.

within Massachusetts of a School (not 'Asylum') for the deaf (not 'deaf-mutes') – a school which would take pupils as young as five, and follow the German method, with sign language strictly forbidden. An oral boarding school eventually opened in Northampton in 1867, under Hubbard's direction, and a day school in Boston in 1869.

The sudden flowering of oral education in Massachusetts happened to come to the attention of the Scottish elocutionist Alexander Melville Bell when he visited Boston in 1868, making a great 'hit', as he put it, with a series of public lectures about a new and scientific method of writing which he called 'Visible Speech'.[7] Bell himself did not touch on the problem of demutization, despite the fact that his wife Eliza was deaf. But back in England their son Alexander Graham Bell was already applying his father's methods to the oral training of two young girls at a small private school for the deaf in London.[8] His reasoning was that, since speech was nothing but 'the mechanical result of certain adjustments of the vocal organs', the girls need only learn to arrange their organs in the ways indicated by his father's scientific notation, and then 'they will speak'.[9]

Three years later, Alexander Graham Bell went out to Boston to pursue his work with the deaf. He scored a notable success with a five-year-old boy, born deaf, to whom he taught writing, a manual alphabet based on Dalgarno's glove, simple vocal drills, and then speech.[10] But he also sought to outdo his father, by developing two pieces of apparatus in the laboratories of the Massachusetts Institute of Technology – devices which would transcribe vocal sounds mechanically rather than manually. In one of them, the supply of gas to a flame was regulated by a membrane sensitive to the sound of a voice, and in the other, the membrane was attached to a bristle which traced

7 Robert V. Bruce, *Bell: Alexander Graham Bell and the Conquest of Solitude*, London, Gollancz, 1973, p. 60. For an explanation of Visible Speech, see below, pp. 258–64.
8 It was Susanna Hull's school in South Kensington. See Bruce, *Bell*, p. 56, and Hull's own recollections of working with Bell in Arthur A. Kinsey, *Report of the Proceedings of the International Congress on the Education of the Deaf held at Milan, September 6th-11th 1880*, London, W. H. Allen, 1880, pp. 72–4.
9 Cited in John Hitz, *Dr A. Graham Bell's Private Experimental School*, Washington, Volta Bureau, 1898, p. 11.
10 Alexander Graham Bell, 'Upon a Method of Teaching Language to a Very Young Congenitally Deaf Child', *American Annals of the Deaf and Dumb*, Vol. xxxviii, April 1883. pp. 124–39.

a wave pattern on a moving smoked-glass plate. (Shortly afterwards Bell improved the apparatus by using real ears taken from a corpse.) He was hoping that these instruments would enable the deaf to see the visible trace of their own voices as they were speaking, and thus monitor their own speech optically, much as hearing people do through their ears. 'If we can find the definite shape due to each sound,' he wrote to his father in 1874, 'what an assistance in teaching the Deaf and Dumb!'[11]

Shortly afterwards, however, Bell's interest in the mechanical transcription of speech was diverted into another channel. As he expressed it, 'the need of developing the speaking telephone took my thoughts away from the subject, and for a number of years I had no practical connection with the deaf.' The invention of the telephone, to which he alludes offhandedly here, was of course distinctly unhelpful to those who could not hear; but as soon as it was completed Bell was able to return – a seriously rich man now – to his primary vocation as a 'teacher of the deaf'.[12]

Mabel Hubbard, whose plight was the original occasion for the implementation of the German method of deaf education in Massachusetts, had been referred to Bell in 1873, when she was nearly 16 and he already 26. She was accomplished and well educated, but despite two years of oral training in Germany, her speech was still very poor. He advised her that her problems arose 'from defective positions of the throat, and from the lack of diaphragm action', and prescribed a course in Visible Speech.[13] It appears to have worked, and they were married in 1877, by which time Bell's technical work on the telephone was more or less complete. On their honeymoon trip round Europe, he started a small 'oral' day school for deaf children in Greenock in Scotland, and said he felt he was teaching articulation not just to three little deaf girls, but to all 'the thirty thousand deaf-mutes of Great Britain'.[14]

When they returned to the United States, Alexander Graham Bell and his deaf wife Mabel took up residence in Washington, close to Edward Gallaudet, a son of the creator of the American Asylum, and

11 See Bruce, *Bell*, pp. 110–11.
12 Cited in Hitz, *Dr A. Graham Bell's Private Experimental School*, p. 6.
13 See Bruce, *Bell*, p. 101.
14 See Bruce, *Bell*, p. 256.

now director of the Columbia Institute for the Deaf and Dumb in Washington DC (later Gallaudet College and then Gallaudet University). In an admirable spirit of scientific collaboration, Bell and Gallaudet resumed the debate over the oral method. Unlike most oralists, Bell had gone to the trouble of learning the 'de l'Épée sign language', as he called it, and was willing to recognize it as 'a distinct language – as distinct from English as French or German or any other spoken tongue'. But he called for its total elimination nevertheless. It was an obstacle to the acquisition of English, and as such – as 'foreign immigrants have found out' – it was 'contrary to the spirit and practice of American Institutions'.[15]

Sign language also tended to isolate the deaf from their fellow citizens, so that they were 'bound to associate together in adult life, and the consequence is they intermarry and their affliction is transmitted to their offspring.'[16] Having undertaken a vast and pioneering statistical inquiry into deafness on Martha's Vineyard, in a vain attempt to identify general patterns of genetic inheritance,[17] Bell wrote an impassioned account of a 'great calamity' which was facing the United States: the short-sighted policy of permitting de l'Épée's system of gestures to be used as a 'special language' by deaf Americans would, he was convinced, lead inexorably to 'the formation of a deaf variety of the human race'. Whereas in Europe 65 per cent of the deaf could speak, in America the proportion was only 9 per cent. The rest, he wrote, 'think in a different language from that of the people at large . . . a language as different from English as French or German or Russian'. This was fostering a 'class-feeling among the deaf and dumb', hare-brained yearnings for separate deaf colonies (there was a new scheme in Manitoba in 1884), and yet more intermarriage, which in its turn further increased 'the production of a defective race of human beings'.[18]

Later, Bell's authority was further enhanced by the public gratitude of Helen Keller, the deaf-blind woman from Alabama who had learned not only to write with great fluency, but also to 'read' lips with her

15 Alexander Graham Bell, '*The Question of Sign-Language*' and '*The Utility of Signs*', Washington, Volta Bureau, 1898, pp. 6, 26–7.
16 Cited in Hitz, *Dr A. Graham Bell's Private Experimental School*, p. 12.
17 See Norah Ellen Groce, *Everyone Here Spoke Sign Language*, p. 8.
18 Alexander Graham Bell, *Upon the Formation of a Deaf Variety of the Human Race*, Memoirs of the National Academy of Sciences, 1883, Vol. 2, Washington, Government Publishing Office, 1884, pp. 172–262, pp. 217–19.

hand, and – thanks in part to Bell's help and advice – to articulate well enough to be understood at least by those accustomed to her voice.[19] Bell also used some of the wealth gained from inventing the telephone to fund the Volta Institute, dedicated to the oralist cause in deaf education. He and his deaf wife made formidable opponents for all those hearing philanthropists, like the brothers Edward and Thomas Gallaudet, who still wanted to defend the collective rights of the deaf and their language of signs.

In Britain and Ireland, the campaign for the oral method as opposed to sign language had little resistance to contend with. Deaf education in the tradition of Braidwood had always attempted to teach speech and lip-reading, and signs were therefore discouraged, if not completely forbidden. An article in the *Encyclopedia Britannica* in 1824 argued that the 'language of pantomime' could be regarded as 'the native language of the Deaf and Dumb', but that, despite de l'Épée and Sicard, it remained exceedingly crude and imprecise, and absolutely incapable of expressing abstract general ideas and instilling spiritual wisdom. 'In Great Britain,' according to the *Encyclopedia*, the method of articulation 'has been at all times cultivated with more assiduity and with greater success than on the continent,' and British deaf schools should continue to encourage the deaf to replace their signs with writing and 'artificial speech'.[20]

And many deaf people agreed. John Kitto, the Cornish missionary who had lost his hearing as a child, was convinced that signs could not express 'abstract ideas' or enable the deaf to form any idea of the Supreme Being. In addition, he had a strong personal aversion to signs, because they attracted attention and excited curiosity: 'as soon, therefore, as a person has attempted to communicate with me by signs, I have ceased to have any other object than to make my escape.'[21] In the same way, the Irish writer Charlotte Elizabeth Tonna, a prolific author of pious Protestant novels, and totally deaf since the age of ten, undertook the reclamation of two poor deaf-mutes in Kilkenny

---

19 Helen Keller's *The Story of My Life*, 1903, is dedicated to Alexander Graham Bell.
20 W. (= Thomas Watson?), 'Deaf and Dumb', *Supplement to the fourth, fifth and sixth editions of the Encyclopedia Britannica*, Edinburgh, 1824, Vol. 3, pp. 467–79.
21 John Kitto, *The Lost Senses: Series I – Deafness*, London, Charles Knight, 1845, pp. 122, 200, 110.

in 1823, affirming that a child was 'necessarily an atheist' until it had learned to spell out the alphabet, and that true spirituality waited on the acquisition of speech.[22]

In 1867, the Reverend Thomas Arnold opened a pure oral school in Northampton, England. He believed that spiritual and intellectual development depended on spoken language, and considered that gestures could express only the 'commonest physical wants'. The voice, after all, made use of air and sound – 'the former necessary to life and the latter the least material of qualities' – and consequently it had 'more than a chance relation to thought'.[23] Gesture was avoided at the Northampton school, and its use was a punishable offence amongst the older pupils.[24] In 1869, the Baroness Meyer de Rothschild opened an oralist Jewish School for the Deaf in London, and later sponsored the Association for the Oral Instruction of the Deaf and Dumb, to foster deaf education in day schools, which she thought would prevent deaf children from associating with each other outside their lessons and thereby regressing to sign language. In 1871, another deaf school opened in London, dedicated to 'the lip-reading system', and its principal impressed the Social Science Congress by exhibiting a deaf gentleman who was able to conduct conversations flawlessly, even with persons wearing a full moustache.[25]

Meanwhile in Doncaster, the principal of the Yorkshire Residential School for Deaf Children instituted daily 'shouting practice' in the school yard for all his pupils, finding that it 'makes them less sluggish, and stimulates the circulation of the blood'. The more able students were taught to articulate, and were given a smart brass badge in the shape of an A, to encourage the others.[26] Many years later, deaf pupils making poor progress in speech would still be threatened with relegation to the 'monkey class', the sink for mental defectives who could not or would

22 Charlotte Elizabeth (C. E. Tonna), *Memoir of John Britt: The Happy Mute*, London, Seeley's, 1850, p. 22.
23 Thomas Arnold, *The Education of the Deaf and Dumb: an Exposition of the French and German Systems*, London, Elliot Stock, 1877, pp. 11–12.
24 Thomas Arnold, *Education of Deaf-Mutes: A Manual for Teachers*, London, Committee of the College of Teachers of the Deaf and Dumb, 1888, p. 128. David Wright, who attended the Northampton school in the 1930s, found that signing was still a punishable offence there, as was the practice of mouthing words without voicing them: see *Deafness, A Personal Account*, pp. 52, 63.
25 *The Times*, 13 October 1871, p. 3.
26 Colin Bingle, 'The Story of a School', *The British Deaf News*, Vol. 12, No 5, Sept-Oct 1979, pp. 142–3.

not be weaned away from the use of signs.[27] And in 1879, the principal of the first English training school for teachers of the deaf, Arthur Kinsey, looked forward to the day when 'an universal education for the deaf shall be decreed in this country', a compulsory system which would 'stamp them with that most characteristic feature of mankind, the greatest gift of the Almighty – Human Speech!'[28]

But Kinsey had no need to worry. By that time, the case against sign language was well-known amongst the British political class. Benjamin St John Ackers, a barrister and later a Member of Parliament, had a daughter who lost all her hearing at the age of three months, and in 1872 he and his wife went on a tour of Europe and North America to investigate remedies for her plight. Uneducated deaf-mutes, in their opinion, were 'often very dangerous to society, more resembling an animal than a human being', and sign language only aggravated their problems. Having observed Alexander Graham Bell at work in Boston, however, they were won over to the oral method: 'many are born deaf,' Ackers wrote, 'but, happily, none need be dumb on that account.'[29]

The Times also took up the cause. Britain, it argued, had pioneered deaf education in the seventeenth century and the eighteenth, but during the nineteenth British traditions had been distorted by French notions, which allowed the deaf to be herded together in residential schools, and confined within the mental prison of sign language. 'The institutions for the deaf have been the great bulwarks of dumbness,' it thundered. It wished good speed to those who were attempting to reverse this other French revolution by restoring the exclusively oral method of deaf education – a method which, by the way, it would refuse to call German, since the Germans had merely taken over, without acknowledgement, what was in truth 'our national system'.[30]

Back in Paris the Fondation Pereire continued to attack the 'French' system from within. They organized a Universal Congress on deaf

---

27 See William Burt's memoir of the Northern Counties School for the Deaf in Newcastle upon Tyne in the 1930s, 'A Century of Deafness', *The British Deaf News*, Vol. 12, No 12, Nov-Dec 1980, pp. 407–8, and Vol. 13, No 7, Jan-Feb 1982, pp. 257–9.
28 Arthur A. Kinsey, *The Education of the Deaf on the 'German' System*, London, W. H. Allen, 1879, p. 16.
29 B. St John Ackers, *Deaf not Dumb*, London, 1876, pp. 27, 21; see also his *Vocal Speech for the Dumb*, London, 1877.
30 *The Times*, 23 June 1880, p. 9.

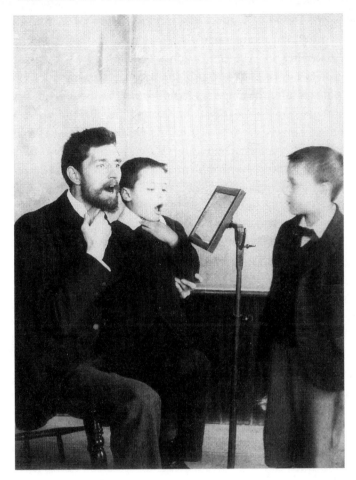

FIG 14. A speech lesson at the Royal School for the Deaf, Exeter, 1899

education in 1878, which resolved to sponsor an international event in Milan where the issue between the French and German systems could be settled once and for all, on neutral soil. More than half the delegates at the Milan Congress in 1880 were Italian, and most of the rest from France. There were a few representatives of the English oralists, too, including St John Ackers, and five Americans, led by Edward Gallaudet, who was determined to defend, if not the 'pure French system' in which speech was not taught at all, at least the 'combined' system, in which the deaf would be taught in sign language and permitted to use it amongst themselves.

But Gallaudet soon realized that the Milan Congress was not going to allow an open discussion of the merits of the rival methods. It was to be a ritual denunciation of sign language. Before the conference began, delegates inspected sixty deaf boys who had received oralist training in the Poor School in Milan. According to the correspondent for *The Times*, their display of 'reading from the lips' was astonishing. Delegates addressed the boys in normal speech, and 'one and all answered in spoken language, though we in our country call them dumb'. In fact the deaf paupers of Milan, who were not allowed to make signs at all, struck the British as rather more civilized than ordinary Italians, amongst whom, as was notorious, 'gesture and action so commonly accompany speech'.[31]

The President of the Congress, Giulio Tarra, explained to the delegates that movements of the lips were the only adequate expression for mental conceptions. When God installed a soul within us, he gave us speech as well, and there was nothing that lay beyond the power of 'that wonderful instrument, the mouth, played upon by the hand of the Deity'. He knew from bitter experience that those who were taught in sign language would never learn abstract ideas, but only 'grossly material images'. And he insisted, despite the lonely protest of Edward Gallaudet, that the two methods could not possibly be combined: 'the method of signs,' he warned, 'stands in deadly opposition to that of speech.'[32]

Herr Hugentobler, German president of a deaf school in Lyon, agreed that sign language should be eliminated; and Signor Fornari of Milan echoed him with emphasis: it must indeed be *abolished*. The only reason for the chronic moral depravity of the deaf was that they had not been weaned from signs. Susanna Hull, the teacher from London who had given Alexander Graham Bell his first chance of working with deaf children back in 1868, maintained that if they were ever permitted to use signs, their spoken and written language would become infected with 'deaf-mutisms', their vocal apparatus would atrophy, and they would soon start to suffer from the lung diseases, distorted shoulders, poor posture, and ungainly carriage characteristic of signing deaf-mutes. Kinsey added theological weight to the medical

31 *The Times*, 10 September 1880, p. 7.
32 Arthur A. Kinsey, *Report of the Proceedings of the International Congress on the Education of the Deaf held at Milan, September 6th-11th 1880*, London, W. H. Allen, 1880, pp. 24, 26.

argument by pointing out that under the German system, 'voices are used as destined by the Good Creator', whereas under the French one they are 'silenced by the prejudiced ignorance of man'. The only possible conclusion, underlined by St John Ackers, was that the use of sign language should be outlawed altogether.[33]

On 11 September 1880, the matter was put to a vote. By 160 to 4, the Congress decided that neither the French Method nor the Mixed Method should henceforth be countenanced in the education of the deaf. If the unfortunate members of this 'neglected class' were to be redeemed, they must be prevented from using signs altogether. The number of deaf delegates at the Congress, Gallaudet noted bitterly, was zero.

33 Kinsey, *Report of the Proceedings of the International Congress*, pp. 21, 23, 34, 71, 81, 39, 95; on the further history of oralism in Britain, see J. G. Kyle and B. Woll, *Sign Language: the study of deaf people and their language*, Cambridge, Cambridge University Press, 1985, Chapter 3.

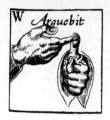

21

The making of the Deaf

In the second half of the nineteenth century, the oralist movement spread through Europe and North America, inspiring politicians, philanthropists and teachers with the dream of converting all deaf children, however poor, into happy and active citizens. Hard-won skills in speech and lip-reading would allow the deaf to merge imperceptibly into hearing society, no longer condemned to a solitary life as sullen outcasts confined to the language of signs. Following the Milan Congress of 1880, the remaining sign-language residential institutions were reformed, and hundreds of new oralist schools were founded – day schools, on the whole, because their aim was to integrate the deaf into the hearing world, rather than allow them to form silent sign-language communities separated from the rest of society.[1]

A hundred years later, however, the old oralist schools would themselves be almost universally condemned, on the grounds that they were paternalistic and violent, catering to the prejudices of hearing adults rather than the needs of deaf children. But still, the oral method had achieved some undeniable successes, especially with pupils who had a little vestigial hearing. In the past, such children would have been

---

1 In 1883, Alexander Graham Bell counted 502 deaf schools in the US, Europe, Japan and Australia, of which 54% were pure oral, 28% combined, and less than 10% manual, the remainder being unknown. See *Upon the Formation of a Deaf Variety of the Human Race*, p. 253.

classified as totally deaf, but with the help of devices like Alexander Graham Bell's 'audiometer', the 'semi-deaf' could now be identified at an early age and equipped with mechanical (or, later, electronic) hearing aids to help them learn speech directly.[2] Even those with very severe hearing loss sometimes benefited from strict oralist regimes, especially if they were 'post-lingually' deaf, and many of them grew up to be grateful to the exacting teachers who, by forbidding them to use signs as children, had forced them to cultivate lip-reading and articulation to the point where their handicap was almost undetectable in much of the everyday business of their lives.[3]

In other ways, however, the new deaf schools did not work out as their founders had hoped. In practice, the deaf would never be able to participate as full equals in the activities of those who could hear; and meantime the schools were encouraging the very tendencies that the oralists most feared – they were allowing the deaf to create a whole new social world for themselves, an exclusive society of the deaf. Local networks of deaf mutual aid, like those which had occasionally established themselves in the past (in Paris, for example, or on Martha's Vineyard), became the rule rather than the exception, and they linked up with each other to form extensive deaf communities – regional, national and even international. For the first time, the deaf came to constitute a conspicuous social group, robust, permanent and sometimes a little defiant. From now on, deaf people were as likely as the rest of the population to marry and have children; and what is more they nearly all chose a deaf partner, usually someone encountered at or through their school. Ironically, then, the oralist opponents of sign language were helping to bring about exactly the kind of separate deaf society they had always wanted to prevent.

Although medical and educational opinion was beginning to regard deafness as a multi-dimensional disability and a matter of degree, for social purposes it was still defined in simple and absolute terms: culturally, everyone had to be one thing or the other, either deaf or hearing. To be truly deaf – or Deaf with a capital D, to follow a

2 See Bruce, *Bell*, p. 394.
3 See for example David Wright, *Deafness, a Personal Account*, and Molly Sifton, 'Fulfilment', in Irene R. Ewing and Alex W. G. Ewing, *Opportunity and the Deaf Child*, London, University of London Press (1947), second edition, 1950, pp. 171–246.

convention introduced in the 1970s[4] – you needed to be brought up in a Deaf community, rather than simply unable to hear. The sociologist Paul Higgins, for instance, is a child of deaf parents, and though his hearing is normal, he can still be accepted as Deaf: 'to be a member of a deaf community,' as he puts it, 'one need not actually be deaf.' The American Deaf world may be riven by deep social divisions – between rich and poor, or black and white, or between those using an elaborate and cosmopolitan version of sign language and those whose repertoire is restricted to a dialect of supposedly rustic and inelegant gestures, or between those who freely use sign language in public and those who regard such conduct as vulgar or obscene – but still it is bound together by a shared sense of unity in opposition to an alien Hearing world. As with sex and sexuality, people who do not fit in with such dichotomies cause embarrassment, anxiety, and even hostility: Higgins explains that the semi-deaf, and those who have lost their hearing 'post-vocationally' or after adolescence, cause 'both ill feelings and amusement', because 'their behaviour does not respect the identity of the deaf community'.[5]

Nevertheless, the utopian aspirations of deaf nationalists like John James Flournoy proved as mistaken as the apocalyptic fears of oralists like Alexander Graham Bell. However much they might want to, the Deaf could never generate the kind of self-reproducing internal structure characteristic of a 'nation', a 'people', or a 'race'. Congenital pre-lingual deafness may be largely hereditary, but that does not mean that it runs in families – that deaf parents have deaf children, and hearing parents do not. So Bell's eugenicist forebodings about marriages between deaf partners turned out to be unfounded. According to a study carried out in the 1970s, in fact, nine out of ten deaf children are born to hearing parents. And even in marriages where both partners are deaf (which account for nine deaf marriages out of ten), more than eight out of ten children have normal hearing.[6]

4 The convention was formally introduced by James Woodward in 'Implications for Sociolinguistics Research Among the Deaf', *Sign Language Studies*, 1, pp. 1–7, 1972; see Padden and Humphries, *Deaf in America*, p. 2, but it has an antecedent in Joanne Greenberg's novel about a poor deaf marriage during the depression: *In This Sign*, New York, Holt, Rinehart and Winston, 1970.
5 Paul C. Higgins, *Outsiders in a Hearing World: A Sociology of Deafness*, Beverly Hills, Sage, 1980, pp. 43, 53–7, 41.
6 See Jerome D. Schein and Marcus T. Delk, *The Deaf Population of the United States*, Silver Spring, Maryland, 1974.

Deaf communities are therefore a very peculiar hybrid from the point of view of social theory: they are unable to perpetuate themselves by family tradition.[7] The collective life of the Deaf is passed from generation to generation not by the family but by the school; in fact deaf school, in some respects, is the Deaf child's family.[8]

Hearing children of deaf parents (Children of Deaf Adults as they have been called, or C O D As) naturally face acute dilemmas of family loyalty. It is not that they are forced to feel like outsiders, though; the problem is that they are liable to cause their own parents to be defined as the cuckoos in the family nest. This is partly because, like the children of adult immigrants, they are likely to be used by their parents as guides and interpreters to the rest of the world; and thanks to casual hearsay, both in the street and from radio and TV, hearing children will soon be much better informed than their deaf parents about the society in which they live.[9] But the main anomaly lies in their relation to grandparents. It is extremely unlikely that the parents of a hearing child's deaf parents will all be deaf; in fact it is very probable that none of them will be. And these hearing grandparents will typically be overjoyed if their grandchild is born with normal hearing: they will experience it as a kind of cancellation or restoration of the aberration that made their own child deaf. Their parental love may then be withdrawn and transferred to the younger generation, so that they are likely to pass family heirlooms straight to their hearing grandchildren as if their own immediate offspring did not exist. 'My grandmother had a beautiful diamond wedding ring,' as one CODA recalled, 'and she kept saying, "Sarah, this is yours! . . ." And my mother put up with years and years of being skipped over.'[10] It has been observed that deaf parents often show a great 'sense of complacency' when a child of theirs turns out to be deaf.[11]

---

7 They can therefore be compared to homosexual communities, or political or artistic ones.

8 As one of the first ethnographers of the deaf puts it, the coincidence of socialization and formal education in deaf communities creates 'a unique situation in complex societies'. See Gaylene Becker, *Growing old in silence*, Berkeley, University of California Press, 1980, p. 29.

9 The torment and anger caused by such problems are eloquently presented in Joanne Greenberg, *In This Sign*.

10 See Paul Preston, *Mother Father Deaf: Living Between Sound and Silence*, Cambridge, Harvard University Press, 1994, p. 41; see also pp. 61–76.

11 Becker, *Growing old in silence*, p. 34.

By constructing separate communities for themselves, based on their schools, the Deaf have been able to live together on their own terms, without having to defer constantly to uncomprehending members of the alien hearing world. They remained objects of curiosity, of course, but by the middle of the nineteenth century they were managing to secure a radical transformation in their reputation: instead of being taken as isolated representatives of natural, pre-social humanity, they were now seen as constituting an enigmatic secret society, rather like non-hereditary Jews or Gypsies – a kind of freemasonry with special social rules adapted to their peculiar condition.[12] One of the first people to recognize the emergence of this new deaf world was Charles Dickens, in a Christmas story for 1865 called 'Doctor Marigold's Prescriptions'. Doctor Marigold is not a doctor, but a travelling trader or 'Cheap Jack', rattling off the story of his life, and telling us how, after losing his little daughter Sophy, and then his wife as well, he adopted a poor abused orphan girl to be a companion to him on his travels. She was 'just the same age that my daughter would have been', he says, and he hoped that if he lavished his love on her, she would grow to be 'like my child'. Whatever she might have been called in her former life, he would always call her Sophy, in order, as he put it, 'to put her ever towards me in the attitude of my own daughter'.

There is a problem with the second Sophy though: she is 'deaf and dumb'. But Doctor Marigold does not despair; indeed he is gratified because it makes the girl all the more dependent on him. He teaches her to read, by pointing out the place names on milestones they pass along the road, and giving her a box of little bone tablets with the letters of the alphabet on them, so that she can spell out words for herself. He even devises a system of home-made manual signs, 'hundreds in number', as he boasts. After ten happy years together, however, he feels obliged to send her to the Deaf and Dumb school in the Old Kent Road to have her education properly completed. 'I want her sir,' he says to the Head Master, 'to be cut off from the world as

12 Both these images are to be found in Carson McCullers, *The Heart is a Lonely Hunter* (New York, Houghton, 1940), which presents its mute character Singer as a strange loner, though it also glancingly recognizes the existence of a deaf community based on signs. Greenberg's *In This Sign* tries to convey the pathos of the deaf community, while Mark Medoff's play *Children of a Lesser God* (first performed 1979, and in 1988 a film by Randa Haines with Marlee Matlin and William Hurt) tries to portray it as seductive as well.

little as can be, considering her deprivations, and therefore to be able to read whatever is wrote, with perfect ease and pleasure.' Having promised that when he got her back he 'wouldn't make a show of her, for any money', Marigold returns to his solitary travelling life for two years, cheered by the knowledge that at the end of the period he will enjoy the companionship of the silent Sophy once again.

At first, their 'reunited life was more than all that we had looked forward to'. But Doctor Marigold had left something out of his calculations. It seemed that he and Sophy were being followed round the country by a strange boy, or rather a young man. One night Marigold observes a tryst between Sophy and her new friend, and is astonished to see that they are conversing in signs. He should have guessed, of course: the young man is deaf, and they had met at the Deaf School in London and fallen for each other. 'I listened with my eyes, which had come to be as quick and true with deaf and dumb conversation, as my ears with the talk of people that can speak.' The boy is imploring her to marry him so that they could go out to China and start a new life together; but she – unaware of being watched by her adoptive father – refuses, tearfully but firmly, for fear of breaking poor old Marigold's heart. Naturally the good Cheap Jack will not allow her to sacrifice her happiness on account of him, so he issues an immediate 'prescription': the two deaf lovers are to marry at once, and build a new life for themselves, with his blessing.

After that Marigold receives occasional letters from China, and before long he learns that Sophy has given birth to a little daughter of her own, though it is too early to tell whether the child is 'deaf and dumb'. Five lonely years later, though, on a solitary Christmas Eve, the old man hears a scuffling noise outside his cart, and then a bright little girl lets herself in, glances around, opens her lips, and says in a clear pretty voice: 'Grandfather!'

'Ah my God! . . . She can speak!' says the tearful trader, welcoming first the perfect child, and then her proud but afflicted parents, noting, with almost as much pleasure, that the little girl is interpreting spoken conversation for them, 'talking . . . in the signs that I had first taught her mother.'[13]

---

13 Charles Dickens, 'Doctor Marigold's Prescriptions' ('To Be Taken Immediately' and 'To Be Taken for Life'), from *All the Year Round*, 1865, in *Selected Short Fiction*, edited by Deborah A. Thomas, Harmondsworth, Penguin, 1976, pp. 343–69.

The signs used by the deaf were becoming an object of popular curiosity, and it was common for the poor deaf to try to make a living by peddling cheap booklets or cards illustrated with engravings of the manual alphabet or sign equivalents of some basic words, and some reverent references to the Abbé de l'Épée.[14] One such booklet, published in Cardiff at the end of the nineteenth century, is adorned by a portrait of the Abbé, and offers homely advice on avoiding deafness (lovers, for instance, must 'beware of kissing the dear one's ears'), along with a few crude pictures of signs. Another, printed in Edinburgh in 1895, gave illustrations of 144 signs, taken from genuine photographs and verified by 'a Deaf and Dumb person well conversant with the various systems in use in almost all the important places of Great Britain'.[15] (See Figures 15, 16 and 17.)

Popular pamphlets like these are the earliest pictorial records of the signs used by the deaf, as opposed to those recommended by their hearing teachers. But they were felt to be an embarrassment by many of the more respectable members of the deaf community, who regarded signing as a kind of family shame. Before long, however, a medium became available which enabled signs to be recorded without vulgarity. In 1902, the American Mutoscope and Biograph Company released a short film (75 seconds) showing a girl from Gallaudet College reciting 'The Star Spangled Banner' in gestural signs.[16] This was in itself a striking demonstration of the contradictions of linguistic nationalism, and in 1913 they were further explored in the film of a lecture given in sign language by George Veditz, a prominent member of the American deaf community. Veditz sought to rally his fellow deaf Americans to the cause of sign language, by describing the plight of their fellows in Europe. 'The French deaf people loved de l'Épée,' he began. 'They loved him because he was their first teacher, but they loved him more for being the father and inventor of their beautiful

---

14 On the role of peddlers in the deaf community in America, see Higgins, *Outsiders in a Hearing World*, pp. 107–22. For the use of such cards in France, see Nicholas Mirzoeff, *Silent Poetry*, p. 209.
15 Anon., *Guide to Chirology*, Cardiff and Chiswick, n.d., (?1899); and Anon., *A Pocket Book of Deaf and Dumb Signs*, Edinburgh, 1895.
16 *Deaf Mute Girl Reciting 'Star Spangled Banner'* (Film), 1902; see Martin F. Norden, *The Cinema of Isolation: a history of physical disability in the movies*, New Brunswick, Rutgers University Press, 1994, p. 18.

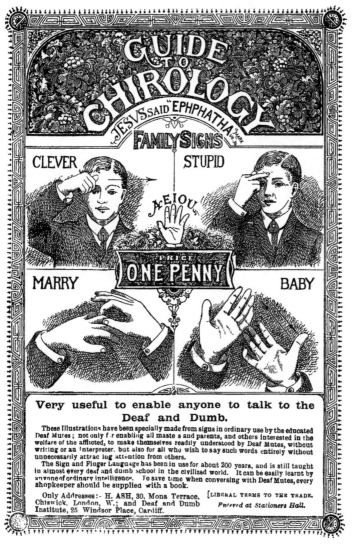

FIG 15. Family Signs, or How to talk to the Deaf and Dumb, 1899

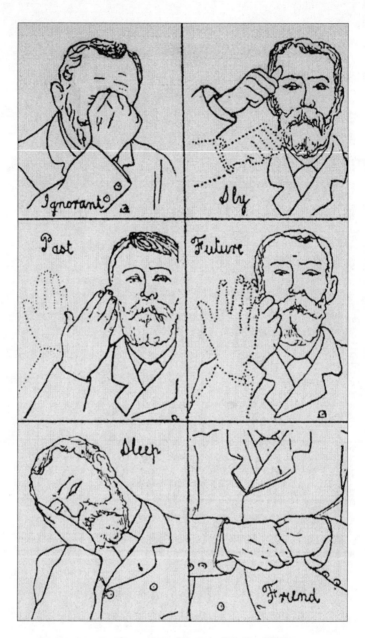

FIG 16. Some signs in use in Britain, 1895

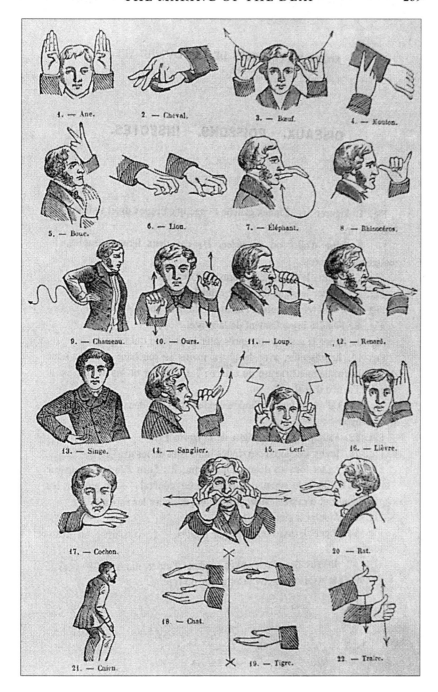

FIG 17. An Iconography of French signs, 1856

sign language.' But then there had been the treachery of the Milan Congress, and

> for the last thirty-three years, the French deaf people have watched with tear-filled eyes and broken hearts this beautiful language of signs snatched away from their schools ... It is like this in Germany also. The German Deaf people and the French Deaf people look up at us American Deaf people with eyes of jealousy. They look upon us Americans as a jailed man chained at the ankles might look upon a man free to wander at will.

Veditz must have know that he was exaggerating the contrast between Europe and America, but it enabled him to emphasize the danger of 'bad times' in the offing. Protagonists of the oral method were once more on the march, he signed, and already 'our sign language is deteriorating'.

> 'A new race of pharaohs that knew not Joseph' are taking over the land and many of our American schools. They do not understand signs, for they cannot sign. They proclaim that signs are worthless and of no help to the Deaf. Enemies of the sign language, they are enemies of the true welfare of the Deaf ... As long as we have Deaf people on earth, we will have signs ... It is my hope that we all will love and guard our beautiful sign language as the noblest gift God has given to Deaf people.[17]

Indirectly at least, Veditz's dream was to come partly true. The prohibition of sign language in oralist schools might continue to intensify, but it was only driving signs underground, creating a sort of linguistic black market in which signing flourished as never before. The oralists were appalled: they thought that if the deaf were allowed to express themselves in gestures, they would exclude themselves for ever from an understanding of the complexities of a proper, historical spoken language such as English. At the Milan Congress, indeed, they had humiliated Edward Gallaudet by making him concede that his pupils at the National College in Washington were often so accustomed to

17 George Veditz, *Preservation of Sign Language* (Film), 1913, passages translated by Carol Padden in Padden and Humphries, *Deaf in America*, pp. 33–6.

thinking in signs that the syntax of their English was deformed by 'mutisms': some of his graduates, he had to admit, were not even 'competent to construct a grammatically correct sentence'.[18]

Gallaudet himself was discomfited by the problem of 'mutisms'; but the newly confident Deaf communities of the twentieth century were able to put a quite different construction on it. The difficulty of expressing signed thoughts in English was not necessarily a proof of the defectiveness of signs, after all. It could just as well be the other way round: sign language might be too precise, subtle or flexible to be interpreted by the clumsy rigidities and unprincipled compromises of conventional speech. Perhaps it was sign language, not speech, that was uniquely beautiful and natural. In due course ordinary signers began to take over the utopian notions that had been projected on to signs by metaphysicians and educators from Plato to Bébian. They saw themselves as inheritors and custodians of an angelic system of communication, purer and truer than speech: their own beautiful language of signs.

In New York in 1913, the five-year-old Mary Bromberg, congenitally deaf daughter of poor Jewish immigrants from Russia, started her special oral education as a weekly boarder at the Lexington School for the Deaf. But her schooling was not a success: all she ever remembered of it was bewilderment and frustration at the endless classroom routines of 'open mouth', 'close mouth', 'feel throat', or 'pick up tongue'. When she ran away eight years later, she could still scarcely read or write, and although she was able to pronounce a handful of isolated English words, the noise she made was embarrassing, and strangers would not understand what she was trying to say anyway.

It was much the same for Benjamin Sidransky, another poor Jew in New York. He lost his hearing when he was two, before learning to speak. At the age of six he was sent to PS 47, a day school for the 'hard of hearing' in Manhattan, where a succession of instructors tried to teach lip-reading by the direct method, together with pronunciation of the easier letters of the alphabet. He too left school with practically no grasp of either written or spoken English.

At PS 47 the pupils were of course forbidden to indulge in any kind of gestural communication; but some of Benny Sidransky's fellow

18 Arthur Kinsey, *Report of the Proceedings of the International Congress*, p. 33.

pupils knew sign language, perhaps from deaf parents, and he picked it up from them when the teachers were not looking. For the rest of his life, he communicated in signs, having drawn almost no benefit from the special education in spoken language which had taken up most of his childhood and youth. Seventy years later, he recalled (in sign) that 'my teacher taught me to name a ball, to name a flower, but she did not teach me what kind of flower was in her hand' – the flower, that is, of gestural language.

Mary Bromberg's experience at Lexington was just the same: her real education took place, she remembered, in the signs she shared with the other girls when out of sight of the teachers. After running away from school she found work in a light bulb factory, and ten years later, thanks to the bonds of sociability which united the working-class deaf community in New York, she met up with Benny Sidransky, who was now employed as an upholsterer, and they married in 1929. The Sidranskys lived in Brooklyn and the Bronx for the rest of their lives, full of hopes and failed enterprises (they even had a stash of books about the Abbé de l'Épée under their bed, belonging to Mary's deaf brother Jack, a relic of his failed attempt to make a living as a peddler on the streets of North America). Mary and Benny Sidransky communicated only in sign language, but they did not use it in public for fear of attracting attention, and in due course they began to feel intimidated by younger signers, who seemed to have acquired a baffling vocabulary of new signs derived from Gallaudet College in Washington.[19]

The Sidranskys had a daughter called Ruth. Her hearing was normal, but she picked up their sign language in infancy and then became their ambassador to the hearing world. Ruth Sidransky recalls the stories her parents told her in their fluent signs: memories of cruel oralist teachers who would hit them if they ever made a gesture, and of uncomprehending parents who tried to prevent their marriage; and traditional tales about the Abbé de l'Épée, his poverty, his chance meeting with two deaf children, and his realization that signs were the natural language of the deaf.

Ruth Sidransky remembered her father explaining sign language to

19 Ruth Sidransky, *In Silence: Growing up Hearing in a Deaf World*, New York, St Martin's Press, 1990, pp. 64, 158, 256.

her, drawing unwittingly on idealized philosophical notions that went back to the French enlightenment and even to ancient Greece:

> He pulled his chair closer to mine, pushed back his thick white hair and signed, 'I tell you language is alive, like a person, like a river, always change, always new words. We make words. Hearing people not try to understand deaf language, but deaf try to understand hearing language. Not need to speak to know language. I late to learn my language, never really learn hearing language, to speak with tongue well, but sign language is real language, separate from English, separate from tongue language. It is first language from God, before man talk with mouth.'
>
> He paused to see if I understood his words. He nodded at my comprehending eyes and continued with his powerful hands. 'I see more in one minute, understand more in deaf sign than you hear in speech words. You must wait for words to speak, one after the other, but I see meaning all at once in a face.'[20]

'He was never confused in his own language,' as Ruth Sidransky puts it; and she herself, though a normal speaker of English, always felt more at home using gestural signs. When she translates the tales her parents told her into a kind of broken telegraphic English, it is not because their language was faulty, but in order to convey its concentrated richness and its haunting gestural rhythms. Her own bilingual experience with English and signs has convinced her that exact translation between the two languages is impossible. 'Signs do not transpose to the printed page,' she says, echoing the Abbé de l'Épée himself: 'they are understood only in the flesh, hand to hand, face to face.' Trying to set down her parents' stories in black and white, using 'universal English', she is constantly dissatisfied – never able to 'conjure the magic of my first language', as she puts it, with its 'sentences, liquid, rising not from the human voice but from the human body'.[21]

20 Sidransky, *In Silence*, pp. 256, 20.
21 *In Silence*, p. 3.

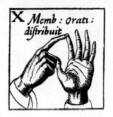

22

Painting the voice

Anyone who watches gestural language fluently used will recognize an enigmatic and unnerving beauty in it – a kind of sublime corporeality, a non-physical physicality, that may well remind you of dancing and the dance. Fluent hearing signers like Ruth Sidransky will often report that they experience gesturing as far more potent than ordinary spoken language: for them, it is essentially connected with love, intimacy and passion rather than the communication of abstract ideas through impersonal grammatical codes. Who can wonder, then, at the bitterness with which the deaf have opposed oralist campaigns to stamp out their language? And who could fail to sympathize with those signers who have angrily turned their backs on every attempt to translate their gestures into speech, and reduce them word-for-sign to the cold, mechanical written form of a primarily spoken language such as English?

On the other hand, the audible utterances of a speaking voice are physical gesticulations too, in their way. They are no less grainy and particular than the signs used by the deaf, and they too can be hauntingly beautiful and erotic. Surely speakers have as much reason as signers to resent the heartless way in which all their tunes and tones, all the rhythms, contours and timbres of their voices, are stripped away and discounted when their utterances come to be written down, offered up to the eye instead of the ear?

Indeed, if writing systems are essentially techniques for making language visible, then speech will presumably suffer more damage from being written down than gestures ever will. A graphic representation of sign language is at least addressed to the same sensory organs as the signs themselves: it is a visible representation of visible facts, whereas ordinary writing makes the inherently implausible promise that it will represent the sounds of speech using a medium which is addressed not to the ear but to the eye. Conventional writing systems may preserve our experience of speech in various ways, but it would seem that they are bound to distort, denature and diminish it as well.

In Plato's *Phaedrus* the relationship between script and speech is compared to that between a portrait and its subject, and the comparison leads Socrates straight to his notorious sermon on the dangers and inconveniences of writing. Texts and paintings are alike, he says, in that they offer the semblance of life instead of the real thing. They cannot speak, and when you ask either of them a question, they remain impassive, and 'preserve a solemn silence'.[1]

The surprise, for modern readers of the *Phaedrus*, is that Socrates does not go on to ask the obvious next question: are some kinds of script more lifelike than others, just as some portraits are? What system of writing, in other words, will give us the least inadequate likeness of the living sounds of speech?

Perhaps it is because the Greek alphabet was still quite new that Socrates, and Plato for that matter, did not apprehend any discrepancy between the writing system at their disposal and the sounds of Greek as they spoke and heard it every day. The script they used was at most four centuries old, having been devised in the ninth century BC, as an adaptation of the Old Phoenician system, which was purely consonantal and had to be augmented with indicators for several vowel sounds before the Greeks could accept it as a means of representing their own language.[2] Later, the Greek alphabet would be adopted by the Romans who altered it once again to accommodate their own very different style of speech. Thus by the time of the Roman Empire different scripts were being applied to different languages: a Greek alphabet for Greek,

1 Plato, *Phaedrus*, translated by Jowett, 275d.
2 See Florian Coulmas, *The Writing Systems of the World*, Oxford, Blackwell, 1989, pp. 162–5.

a Latin alphabet for Latin, and of course further alphabets for Hebrew or Arabic or Persian, not to mention Sanskrit or Chinese. So it was easy to assume that each separate script was perfectly suited to the particular language which it served.

But language inevitably changes from one generation to the next. And habits of speech, being embodied in the transient medium of sound and therefore leaving no permanent trace of themselves, naturally change much faster than corresponding written forms. The ageing sitter no longer resembles the young portrait, and spoken language outgrows its scriptural garments, however perfectly they used to fit. With the decline of the Roman Empire, spoken Latin started to break up into several dialects, diverging in the process from the written language – the Latin that enshrined the principles of law and administration, not to mention the rituals of the Christian church and the canonical word of God. At the beginning of the seventh century, for example, Isidore of Seville noticed that the inhabitants of Italy were substituting /z/ for /d/ in their speech, so that they now pronounced the word *hodie* ('today') as if it were written *ozie*.[3] In the eighth century, officials in the Frankish court began to express alarm at the growing mass of grammatical anomalies in the correspondence of Bishops and Abbots – departures from traditional spelling, incorporations of alien, germanic words, neglect of case-endings, or confusions between feminine singulars and neuter plurals – and Charles (the future Charlemagne) initiated a drastic programme of linguistic repair. From 782 onwards he summoned scholars from England, Ireland, Italy and Spain to join his travelling court, and they came bearing manuscripts to be compared, improved, copied and redistributed, so as to enforce a linguistic 'norm of correctness' throughout Christendom.[4] Latin should henceforth be written in accordance with classical or early Christian models; and conversely, it should be spoken as it was written – *ad litteras*, with each letter distinctly enunciated – so that it would sound as it was presumed to have done five hundred years earlier, before the growth of the new vernaculars.[5]

3 Isidore of Seville, *Etymologiarum sive originum libri xx*, edited by W. M. Lindsay, Oxford, Clarendon Press, 1911, XX, ix, 4.
4 See Josef Fleckenstein, *Die Bildungsreform Karls des Grossen als Verwirklichung der Norma Rectitudinis*, Freiburg-im-Breisgau, 1953, pp. 20–1, 48–9, 75–7, and Judith Herrin, *The Formation of Christendom*, Oxford, Blackwell, 1987, pp. 400–5.
5 See Coulmas, *The Writing Systems of the World*, p. 249.

Literacy in medieval Europe was of course basically literacy in Latin; but the Latin alphabet was also used, on occasion, for transcribing the names of foreign places, people or events, or to make records of debates or agreements transacted in other languages, or to preserve vernacular poetry. But these early non-Latin texts constituted sporadic colonial excursions into the speech-worlds of foreign languages, rather than independent written traditions.[6] Spellings were improvised and in some regions extra characters ('wynn' and 'thorn' for instance) were invented to represent sounds that the Latin alphabet could not express. From the twelfth century on, however, most European languages began to aspire to standardized written forms of their own. New compromises about spelling were devised (novel consonant groups like *wh* and *gh* for example, comparable to the *th*, *ph* and *ch* used in Latin transcriptions of Greek), and readers were also supplied, for the first time, with a systematic collection of non-alphabetic aids: breaks between words, and punctuation marks for grouping words into sentences and clauses, or distinguishing statements from questions – marks which derived from the acute, grave and circumflex accents which marked pitch changes in the notation of Gregorian chant.[7]

But the Latin alphabet itself came under strain as it was forced into the service of several different vernaculars: the same letters were being standardized to different sounds in different languages. The case of English was most notorious. Compromises which may have seemed a good idea in the thirteenth and fourteenth centuries led to spellings which, by the seventeenth, looked decidedly perverse. Words like *plough*, *through*, *thorough*, and *enough* were deeply discouraging for young scholars trying to read and write their mother tongue, and humiliating for foreigners whenever they opened their mouths and started to pronounce English as it was spelt. The eccentricity of the Latin writing-system became even more apparent in the eighteenth century when oriental linguists like Sir William Jones compared it

6 See Dick Leith, *A Social History of English*, London, Routledge, 1983, pp. 7–49.
7 The conventions, first developed in Ireland before the seventh century, and then taken up by Carolingian scribes, were regularized in the twelfth century: see M. B. Parkes, *Pause and Effect: An Introduction to the History of Punctuation in the West*, Aldershot, Scolar Press, 1992, pp. 23–6, 41 ff. On the musical associations of the virgule, the punctum, and the clivis see C. F. Abdy Williams, *The Story of Notation*, pp. 51–8, and Leo Treitler, 'The Early History of Music Writing in the West', *Journal of the American Musicological Society* 35, 1982, pp. 237–79.

systematically with Arabic, Persian and Sanskrit, and demonstrated the extreme difficulty of writing Eastern words in the Western alphabet.[8]

Although there were continuing piecemeal spelling reforms in all European languages, they only exacerbated the problems of the old Latin alphabet. W and U were increasingly distinguished from the Latin V, and I was separated from J, while different values could be given to the same letter by calling again on the old musical accents (acute, grave and circumflex), and instituting new devices like tremas, cedillas and tildes. The resulting modern texts were a horrid mess compared with elegant old Roman inscriptions, and the complexity and international discord were alarming for printers and readers alike. Voltaire recommended urgent action, suggesting for example that the 'double V' used by the Germans should be transposed into a simple 'V-consonant', and their 'O with two dots above it' replaced by a straightforward 'E'. But the English were the worst, he thought: they were 'even more inconsistent – they have perverted all the vowels, and they pronounce them quite differently from all other nations.' A thorough reform of European alphabets was needed, according to Voltaire; after all, he reflected, 'writing is a painting of the voice: and the closer the likeness, the better it will be.'[9]

There were others, however, who believed that the crisis of the Latin alphabet – its variable application to diverse languages, the survival of bizarre, obsolete forms within it, and its vagueness as a means of capturing the particular qualities of a speaking voice – called for more radical changes. Considered as techniques for identifying the sounds of speech, traditional alphabets are, after all, somewhat circular and inconstant. You may chant your A B C with fluent confidence, and agree with all your acquaintances in your pronunciations; but who is to say if you are really getting them right? The whole system of sounds that you share with other speakers of your language could have drifted far away from its origins, but the sounds of the alphabet would have changed along with it, so how would you ever know?

8 William Jones, 'A Dissertation on the Orthography of Asiatick Words in Roman Letters', *Works*, 1799, Vol. 1, pp. 175–228.
9 Voltaire, *Questions sur l'Encyclopédie*, Part 8, 1771, pp. 161–2, s.v. 'Orthographe', reprinted in *Dictionnaire Philosophique*, Paris, Ménard and Desenne, 1827, Vol. 11, pp. 181–2.

The first inquirers to attempt an absolute notation for speech, tied down to invariant standards of sound, were the early oral educators of the deaf. The basic problem that confronted them was to find a way of teaching language to a child who could not take it in 'through the ear'. The obvious solution had been to work through written language addressed to the eye, so they immediately found themselves wrestling with the inadequacies and irrationalities of the received alphabet. Hence Bonet's pioneering *Simplification of the Alphabet and Method of Teaching the Dumb to Speak*, which reduced speech to 21 different letters, each corresponding to a specific configuration of mouth, tongue, teeth and lips. Hence too John Wallis's progression from theoretical investigations of the 'true sound of letters' in the early 1650s, to experiments in training two deaf boys in the 1660s. And hence also the warnings of his rival, William Holder, who noted that the biggest obstacle confronting deaf pupils and their teachers was 'the inconvenience of faulty Alphabets and Usages of writing'.[10]

But these early teachers of the deaf were willing to acknowledge other forms of writing apart from mere scripts, whether traditional or reformed. There were various methods of finger-spelling, for instance, which could be regarded as writing in the sense that they presented language to the eye, even though they did not involve permanent marks on fixed surfaces. And then there was the direct 'seeing of words' on a speaker's face, as described for the first time by Kenelm Digby in 1644.[11] Although many teachers had practical doubts about the idea that (as Dalgarno put it) 'words might be gathered, and read from the transient motions, and configurations, of the mouth . . . as readily as from permanent Characters upon paper', they all accepted that the visible facial movements associated with speech must, in theory at least, be the most perfect, natural and direct kind of writing.[12] Our lips spell out visible letters to the eye just as alphabetic scripts do, but entirely naturally and without reference to variable and artificial conventions. In this sense, speakers are always writing with and on their own faces, albeit in a fleeting script, and, as the Abbé de l'Épée put it, the deaf need only learn this natural alphabet in order to 'hear with their eyes',

10 Juan Pablo Bonet, *Simplification of the Alphabet*, p. 77; John Wallis, *De Loquela* (1653); William Holder, *Elements of Speech* (1669), pp. 133–4.
11 Kenelm Digby *Two Treatises*, pp. 234–5; see above p. 100.
12 George Dalgarono, *Didascalocophus*, p. 32; see above p. 104.

read the lips of others, and even start spelling with their faces just as hearing people do.[13]

Back in the seventeenth century, Francis Mercury van Helmont had argued that alphabetic script originated in pictorial representations of the vocal organs, and this theory continued to attract adherents through the eighteenth century. In 1772, for instance, Charles Davy described the alphabet as fundamentally a 'kind of picture-writing . . . that served to point out sounds instead of things'. Its letters were essentially 'representations' of the 'positions of the organs in their utterance' – the character 'B' for instance a profile of the lips saying the letter 'B' – and that was how it had first been possible to make our 'vocal powers in some measure the objects of our sight as well as hearing'.[14] Sir William Jones was also inclined to favour the opinion – 'entertained by many' – that every alphabetic writing system could be traced back to an ancient method of recording 'rude outlines of the different organs of speech',[15] and the Dutch poet and linguist Willem Bilderdijk applied the theory directly to the modern alphabet: 'M' and 'W', for instance, simply traced the shape of the lips in full face.[16]

But there was no need to embark on speculative etymologies concerning the existing alphabet: a bold inventor could simply abandon it and replace the whole thing with a new system of graphic vocal diagrams. John Wilkins made a start with the table of 'natural Pictures of the Letters' that he casually proposed in 1668.[17] (See Figure 18.) But it was not till the nineteenth century, with the development of mechanical techniques of graphic representation, that the last elements of arbitrariness and convention could finally be eliminated from visible representations of speech. Alexander Graham Bell was still trying to perfect a 'phonautograph' – an automatic sound-writer, intended to

13 Charles-Michel de l'Épée, *Institution*, p. 155; see above, p. 176.
14 Charles Davy, *Conjectural Observations on the Origin and Progress of Alphabetic Writing*, London, 1772, pp. 83, 74, 80.
15 William Jones, 'Discourse on the Hindus' (1786), *Works*, 1799, Vol. 1, pp. 19–34, 27.
16 Willem Bilderdijk, *Van het letterschrift*, Rotterdam, 1820; see Nicholas Rupke, 'Romanticism in the Netherlands', in Roy Porter and Mikulás Teich, *Romanticism in National Context*, Cambridge University Press, 1988, p. 196.
17 John Wilkins, *An Essay Towards a Real Character and a Philosophical Language*, London, 1668, pp. 375, 380. This 'natural character' was not taken very seriously by Wilkins, as he preferred to concentrate on a 'real character', a system of writing which would record the natures of things, not the sounds of words.

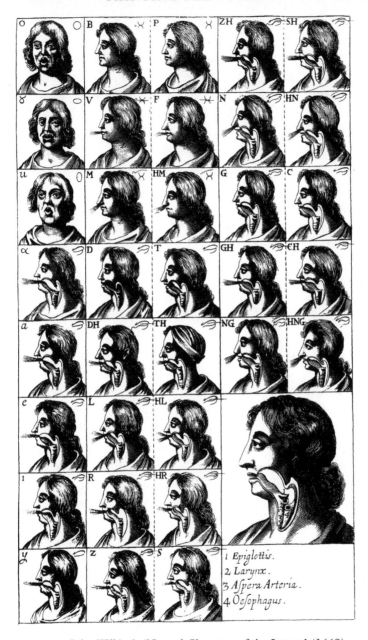

FIG 18. John Wilkins's 'Natural Character of the Letters' (1668)
(Each engraving depicts the configuration of vocal organs required to
produce the sound conventionally represented by the alphabetical
character at the top left; the figure at the top right is a schematic
'picture' of the same configuration.)

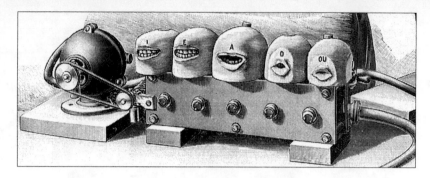

FIG 19. Marage's voice machine, 1908
(Vowel sounds, synthesised by pumping air past rotating perforated discs, are
piped through rubber replicas of real human mouths to reproduce the timbre of
individual voices.)

give deaf children immediate optical feedback on their attempts at articulation – when he turned away to develop methods of synthesizing speech in 1875.[18] That same year, in Paris, a French physiologist called Étienne-Jules Marey, who specialized in designing machines for generating graphic records of variations in pulse rate, blood pressure and other bodily functions, was invited by Léon Vaïsse of the Paris Institution to apply his 'graphic method' to speech, with a view to assisting the education of the deaf. And Marey's laboratory was soon developing techniques of 'optical acoustics' or 'phonetics of the eyes' through which speech sounds could be recorded as undulating lines on sheets of paper, thus giving an enduring 'material expression', as Marey put it, to the 'essentially fugitive phenomena' of sound, which the ear alone could 'never analyse or compare with any certainty'.[19]

During the 1880s, Marey started to develop a new medical technique called 'chronophotography'. He built machines which took high-speed photographs of moving objects at a rate of about fifteen frames a second, and was able to use the results to analyse physiological movements that were too rapid to be followed optically at normal speed. One of Marey's assistants, M. G. Demeny, then took the initiative of applying chronophotography to the analysis of the facial movements associated with speech, so as to produce what he called

18 See Bruce, *Bell*, pp. 110, 121; see also above, p. 222.
19 E. J. Marey, 'Inscription des mouvements phonétiques,' in *La méthode graphique dans les sciences expérimentales*, Paris, Masson, 1878, pp. 390–2.

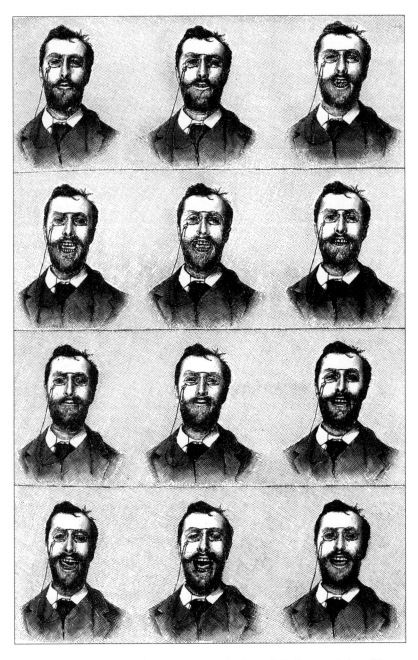

FIG 20. Photography of the voice: 'Vive la France!' in Demeny's 'speaking photographs' (1892)

'photographs of the voice'. The knowledge gained through vocal photography could then be applied to the design of synthetic voice-machines—such as those designed by Marage in 1905, using rubber models of a human mouth—which for a while promised to give more faithful imitations of the human voice than ordinary phonographs. (See Figure 19 page 252.) But more immediately, the technique could be used for speaking directly to the eyes of the deaf. In 1891, Demeny explained how the separate photographs could be attached to the rim of a rotating drum to create an illusion of continuous movement, and reported that deaf students from the Institution in the Rue St Jacques, already adept at 'reading from the mouth', had been able to transfer their lip reading skills directly to the sequences of photographs displayed on his 'phonoscope'.[20] (See Figure 20 page 253.) Photography, he argued, would at last provide a perfect method for 'deaf-mute education through the eyes'.[21]

20 The technique of speech photography played an obvious role in the early development of cinema, as well as permitting increasingly detailed analyses of voice-production, which were followed closely by certain teachers of elocution and singing. See Charles Duffart, 'L'art de la bonne diction et la chronophotographie de la parole', La Nature, Vol. 33, No 1680, 5 August 1905, pp. 145–7.
21 M. G. Demeny, 'La photographie de la voix', La Nature, Vol. 19, No 949, 8 August 1891, p. 158. See also his 'Les photographies parlantes', La Nature, Vol. 20, No 985, 16 April 1892, pp. 311–15.

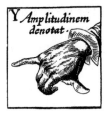

23

Writing and
the analysis of speech

But the old Platonic idea of writing as a picture of the speaking voice did not need to be taken quite so literally. In the last part of the eighteenth century, in fact, and throughout the nineteenth, most linguists were more interested in tinkering with conventional alphabetic scripts to improve their phonetic accuracy than in replacing them with techniques of mechanical transcription such as Demeny's 'photography of the voice' and Marey's 'phonetics of the eyes'.

It was in 1775 that Joshua Steele, an admirer of the London stage, first suggested supplementing ordinary alphabetic script with a five-line musical stave complete with bar lines and time signatures, and sinuous curves to indicate swoops and glides between tones, so that great theatrical declamations could be recorded for posterity 'as accurately . . . as musical compositions'.[1] (See Figure 21 overleaf.) Although the method did not really catch on, Charles Dickens was to experiment with it on occasion, in an attempt to capture the absurdities of parliamentary oratory which would otherwise, as he put it, be 'barely

1 Joshua Steele, *An Essay Towards Establishing the Melody and Measure of Speech to be Expressed and Perpetuated by Peculiar Symbols*, London, Almon, 1775, pp. 14, 28, 40–6. See also David Abercrombie, 'Steele, Monboddo and Garrick', in *Studies in Phonetics and Linguistics*, pp. 35–44.

expressible to the eye'.[2] In addition, the use of musical notation to describe ordinary speech sounds inspired important innovations in musical composition at the beginning of the twentieth century.[3]

But the most popular remedy for the evident shortcomings of the Latin alphabet as a means of depicting speech was simply to extend or modify it. The simplest approach was the one pioneered in John Walker's *Pronouncing Dictionary* of 1791, which attached superscript numerals to the five vowel characters, and used hyphens and apostrophes to indicate rhythmic units. (For instance, *pronunciation* is

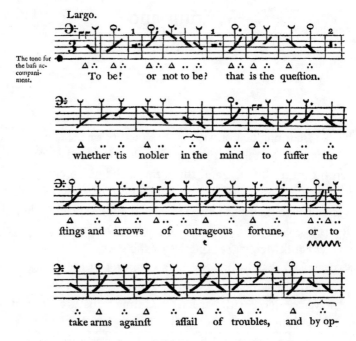

FIG 21. The 'melody and measure' of a Shakespearean performance, recorded by Joshua Steele, 1775

2 Dickens used the stave to satirize parliamentary orators in *Household Words*, 28 June 1851. See Norman Page, *Speech in the English Novel*, second edition, London, Macmillan, 1977, pp. 157–8, where some examples are reproduced.
3 Leoš Janáček's work in particular was closely connected with his experiments in describing speech (including his daughter's dying words) in musical notation: see *Janáček's Uncollected Essays on Music*, edited and translated by Mirka Zemanová, London, Marion Boyars, 1989, pp. 33–61.

noted by Walker as pro[1]-nu[2]n-she[1]-a[1]'shu[2]n and *language* as la[4]ng'gwi[2]dje.)[4]

This unpretentious compromise combined a reasonable exactness of description with relative ease of comprehension, and it was to be imitated in most subsequent pronouncing dictionaries. But many reformers dreamed of more radical improvements in the verisimilitude of written representations of speech, drawing their inspiration from the practice of shorthand – special rapid writing systems, that is to say, suitable both for speedy composition (as in Pepys's diaries) and for recording live speeches, such as sermons or legal and political debates.

Shorthand had been widely used in Europe since the seventeenth century, and was regularly taught in English schools. There were dozens of rival techniques, based on various principles for contracting recurrent groups of letters into single easily-executed graphic marks.[5] In the 1830s, however, an idealistic young schoolmaster called Isaac Pitman, convinced that the Latin alphabet contained 'not one single principle of truth',[6] proposed an entirely new kind of shorthand, in which conventional spelling would be ignored, and 'words . . . written exactly as they are pronounced'. In the system of *Stenographic Sound-Hand*, published in 1837, Pitman gratefully adopted Walker's analysis of English speech sounds, but instead of recording them in an inflected alphabet, he proposed to give 'every sound in the language' a simple mark or 'phonograph' of its own. He believed that this 'system of *Phonetic* shorthand', with its repertory of just over a hundred strokes and loops, would add 'a sevenfold celerity' to the practice of writing. The productivity of authors would be so much improved that they would be able, within the span of an ordinary lifetime, to write bodies of work that would otherwise have taken them at least three hundred years. The art of 'Phonography' was, above all, efficient: 'the plainest practical plan of putting pen to paper for the production of peerless poems or profound and powerful prose for the press or private pursuits,

---

4 John Walker, *A Critical Pronouncing Dictionary and Expositor of the English Language*, London, Robinson, 1791. Walker's key, printed at the head of each page, runs: 'Fa[1]te, fa[2]r, fa[3]11, fa[4]t; – me[1], me[2]t; – pi[1]ne, pi[2]n; – no[1], mo[2]re, no[3]r, no[4]t; – tu[1]be, tu[2]b, bu[3]11; o[3]i[2]1; – po[3]u[3]nd; *th*in, T*H*is.'
5 See Vivian Salmon, *The Works of Francis Lodwick: a Study of his Writings in the Intellectual Context of the Seventeenth Century*, London, Longman, 1972, pp. 60–3.
6 Isaac Pitman, *A Brief Exposition of English Orthography and Phonotypy*, London, 1847, p. 1.

ever published,' Pitman proudly proclaimed.[7] By the end of the nine-teenth century, Pitman's method had been adapted to a dozen different languages, and was established as by far the most popular shorthand system in the world.

Pitman promoted his phonetic shorthand as an 'exact picture' of 'speech itself'.[8] But the elocutionist Alexander Melville Bell was unper-suaded, and responded in 1849 with a proposal for a radically new approach to the 'Science of Universal Alphabetics'. Whereas Pitman's Phonography was based merely on intuitive perceptions of the sounds of English, Bell's radical new script would be grounded in the facts of human vocal physiology, scientifically established with the help of rep-licas of Kempelen's *machine parlante* built by Bell's enthusiastic children.[9]

It was on this experimental foundation that Bell constructed the system of 'self-interpreting physiological letters' known as 'Visible Speech'. By describing the 'actual movements of the organs of speech', Bell's symbols would provide 'invariable marks for every appreciable variety of vocal and articulate sound'. (See Figures 22 and 23.) The new Physiological Alphabet would be immediately intelligible 'to readers of whatever country or tongue', serving to 'represent not merely every language, but every dialect, and even every idiosyncrasy of speech'.[10]

Bell took fifteen years to perfect the notation, and it was, in its way, an outstanding technical success. For instance he could invite foreigners to speak to him in languages he did not know, transcribe the result in Visible Speech, and then summon his son to read the transcript to his guests; and the young Alexander Graham Bell would pronounce the passage flawlessly, like a native. For Visible Speech, unlike Pitman's Phonography, was truly an absolute and universal notation: its letters, as the elder Bell explained, were not so much alphabetic as physiological, and therefore musical and arithmetical too.

7 Isaac Pitman, *Stenographic Sound-Hand*, London, Samuel Bagster, 1837, pp. 1–3, 5, 11; *A Manual of Phonography or, Writing by Sound* (1840), seventh edition, 1845, p. 19.
8 Isaac Pitman, *A Persuasive to the Study and Practice of Phonography or Phonetic Shorthand*, London, Pitman, 1854, p. 5.
9 See Robert V. Bruce, *Bell*, pp. 35–7.
10 Alexander Melville Bell, *Visible Speech: The Science of Universal Alphabetics or Self-Interpreting Physiological Letters, for the writing of all languages in one alphabet*, London, Simpkin, Marshall, 1867, pp. 14, 15, 18.

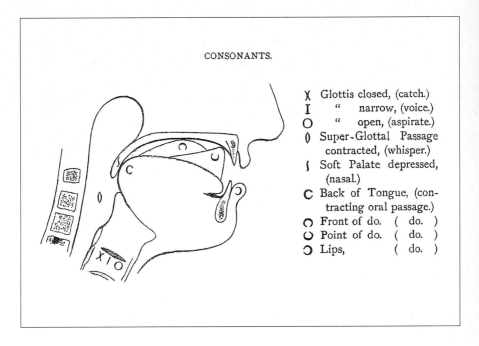

CONSONANTS.

Ɣ Glottis closed, (catch.)
I   "   narrow, (voice.)
O   "   open, (aspirate.)
Ɵ Super‑Glottal Passage contracted, (whisper.)
ʃ Soft Palate depressed, (nasal.)
Ϲ Back of Tongue, (contracting oral passage.)
Ω Front of do.   (do.)
ᴜ Point of do.   (do.)
Ɔ Lips,   (do.)

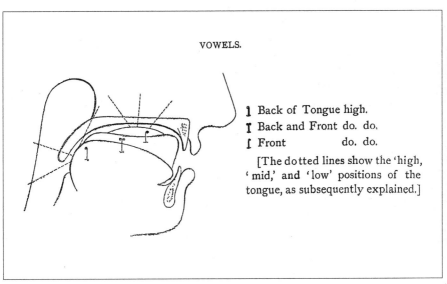

VOWELS.

𝟏 Back of Tongue high.
Ɪ Back and Front do. do.
ᶴ Front   do. do.

[The dotted lines show the 'high,' 'mid,' and 'low' positions of the tongue, as subsequently explained.]

FIG 22. The key to Visible Speech, 1867

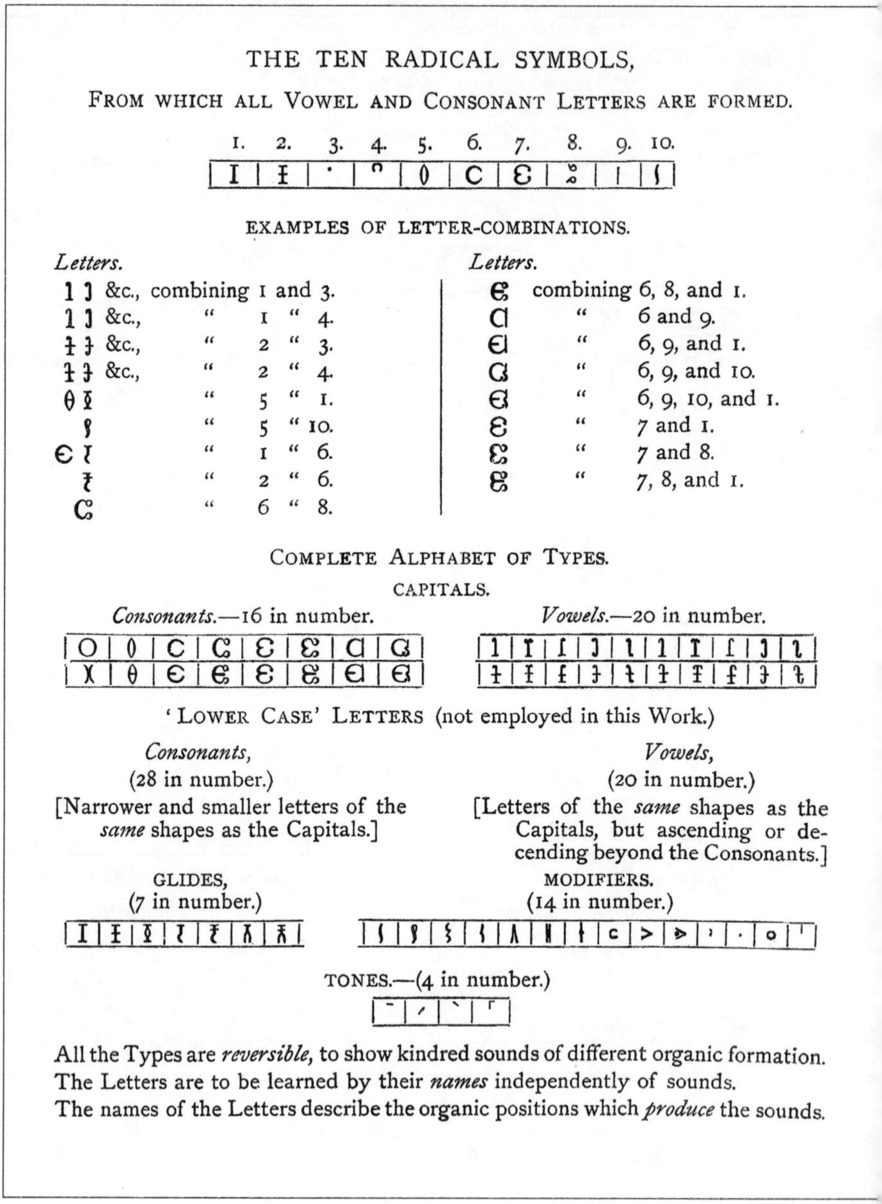

THE TEN RADICAL SYMBOLS,

FROM WHICH ALL VOWEL AND CONSONANT LETTERS ARE FORMED.

I.   2.   3.   4.   5.   6.   7.   8.   9. 10.

EXAMPLES OF LETTER-COMBINATIONS.

Letters.

1] &c., combining I and 3.
1] &c.,   "   I " 4.
‡ ‡ &c.,   "   2 " 3.
‡ ‡ &c.,   "   2 " 4.
θ ɪ   "   5 " I.
ʃ   "   5 " IO.
ɛ ɩ   "   I " 6.
ʒ   "   2 " 6.
Ꮯ   "   6 " 8.

Letters.

ɛ   combining 6, 8, and I.
ɑ   "   6 and 9.
ɘ   "   6, 9, and I.
Ꮐ   "   6, 9, and IO.
ɘ   "   6, 9, IO, and I.
ɛ   "   7 and I.
ɛ   "   7 and 8.
ɛ   "   7, 8, and I.

COMPLETE ALPHABET OF TYPES.

CAPITALS.

Consonants.—16 in number.

Vowels.—20 in number.

'LOWER CASE' LETTERS (not employed in this Work.)

Consonants,
(28 in number.)
[Narrower and smaller letters of the *same* shapes as the Capitals.]

Vowels,
(20 in number.)
[Letters of the *same* shapes as the Capitals, but ascending or decending beyond the Consonants.]

GLIDES,
(7 in number.)

MODIFIERS.
(14 in number.)

TONES.—(4 in number.)

All the Types are *reversible*, to show kindred sounds of different organic formation.
The Letters are to be learned by their *names* independently of sounds.
The names of the Letters describe the organic positions which *produce* the sounds.

FIG 23. The roots of the Organic Alphabet, 1867

'Like musical notes,' he said, 'they have a uniform value in relation to sound in all countries; and like Arabic numerals, they have an absolute value in relation to meaning in all languages.'[11] Traditional alphabets could be used to spell words, whereas Visible Speech – to use a phrase that Bell was fond of – 'spells spelling'.[12]

Bell the elder had hoped that Visible Speech might prove useful for 'teaching articulate speech to the Deaf and Dumb'.[13] But when his son Alexander Graham tried to implement the plan in the late 1860s, his deaf pupils found the notation too difficult, and despite the disappointment it caused his father, he went back to using the ordinary alphabet instead.

The elder Bell had also imagined that his invention could be applied in telegraphy. If operators understood Visible Speech, he thought, and were trained to convert it into telegraphic code, then they could send exact representations of spoken messages down the wire, even if they did not understand the language in which they were expressed. They would 'transmit the *ipsissima verba*, and the very sounds of the original, as a *viva voce* utterance to the receiver', he said.[14] Within a few years, of course, his son had deflated this scheme too, since the telephone was able to meet these requirements with infinitely more efficiency than a Visible Speech telegraph. But despite being overshadowed by his own offspring, Bell could still keep faith with his old ideals. Visible Speech had 'no nationality', and would eventually show the world how to avoid the time-wasting vagaries of traditional alphabets, and thus 'convert the unlettered millions in all countries into readers'. Moreover, by 'macadamizing the linguistic highway between nations', Visible Speech would lead to the 'Linguistic Temple of Human Unity' and thence to a United States of the World, guaranteeing a peaceful future for us all.[15]

Melville Bell published a shorthand version of Visible Speech in 1869, but despite its technical excellence, 'Steno-Phonography' was unable

---

11 Alexander Melville Bell, *Explanatory Lecture on Visible Speech*, London, Simpkin, Marshall, 1870, pp. 3–4.
12 Alexander Melville Bell, *Visible Speech*, pp. 30, 99.
13 Alexander Melville Bell, *Universal Line Writing and Steno-Phonography, on the basis of 'Visible Speech'*, London, Simpkin, Marshall, 1869, p. 1, and *Explanatory Lecture*, p. 4.
14 Alexander Melville Bell, *Visible Speech*, p. 101.
15 Alexander Melville Bell, *Visible Speech*, pp. ix, 21; *Explanatory Lecture*, p. 15.

to compete with Pitman's well-established Phonography. And Visible Speech also suffered from the success of Pitman's other great enterprise: a system of 'Phonotypy' pioneered by his associate Alexander Ellis in the early 1840s. Phonotypy was a pragmatic compromise between the high principles of phonetic shorthand and the abilities of ordinary printers and readers, its phonetic characters being modelled on the Latin alphabet, and capable of being printed by conventional techniques in lines of type, with 43 characters for English, and a further 39 to extend the system to Sanskrit, Greek, German, Dutch, Russian, Persian, Arabic and Hebrew. This scheme was an essential part of Ellis's chosen mission in life: to transform British culture by eradicating all the evils of English spelling or orthography. (The very word 'orthography' was self-incriminating, as Ellis explained, because it could just as well be written *eolotthowghrhoighuay*, by analogy with the spellings found in *George, colonel, Matthew, knowledge, ghost, rheumatic, Beauvoir, laugh,* and *quay.*)[16] He even tried to make phonetic script into a means of popular communication, by publishing Phonotype editions of the classics, and launching a monthly 'jurnal' called the *Fonetic Frend.*[17] (See Figure 24.)

In the early 1870s, these controversies over Universal Alphabetics attracted the attention of George Bernard Shaw, then an office boy in Dublin, and he soon mastered Melville Bell's Visible Speech for himself.[18] Bell had already used his notation to record regional varieties of speech – for example, the different ways in which English numerals were pronounced in London, Teviotdale, Peebles, Midlothian, Dunfermline and Strathbogie. (See Figure 25 page 264.) This opened the young Shaw's eyes to the phonetic inadequacy of alphabetic writing – a defect which, as he was to observe later, 'makes the art of recording speech almost impossible'. The English language, in particular, was 'inaccessible' even to the English, because 'they have nothing to spell it with but an old foreign alphabet'. Having satisfied himself that 'nothing annoys a native speaker of English more than a faithful setting down in phonetic spelling of the sounds he utters', he took to writing English phonetically, rather like Professor Higgins in *Pygmalion*, who

16 Alexander John Ellis, *A Plea for Phonotypy and Phonography, or, Speech-Printing and Speech-Writing*, Bath, Pitman, 1845, pp. 16, 4 fn.
17 Alexander Ellis (Alecsander J. Elis), ed., *Fonetic Frend*, London, 1849–50.
18 Michael Holroyd, *Bernard Shaw*, Vol. 1, p. 54.

Not isheud eedher by dhe Speling Reform Asoasiaishun, or dhe Filolodjicul Soseiety,

Comeunicaishunz respectfuuly solisifed from aul hoo se a copy ov dheez paijez, ritn, if posibl, in dhis Speling, az dhe best meenz ov testing its valew, and adrést too dhe Auther, at 25 Argeil Road, Kenzingtun, W. Aul such comeunicaishunz wil be cairfuuly studid, and prezurvd for feuteur eus, but oaing too dhe Autherz neumerus engaijments, it wil not jéneruly be posibl too send a repley.

DIMIDIUN SPELING
or
HAAF OV WHOT IZ NEEDED.

A SUJESCHUN FOR A SISTEMATIC REVIZHUN OV OUR
PREZENT UNSISTEMATIC ORTHOGRAFY,

Submit·ed too dhe consideraishun ov dhe Speling Reform Asoasiaishun,

DHE FILOLODJICUL SOSEIETY,

AND UDHERZ IN·TERESTED IN EDEUCAISHUN AND FILOLOJY.

By ALECSAANDER JON ELIS, B.A., F.R.S., F.S.A.,

PREZIDENT (FOR DHE SECUND TEIM) OV DHE FILOLODJICUL SOSEIETY,

A Veis-Prezident ov dhe Speling Reform Asoasiaishun,

Felo and formerly wun ov dhe Veis-Prezidents ov dhe Colej ov Presépterz,

AUTHER OV " URLY INGGLISH PRONUNSIAISHUN," " QWON·TITAITIV PRONUNSIAISHUN

Ov Latin," "Ingglish, Deionishiun and· Helenic Pronunsiaishunz ov Greek,"

"PRONUNSIAISHUN FOR SINGERZ,"

" Speech in Song," " Alfabet ov Naiteur," " Esenshulz ov Fonetics," " Reeding Aloud,"

"Dhe Acqwisishun ob Lungglwejez,"

"A PLEE FOR FONETIC SPELING," ETSETERA.

Editer and Propreieter ov " Dhe Fonetic Neuz."

MOTO.

LATIN ((DIMIDIUM FACTI QUI BENE COEPIT HABET)).

Ingglish Latin, Deimidium factey qwey beeny seepit haibet

Ingglish: Wel begu'n Iz haaf dun.

LUNDUN:

F. PITMUN, 20, PAT·ERNOSTER RO, AND DHE AUTHER AZ ABUV·.

Preis Sixpens, poast fre.

FIG 24. Haaf ov whot iz needed: a plea for spelling reform, 1880

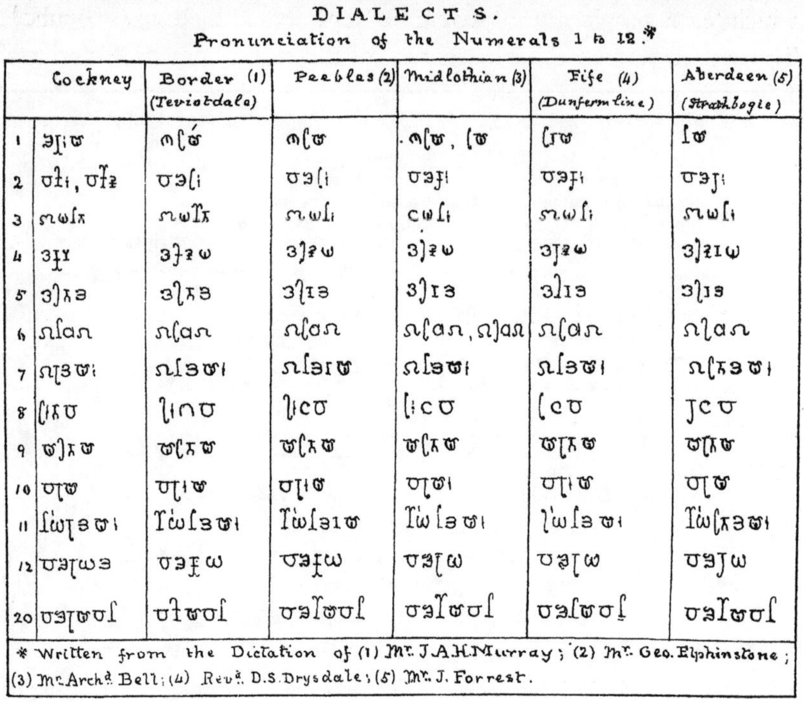

DIALECTS.

Pronunciation of the Numerals 1 to 12.[*]

	Cockney	Border (1) (Teviotdale)	Peebles (2)	Midlothian (3)	Fife (4) (Dunfermline)	Aberdeen (5) (Strathbogie)
1						
2						
3						
4						
5						
6						
7						
8						
9						
10						
11						
12						
20						

[*] Written from the Dictation of (1) Mr. J.A.H. Murray; (2) Mr. Geo. Elphinstone; (3) Mr. Archd. Bell; (4) Revd. D.S. Drysdale; (5) Mr. J. Forrest.

FIG 25. Local pronunciations recorded in Visible Speech, 1867

recorded Eliza Doolittle's 'Lisson Grove lingo' in Bell's Visible Speech.[19]

But Shaw himself soon tired of Bell's notation, and turned to Pitman's shorthand instead, even though he disparaged it as the 'Pitfall system'. At length, however, he accepted that for ordinary purposes a 'complete and exact phonetic script' was quite unnecessary, and a simple enlargement of the traditional alphabet would be sufficient for the representation of English speech.[20]

The same conclusion was reached by James Murray in the work which became the *Oxford English Dictionary*. Murray was an associate of Ellis in the movement for spelling reform, and his Dictionary, which started publication in 1884, was designed to describe 'the living word' (or 'sound cognizable by the ear') by means of a phonetic script in

19 George Bernard Shaw, Notes to *Captain Brassbound's Conversion* (1900), Preface to *Pygmalion*, and *Pygmalion* (1913), in Dan H. Laurence, ed., *Collected Plays with their Prefaces*, London, Bodley Head, Vol. 2, 1971, pp. 421–2; Vol. 4, 1972, pp. 659, 686–7.
20 Preface to *Pygmalion*, *Collected Plays*, Vol. 4, pp. 660–1.

which 'each simple sound' would be 'represented by a single symbol'. The system was an eclectic mixture of the techniques of Walker and Ellis, explained empirically by means of examples. Murray promised that he would shortly tie it down to 'a permanent standard, such as the *Visible Speech* of Mr A. Melville Bell', but it seems he never got round to doing so.[21]

Phonetic notation was then re-launched on a slightly different basis by an organization of French teachers of shorthand and English, founded in Paris in 1886. The aim of the French Phonetic Teachers' Association (or as they wrote it, Dhi Fonètik Tîtcerz' Asòciécion) was to promote phonetic spelling in French schools, and they soon internationalized the cause by forming the Association Phonétique Internationale, also known as the Weltlautschriftverein, or the International Phonetic Association. From 1889 onwards, the Association assumed responsibility for an international standard in phonetic notation, and, while acknowledging the inspiration of Alexander Melville Bell's Visible Speech, they preferred to work with Ellis's Phonotypy, which was more convenient to write and print and considerably easier to learn. In the early years, the Association's journal (*Dhi Fonètik Tîtcer*) concentrated on educational reform through phonography and all the articles, in French, German and English, were written in phonetic notation. (The exceptions were that titles of 'pîryodiklz' and 'buks risîvd' were given in conventional spelling; and, to avoid misunderstandings, subscription rates were given in arabic numerals.) Gradually, however, the movement fell into the hands of historical linguists rather than language teachers. The Association started to regard the International Phonetic Alphabet as an instrument of scientific research, rather than an engine of educational, cultural and political reform, and the journal slowly relaxed its rules and began to publish articles in ordinary spelling.[22]

The collapse of the nineteenth-century infatuation with phonetics –

---

21 J. A. H. Murray, 'General Explanations', in *A New English Dictionary on Historical Principles*, Part One, Oxford, Clarendon Press, 1884, p. xiv.
22 The journal carried articles in phonetic script until 1971. See M. K. C. MacMahon, 'The International Phonetic Association: The First 100 Years', *Journal of the International Phonetic Association*, Vol. 16, 1986, pp. 30–8, and Geoffrey K. Pullum and William A. Ladusaw, *Phonetic Symbol Guide*, Chicago, University of Chicago Press, 1986, pp. xix-xxiv.

the forlorn retreat from magnificent promises of international understanding to humble ancillary tasks in systematic lexicography – was
not a mere historical accident. It was due to an inherent flaw at the
root of the old phonetical dream, a long-hidden theoretical fault in
the very idea of writing as a kind of portraiture, a 'painting of the
voice', a visible manifestation of vocal sound. The mistake did not
become evident until the end of the century, with the formulation of
an entirely different theory of the speaking voice: a genuine scientific
revolution, if ever there was one, which was to drive a wedge between
the old phonetic conception of speech, and a new approach which
would be called *phonology* as opposed to phonetics.[23]

The basic principle of the new phonology was first promulgated by
the Polish linguist Baudouin de Courtenay in 1894. His contention
was that spoken words ought not to be regarded as streams of sound
issuing from an individual speaker's lips, but as sequences of repeatable
abstract sound-types, or *phonemes*. A phoneme, as de Courtenay conceived it, was not an actual noise in the mouth or the ear; rather it
was its 'mental equivalent' in the mind of a speaker or listener. Any
given phoneme – for example the vowel sound at the beginning of
the word 'any' – can be pronounced in a vast range of different ways;
but to grasp the phoneme is not a matter of knowing each of these
possible pronunciations individually, but of understanding their overall
range and how it is defined.

Human voices from around the world are naturally capable of much
the same vocal sounds, as de Courtenay realized; but each different
language selects for itself its own collection of abstract sound-types –
usually around forty or fifty altogether – which will constitute the set
of phonemes out of which all its words will be composed. Phonemes
are thus, as de Courtenay put it, the conventional linguistic targets
which speakers and listeners 'aim at' in a given language: repeatable
phonological units picked out from the flowing stream of vocal sound.[24]

23 Saussure failed to make a clear contrast between the terms *phonetics* and *phonology*; it
was read into his work, rather, by the members of the Linguistic Circle of Prague, which
was formed in 1926. See N. S. Trubetzkoy, *Grundzüge der Phonologie* (1939), translated
as *Principles of Phonology* by Christiane A. M. Baltaxe, Berkeley, University of California
Press, 1969, Introduction, esp. pp. 4, 13.
24 See J. I. N. Baudouin de Courtenay, *Versuch einer Theorie phonetischer Alternationen,
Ein Capitel aus der Psychophonetik*, Strasburg, Trübner, 1895 (translated by the author
from the Polish of 1894), p. 9. See also p. 7 n. 1, where the distinct conception of the
phoneme is attributed to de Courtenay's pupil M. H. Kruszewski.

The most thorough and influential expositions of the new 'phonemic' phonology were given by Ferdinand de Saussure in lecture courses delivered in Geneva from 1906 to 1911 and posthumously edited and published as the *Course in General Linguistics*.[25] Saussure's principal argument was that every language is, first and foremost, a 'system'. Languages are organic rather than atomic; they are not built up out of pre-existing words, in the way a wall is composed of pre-existing bricks. You do not learn first one word, then another, until you have eventually amassed enough to speak the language. On the contrary: you do not know any words at all unless you understand the language to which they belong.

The idea of languages as systems implied, Saussure argued, that speech was something other than mere 'material sound, a purely physical thing'. Speech was cultural rather than natural: it depended, as de Courtenay had already discovered, on laying an artificial grid over the vocal continuum, and partitioning it into a small number of separate, discontinuous areas, corresponding to 'well-differentiated phonemes'. Minute phonetic inquiries were therefore pointless and even 'antilinguistic'. The system or 'gamut' of phonemes was 'the only reality which concerns the linguist', so there was no linguistic purpose in putting real vocal sounds under a phonetic microscope. Phonemes were not 'positive' material entities at all, but 'differential' ones, whose essential property was simply that 'they should not be confused with each other'.[26]

Or, as Edward Sapir was to put it, phonemes create 'definite psychological barriers . . . between various phonetic stations, so that speech ceases to be an expressive flow of sound and becomes a symbolic composition with limited materials or units'.[27] It is like having a system of signalling which depends on displaying either red, yellow or green lights. The exact shades of each colour are irrelevant: the red light can be pink, crimson or scarlet as long as it is clear that it is meant to be

---

25 Ferdinand de Saussure, *Cours de Linguistique générale* (1916), edited by Tullio de Mauro, Paris, Payot, 1972. Confusingly, the original editors of the *Cours* included (pp. 63–95) a text of 1897 which discusses 'phonology' and 'phonemes' in terms which do not harmonize with those adopted by Saussure a few years later. See Leonard Jackson, *The Poverty of Structuralism*, London, Longman, 1991, pp. 49–51, 281–4.
26 Saussure, *Cours de linguistique générale*, pp. 98, 32, 58, 302–3.
27 Edward Sapir, 'Language' (1933), in *Selected Writings*, edited by David G. Mandelbaum, Berkeley and Los Angeles, University of California Press, 1949, pp. 7–32, p. 8.

red rather than yellow or green. And the same applies to the sounds of speech. In Wonderland, when Alice has told the cat what became of the baby, it returns with the question: 'Did you say "pig" or "fig"?' But this is not an inquiry about the precise noises that issued from Alice's lips. In fact when she gives her reply ('I said "pig"') she will probably utter a quite different sound, pronouncing the word with exaggerated distinctness and perhaps some petulance too. Still, she has answered the cat's question correctly, since the purpose of repeating the word was not to reproduce the original shading of her voice, but only to indicate which of two sound-types or phonemes the vital word began with – /p/ or /f/.[28] Speech, the cat knew, is composed of a sequence of linguistic units, not a stream of vocal sounds.

As Saussure realized, the phonemic theory of speech was destined to awaken linguists from their voluptuous dreams of a perfect inter-national spelling system capable of representing the sounds of any language with the last degree of accuracy. It was in the nature of languages, he pointed out, to permit 'latitude of pronunciation'. This tolerance was a linguistic virtue and not a fault, and spelling systems should be designed accordingly. The same phoneme can have innumer-able 'non-distinctive features' or 'allophones' (to use a later terminol-ogy), allowing it to be spoken in any number of different ways without ceasing to be the same phoneme; but what was linguistically significant in speech, and therefore worthy of being written down, was not the prodigious variousness of the phonetic surface, but the austere sim-plicity of the phonemic structure underlying it.[29]

Against the background of the nineteenth-century obsession with phonetic accuracy, the concept of the phoneme stands out as an inspired scientific advance, providing a basis for all the extraordinary achievements of twentieth-century linguistics. In a longer historical perspective, however, the phonological revolution is perhaps a little

28 Lewis Carroll, *Alice's Adventures in Wonderland* (1865), Oxford University Press, 1971, p. 59. As Roman Jakobson put it, 'the feline addressee attempts to recapture a linguistic choice made by the addresser.' See 'Two Aspects of Language and Two Types of Aphasic Disturbances' (1956), in *Language and Literature*, edited by Krystyna Pomorska and Stephen Rudy, Cambridge, Harvard University Press, 1987, pp. 95–114, p. 97.
29 Saussure, *Cours de linguistique générale*, pp. 58, 164, 303; see also Leonard Bloomfield, *Language*, New York, Henry Holt, 1933, p. 77.

disappointing: for what was phonemic phonology, really, except a laborious reinvention of the alphabet – theory catching up with practice, formal science with tacit technique, some twelve thousand years later?[30]

The apparent looseness for which traditional writing systems had so often been reproached was, we might now say, a sign of phonological insight rather than phonetic laxity. The great phonetic transcription systems of the nineteenth century, however successfully they might record the details of a speaking voice, did nothing to remove the risks of linguistic misunderstanding; indeed they greatly magnified them. Readers of books and magazines printed in Phonotype or the International Phonetic Alphabet had terrible difficulty figuring out which words were actually meant, or even what language was being used. And Melville Bell's Visible Speech was equally self-defeating: when he boasted that it could discriminate dozens of different regional pronunciations of the English numerals, he was actually demonstrating its limitations, not its versatility. After all, when you inquire how much something is or how heavy or how large, you are not interested in learning about the differences between local dialects. Bell's efforts to do away with the Latin alphabet only showed how remarkably efficient it is, even in its application to English, as a way of identifying the linguistic units behind the sounds of speech.[31]

It was always misleading, therefore, to regard writing as a 'portrait of the voice'. If written texts are representations of speech, then they are more like abstract plans or architectural designs than exact likenesses. They project what a structure is meant to be, rather than showing how a particular realization of it might appear on an individual occasion. Writing systems, that is, are theoretical conjectures about the structures of the languages they apply to, rather than mechanical records of their audible features. They are hypotheses that attempt to

30 As David Abercrombie put it, 'It may . . . be questioned whether, if *letter* had been retained in something like its traditional functional sense, the need for a phonemic theory would ever have arisen.' See *Studies in Phonetics and Linguistics*, p. 84.
31 See Émile Benveniste, *Problèmes de linguistique générale*, Paris, Gallimard, 1966, p. 24: 'the Latin and Armenian alphabets are admirable examples of what might be called a phonematic notation . . . a modern analyst would find almost nothing to change in them.' As Noam Chomsky and Morris Halle put it, 'conventional orthography is . . . a near optimal system for the lexical representation of English words.' See *The Sound Pattern of English*, New York, Harper and Row, 1968, p. 49.

recapitulate the linguistic perceptions of ordinary users of the language in question, whether or not they can read and write. They set out the discriminations made by all of us when we treat passages of vocal sound as combinations of a small number of repeatable elements, in other words when we perceive them as language. Or, as Rousseau noted long before Saussure, the function of writing is 'not so much to paint speech, as to analyse it'.[32] It was inside this theoretical gap between description and analysis, portraiture and plan, that a new understanding of sign language was eventually able to take shape.

32 Alphabets, according to Rousseau, 'decompose the speaking voice into a number of elementary parts ... out of which all imaginable words and syllables can be formed ... To write in this way is not so much to paint speech, as to analyse it.' See Jean-Jacques Rousseau, *Essai sur l'origine des langues*, p. 57.

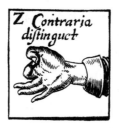

24

Signs and primitive culture

The founders and leaders of nineteenth-century scientific linguistics regarded their discipline as fundamentally historical. Franz Bopp and Jacob Grimm, for example, held that a language consisted not only of sounds and meanings and perhaps a script for recording them; it was also profoundly old and essentially traditional. In learning to speak your first language, therefore, you were not only acquiring a useful communicative skill; you were also joining an institution built up by the patient intelligence of your ancestors over dozens and dozens of generations: you were becoming part of a venerable collective heirloom.

From this point of view, historical etymology was not a quest for curious and amusing antiquities, but a form of intellectual self-knowledge. Thus when the German linguist Max Müller – a pupil of Bopp, translator of Kant, and the first Professor of Comparative Philology at Oxford – traced the links in Greek between *logos* in the sense of 'saying', and *legein,* or the act of 'gathering to-gether', and noted their echo in the Anglo-Germanic notions of *zählen* and *counting* and *telling,* he was aiming not only to record an objective fact about Western languages – that they all presume some kind of connection between speech, intellectual synthesis and the telling of tales – but also to expound an important element of our inherited intellectual constitution, and indeed his own.[1]

The history of our languages was the history of ourselves, therefore; and, as Müller put it, 'the growth of language and the growth of the mind are only two aspects of the same process.' At the same time, the histories of different languages were the histories of the races that spoke them, and national traditions propagated themselves along lines of speech as much as blood. Moreover the linguistic history of the human race was exactly recapitulated in the linguistic development of the individual. At the beginning of history – in the epoch of 'the first poesy of mankind' – linguistic expressions had, Müller surmised, been semantically indistinct and grammatically unstructured, like those of human infants even today. In some parts of the world, especially Europe, this raw material had been 'elaborated by successive generations of rational men' and wrought into those 'inflectional and highly refined languages' which are the medium of Western science and philosophy. Elsewhere, however – in China and Polynesia in particular – language was still stuck at an infantile stage, incapable even of differentiating between a subject and a predicate. It followed, according to Müller, that 'a Chinese child [or a Polynesian] speaks the language of a child, an English child the language of a man'.[2]

What then of the sign language of the 'deaf and dumb'? Müller hardly needed to study the evidence in order to be confirmed in the received opinion. 'There never was an independent array of determinate conceptions,' he claimed, outside the 'articulate sounds' of a historical language, and the maxim *without speech no reason, without reason no speech* was 'one of the fundamental principles of our science'. This implied that schemes for the linguistic education of the deaf were, though kindly conceived, a complete waste of effort. For what did the deaf really learn in deaf schools?

> They are taught to think the thoughts of others, and if they can
> not pronounce their words, they lay hold of these thoughts by
> other signs, and particularly by signs that appeal to their sense
> of sight, in the same manner as words appeal to our sense of
> hearing. These signs, however, are not the signs of things or

1 Max Müller, 'Language and Reason', in *Lectures on the Science of Language*, Second Series, London, Longman, 1864, p. 63.
2 Müller, 'Language and Reason', pp. 84–6, 70.

their conceptions, as words are: they are the signs of signs, just as written language is not an image of our thoughts, but an image of the phonetic embodiment of our thought.[3]

Linguistic training brought no more benefit to the deaf than to parrots: they might imitate, but they could never understand. They would never be able to participate in a great linguistic tradition, and they were therefore irremediably isolated from the intellectual sources of civilization. The signs used by the deaf were orphans, barren listless transients without chronological, cultural or political depth, and they scarcely merited the attention of a scientific linguist.

Except for one thing: might not the linguistic rootlessness of the deaf, and their consequent intellectual backwardness, furnish useful scientific evidence about life in primitive or prehistoric times – about the thinking that preceded thought, the culture that came before civilization, the language that was used before speech?

Studying Sanskrit in Bombay in the 1780s, Sir William Jones was impressed by its similarities to Greek and Latin, and possibly Gothic and Celtic as well. Having pursued his textual inquiries 'upwards, as high as possible, to the earliest authentick records of the human species', he had come to the conclusion that 'no philologer could examine them . . . without believing them all to have sprung from some common source, which, perhaps, no longer exists'.[4]

Jones's hypothesis had profound intellectual consequences. The idea of a single Indo-European linguistic origin – a lost primitive mother-tongue common to East and West – was to upset the traditional cultural geography of Europe, centred on the Mediterranean. And when it was developed by the next generation of comparative linguists (notably Bopp and Grimm), it also opened up chronological vistas in the history of language – and indeed in historical inquiry in general – far vaster than any that had previously been imagined.

The new time-scales of linguistic scholarship gave an extra impetus to European fascination with ancient Egyptian civilization, and especially the 'hieroglyphic' inscriptions which – together with Chinese script – had been regarded by philosophers from Bacon to Vico and Warbur-

3 Müller, 'Language and Reason', pp. 44–84, pp. 69, 62, 75, 69–70.
4 William Jones, 'Discourse on the Hindus' (1786), *Works*, Vol. I, pp. 22, 26.

ton as essentially pictorial, and hence as diametrically different from the alphabetic writing systems of the occident.[5] Jean François Champollion, drawing on sources made available by Napoleon's Egyptian expedition of 1798, managed to identify the language spoken by the ancient Egyptians as a precursor of the Coptic that was still spoken in some parts of the region: the 'extreme antiquity' of Coptic was proved, to Champollion's satisfaction, by the noble simplicity of its grammar, which was 'truly philosophical' and embodied 'the highest perfection to which the mechanism of language can attain'. Champollion then took this conjecture as the basis for a bold new attempt at deciphering Egyptian texts: he would argue that the Egyptian writing system was not pictorial at all, but purely phonetic or alphabetic. 'And this is no paradox,' he added defiantly.[6]

No doubt the Egyptian hieroglyphic characters had originally functioned as schematic pictures of the birds, animals, and other physical objects that they manifestly resembled; but they had then been transformed, according to Champollion, into phonetic characters which represented the initial sound of the object's name in Coptic. With the help of the triple inscription on the large stone which the Egyptologists had taken from the town of Rashid (or 'Rosetta'), Champollion eventually succeeded in matching the apparently pictorial Egyptian symbols to the letters of the Greek alphabet, in what he called a 'series of phonetic hieroglyphs'.[7]

As far as the status of gestural means of communication was concerned, the phonetic interpretation of hieroglyphic script – soon recognized as one of the great scientific triumphs of the age – was in the first instance decidedly unfavourable. For one thing, it tended to discredit the flattering old philosophical speculation that gestures might be the fluent living analogues of ancient Egyptian picture-writing, and therefore of ancient Egyptian wisdom.[8] And at the same time, by pushing

5 See above, chapter 12; see also Martin Bernal, *Black Athena: The Afroasiatic Roots of Classical Civilization*, Vol. 1, London, Free Association Books, 1987, pp. 151–5, 161–88.
6 Jean François Champollion, *L'Egypte sous les Pharaons*, Paris, Didot, 1811, pp. 23–4.
7 Jean François Champollion, *Lettre à M. Dacier relative à l'alphabet des hiéroglyphes phonétiques*, Paris, Didot, 1822, pp. 5, 34.
8 The hypothesis was developed by Bacon, for example, and seconded by Vico, Warburton, and Diderot; see above pp. 122, 132–3, 135.

the origins of speech back beyond Hebrew, Greek, Latin and Sanskrit, it seemed to confirm the relative rootlessness of gestural systems of communication.

There were other ways, however, in which Champollion's solution to the riddle of Egyptian hieroglyphs helped gestural languages to be taken more seriously. Philological scholars could no longer base themselves entirely on the written records of identifiable spoken languages, and they had to rely increasingly on hypothetical constructions to carry them over the gaps in their sources. And in doing so, they found themselves reviving the old philosophical tradition, running from Plato to Rousseau, which postulated that gestural communication, though it had left few traces in historical documents, might nevertheless be supremely ancient, even perhaps the begetter of speech itself.

Ever since the Renaissance, classical scholars (including John Bulwer in England) had been seeking to revive the chironomical or manual rhetoric which had been an integral part of ancient oratorical training, and also to reconstruct the pantomimic elements of Greek and Roman theatre.[9] In Italy at the beginning of the seventeenth century, for instance, Giovanni Bonifaccio set out to vindicate the 'dignity of this most noble and ancient of arts'. Making resourceful use of scant evidence, Bonifaccio speculated on the original classical definitions of many hundreds of gestural signs, maintaining their lasting validity in all fields of human knowledge, from metaphysics and arithmetic to agriculture and hunting.[10]

Such attempts to rediscover the gestural codes of the distant past were inevitably conjectural, but by the end of the eighteenth century inquiries into ancient theatre and oratory could, by employing new models of historical progress, avail themselves of new kinds of evidence. According to Vincenzo Requeno, writing in 1797, the immortal arts of pantomime and *chironomia* must have originated in a set of gestures belonging to the 'extreme rudeness of a most ancient nation'. But he pointed out that infants use gestures before learning to speak; and the same applied, he would presume, to the human race itself in the early stages of its development. 'Nations that are still in a state of savagery,'

9 See above, pp. 125–4.
10 See Giovanni Bonifaccio, *L'Arte de' Cenni*, Vicenza, 1616, esp. pp. 9, 497.

Requeno said, 'are, like little children, in the first infancy of their culture.' So although direct evidence about the signs used in ancient theatre might be sparse, it could be supplemented by reports from travellers in America where, it appeared, the natives were so backward in spoken language that they still had to rely extensively on gestures.[11]

The first systematic dictionary of the hypothetical primitive sign language that preceded the historical origins of speech was published in 1832 by a Neapolitan connoisseur of ancient art called Andrea de Jorio. De Jorio described the manual equivalents of about a hundred words – MONEY, for instance, could be translated into signs in two ways: either 'the tips of the thumb and forefinger rubbed solicitously against each other' or 'the half-closed hand striking against the pocket'. (See Figures 26 and 27.) In establishing his definitions, de Jorio drew on the depiction of gestures in Greek and Roman art, as well as travellers' tales (the use of thumb and forefinger to signify money was attested by missionaries in Canada and Quebec, it seems). But above all he was guided by the local poor: the gesticulations used by uneducated Neapolitans might be despised by refined northerners, but in truth they were 'full of philosophy', almost unspoiled survivals of the pristine gesture language of the ancient Romans and Greeks. Archeologists wishing to decipher classical languages and antique art, according to de Jorio, must start with the gestural signs of the *basso popolo* of Naples.[12]

Champollion's alphabetical interpretation of the Egyptian hieroglyphs might have been expected to put an end to philosophical speculation about Egyptian mysteries, but de Jorio was still attracted by Bacon's comparison between manual gestures and Egyptian pictorial writing.[13] In any case Champollion was now widely regarded as a dangerously radical adherent of Ideology, and his conclusions were being tenaciously opposed by conservative Christians.[14]

One such was a French amateur Egyptologist called Joseph Barrois, whose reverence for the classical world was affronted by Champollion's view that the glory of ancient Greece might be no more than a reflec-

11 Vincenzo Requeno, *Scoperta della chironomia ossia dell'arte di gestire con le mani*, Parma, 1797, pp. 16–17.
12 Andrea de Jorio, *La Mimica degli Antichi investigata nel Gestire Napoletano*, Naples, Fibreno, 1832, pp. 126, vii, xii.
13 *La Mimica degli Antichi*, p. 2.
14 See Martin Bernal, *Black Athena*, Vol. 1, p. 225.

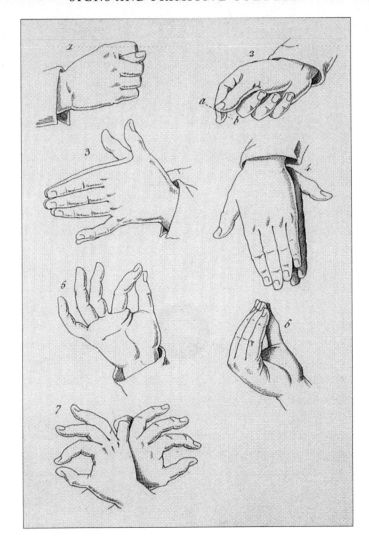

FIG 26. Primitive manual signs used by the Neapolitan poor, 1832
(1. cunt, fuck off (*Mano in Fica*), 2. Cash (*Danaro*), 3. Idiot
(*Stupido*), 4. Idiot (*Stupido*), 5. Love, beg (*Amore, chiedere*), 6. Beg,
Kiss (*Chiedere, Bacio*), 7. Low cunning (*Condotta versipelle*)

tion of the achievements of a still more archaic Egyptian civilization;
still worse, his piety was offended by the implication that Egypt existed
four or even five thousand years before Christ, which took it back
beyond the date to which Christian chronographers, on good scriptural
grounds, assigned the creation of the world.

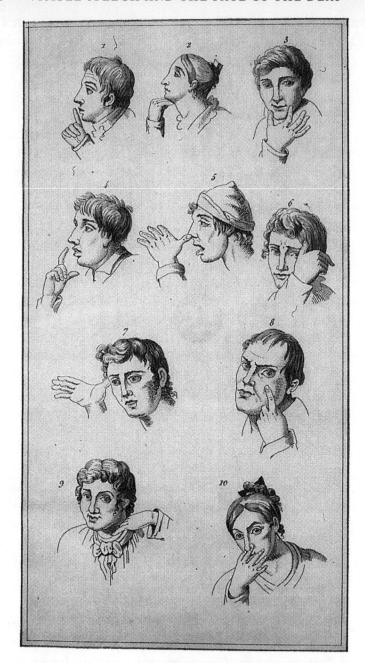

FIG 27. Primitive gestural signs used by the Neapolitan poor, 1832
(1. Silence (*Silenzio*), 2. No (*Negativa*), 3. Prettiness (*Bellezza*), 4.
Hunger (*Fame*), 5. Mockery (*Beffegiare*), 6. Toil (*Fatica*), 7. Fool,
dupe (*Stupido*) 8. Squint, hypocrisy (*Guercio*) 9. Deceive
(*Ingannare*), 10. Clever, crafty (*Astuto*)

Barrois's attacks on the 'ideological interpretations of the egyptologists', published in the 1850s, rested on a claim that all conventional human languages could be traced back to a single source, which he called 'Patriarchal'. Patriarchal was a rough, uninflected and simple means of communication based on just sixteen elementary signs. It was invented by Noah, and adopted by all the people on his ark, so that it was the universal language of mankind between the flood and the construction of the tower of Babel.[15] But Patriarchal was not destroyed in the ensuing catastrophe, merely withdrawn from general circulation, and reserved for the cultivation of sacred wisdom amongst priestly castes.

Patriarchal had been the language not only of the Old Testament prophets, but also of the holy men of ancient China, India, Mexico and Egypt. It then became the model for classical Greek, and for this reason Barrois also referred to it as 'Prohellenic'. Indeed, spoken Prohellenic or Patriarchal was so similar to Greek that, providentially, it was 'already familiar to all those who have had the advantage of a classical education'.[16] The language had remained in use amongst the European priesthood until the Reformation, when, like most other venerable traditions, it was driven out by the twin misfortunes of printing and Protestantism; but Barrois was pleased to find that in India, China and Japan 'the traditional Prohellenic language is still the sacred language of learning to this day'.[17]

Barrois realized that his claims might seem extravagant and implausible; but that, he thought, was only because scholars had overlooked the most striking peculiarity of the Patriarchal or Prohellenic system of communication. Unique amongst languages, it could be expressed in two different primary modes, one audible and vocal, the other visible and manual or 'dactylological'. Each of its sixteen elements could be embodied either in a special sound of the voice, or in a distinctive shape of the hand. The sounds and gestures of the Prohellenic alphabet corresponded to each other one for one and Moses and all the patriarchs had used speech and gesture interchangeably. In Old Testament times, indeed, God himself addressed his people in the gestures of

---

15 Joseph Barrois, *Lecture littérale des hiéroglyphes et des cunéiformes*, Paris, Didot, 1853, pp. ii, 24.
16 Joseph Barrois, *Dactylologie et Langage Primitif restitués d'après les monuments*, Paris, Didot, 1850, pp. 58, 235.
17 Joseph Barrois, *Lecture littérale*, pp. 4–5; *Dactylologie*, p. 70.

Dactylological Prohellenic ('the people saw voices', as it is written in Exodus), leaving it to the prophets to translate his gesticulated commandments into vulgar Hebrew speech.[18]

Barrois surmised that before the rise of the Patriarchal or Prohellenic language – during the seventeen centuries from the first creation to Noah's flood – the only means of human communication had been 'the language of action' or natural pantomime, in which the sounds of the voice played no essential part. But once the gestural and vocal conventions of Patriarchal had been drawn up by the weary Noah on his ark, natural mimic signs were displaced by artificial dactylology, rather like the system 'recently invented' by the Abbé de l'Épée and used thereafter by the deaf-mutes of Paris, Barrois said.[19]

Barrois's contention that the original conventional language of mankind was dactylological as well as phonetic was intended to throw a completely new light on the history of writing systems. The old problem of how visible marks could ever be used to describe audible sounds became irrelevant, since if Barrois was right, the letters of the alphabet were originally just drawings of the sixteen handshapes of Dactylological Prohellenic, which Noah had appointed as the equivalents – or 'protophonetic interpretants' – of the letters of his spoken alphabet.[20] (See Figure 28.) Through a prodigious comparative study of the representation of hands in the art of ancient Egypt, as well as in Greek, Roman, Etruscan, Christian, Indian and Mexican traditions, Barrois was able to identify thousands of examples of protophonetic handshapes, each representing a letter of the alphabet corresponding to the initial sound of a Prohellenic word. With the help of this powerful translation scheme, Barrois induced works of art from every corner of the globe to speak to him 'acrologically' – that is to say by spelling initial letters only – in clear but simple classical Greek. (See Figure 29.)

A method of writing that relied on the portrayal of people with gesturing hands was subject to a severe limitation, however: it was impossible for a normal human figure to express more than two letters

18 *Lecture littérale*, p. 45; *Dactylologie*, pp. 267–8. Barrois refers to Exodus 20:18 in the Vulgate: 'Populus videbat voces.' The Hebrew for *voice* is translated by 'noise' in the Authorised Version.
19 *Dactylologie*, pp. 30, 11.
20 *Dactylologie*, p. 160.

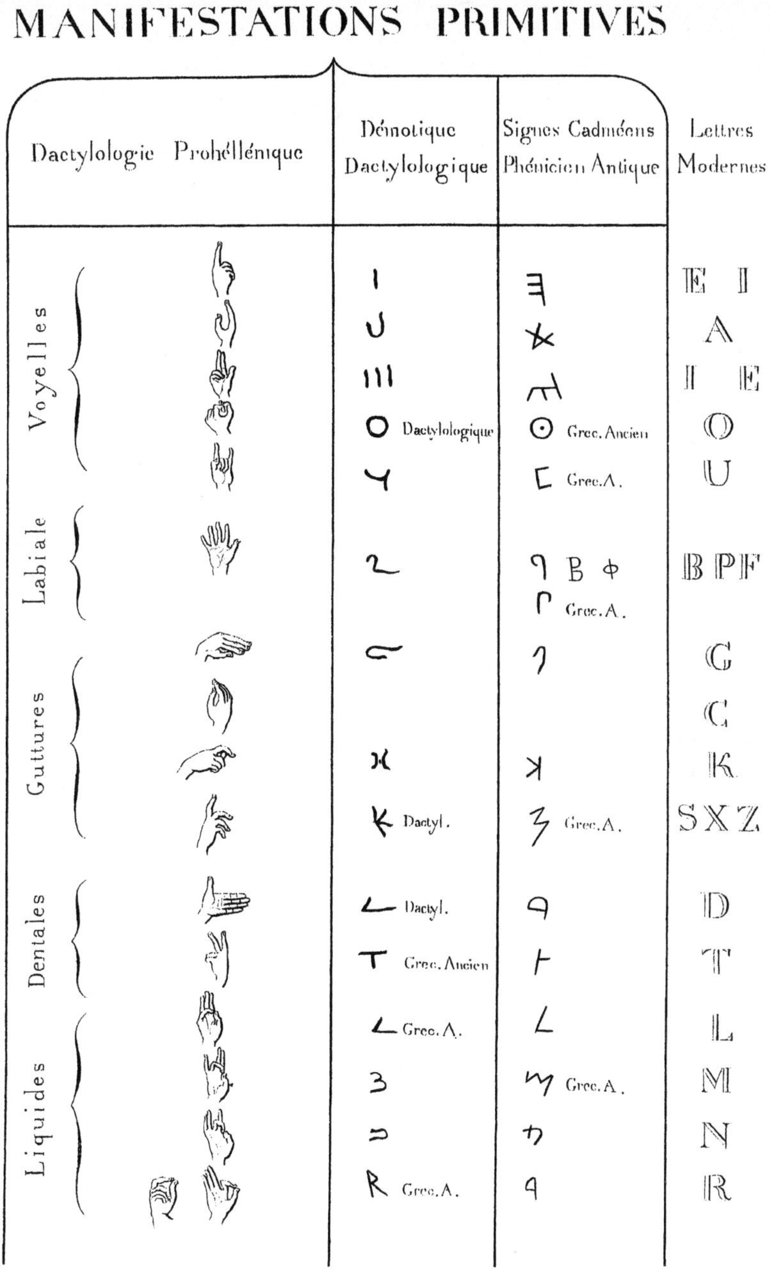

MANIFESTATIONS PRIMITIVES
Dactylologie Prohéllénique
Démotique Dactylologique
Signes Cadméens Phénicien Antique
Lettres Modernes
Voyelles
Labiale
Guttures
Dentales
Liquides
Dactylologique
Grec. Ancien
Grec. A.
Dactyl.
E I
A
I E
O
U
B P F
G
C
K
S X Z
D
T
L
M
N
R

FIG 28. The handshapes of Dactylological Prohellenic and the origins of the alphabet according to Joseph Barrois

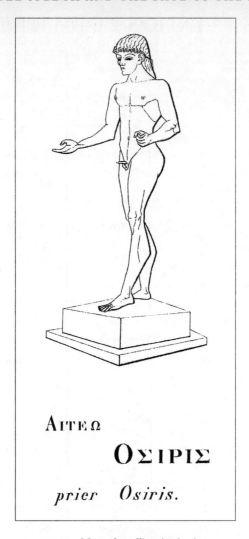

FIG 29. Manual spelling in Ancient
Sculpture (1850)
(Barrois invites us to see an A in the right
hand and an O in the left, forming an
acrological sign for *Aiteo Osiris* – 'Pray to
Osiris'.)

at a time, one with each hand. The technique was exceedingly incon-
venient therefore, if beautifully laconic.[21] No doubt it was for this reason
that the Egyptians had resorted to the hieroglyphic script, in which

21 *Dactylologie*, p. 159.

they depicted objects in order to evoke the initial sounds of their spoken names. (On this particular point Barrois found himself in agreement with the godless Champollion, except that his Egyptians spoke Prohellenic rather than Coptic.)[22]

The other Egyptian writing system, however – the demotic script – represented Prohellenic in its gestural rather than its spoken form: with this writing system ('finger speech in action,' Barrois called it) each character depicted an isolated gesturing hand, detached from any arm or body, which made it possible to write down as many letters as might be desired.[23] Barrois argued that the wedge-shaped marks of Assyrian or cuneiform script were simply alternative ways of drawing the sixteen basic handshapes of Prohellenic dactylology. This stylized form of hand-portraiture was then developed into the Hebrew and Phoenician writing systems, before becoming the fully explicit alphabet of the Greeks, and eventually the Latin alphabet that we still use today – though under the constant misapprehension that it is essentially a means of portraying the sounds of speech, rather than a set of drawings of the manual signs invented by Noah on his ark.[24]

Unfortunately Barrois was always regarded as mad, and his highly original work has failed to find a place amongst the classics of historical linguistics. Still, the task of rehabilitating the history of gesture was soon taken up again, this time by Edward Burnet Tylor, as part of his lifelong quest for a scientific account of what he called 'primitive culture'. Tylor, who later became the first Professor of Anthropology at Oxford University, intended to trace back the roots of 'culture or civilization' far beyond the oldest surviving literary and monumental records – a limit which had hitherto marked the absolute boundary of disciplined historical inquiry. In the light of the new scientific principles of 'evolution', 'development', and 'survival', he thought, anthropologists could now reconstruct the 'pre-history' of human culture not by excavating ancient buried artefacts, but by studying 'modern savage tribes' in far-flung parts of the globe.[25]

22 *Dactylologie*, pp. 235–6.
23 *Dactylologie*, p. 96.
24 Barrois, *Lecture littérale*, pp. 11, 50–52, 78.
25 Edward B. Tylor, *Primitive Culture: Researches into the Development of Mythology, Philosophy, Religion, Art and Custom*, London, John Murray, 1871, Vol. 1, pp. 1, 19; Vol. 2, p. 401.

Tylor believed that the principal instrument of civilization was spoken language. But it was well known that the aboriginal inhabitants of both North and South America communicated by means of gesture as well as speech; indeed, despite their rude savagery, the American Indians were able to execute gestural signs 'better and more easily than the educated man'. The inference was irresistible: the gestures they employed must be 'primitive signs' which had survived intact from 'prehistoric' times.[26]

Tylor was unable to conduct his own fieldwork on American Indians, so he made use of a class of Europeans who had the misfortune to be stuck at much the same stage of cultural evolution. His studies of pupils in 'Deaf and Dumb' schools in Exeter and Berlin confirmed his hypothesis that authentic gestural language is essentially 'a system of representing objects and ideas by a rude outline-gesture, indicating their most striking features'. Within such a system, meanings were more or less self-evident, and 'the relation between idea and sign . . . is scarcely lost sight of for a moment'. Civilized language, in contrast, by deploying grammatical distinctions between parts of speech, together with logical conjunctions and the highly abstract verb 'to be', had developed a vast network of artificial meanings in which the 'connection between word and idea' was greatly attenuated, if not actually broken and effaced. The 'natural grammar and dictionary of the deaf-and-dumb', conversely, was exceedingly restricted: 'horse-black-handsome-trot-canter', Tylor found, would be the literal English translation of the signs used to describe a handsome black horse as it trotted or cantered along: 'the gesture-language,' he concluded, 'has no grammar, properly so-called.'[27]

Tylor was aware, however, that his European deaf-mutes were not absolutely uncontaminated specimens of humanity in its most primitive stage of development. Their teachers, following the Abbé de l'Épée, were constantly trying to 'graft' the grammar and vocabulary of spoken language on to the 'real deaf-and-dumb language of signs', producing 'curious hybrid systems' as a result. But their 'factitious grammatical signs' were not viable in the natural state of gesture-language, and could scarcely withstand even 'the short journey from the schoolroom

---

26 Edward B. Tylor, *Researches into the Early History of Mankind and the Development of Civilisation*, London, John Murray, 1865, p. 21.
27 *Researches into the Early History of Mankind*, pp. 15–16, 24.

to the playground'. Still, he had to admit that it was not always easy to separate 'real gesture language' from alien speech-based elements that 'do not fairly belong to it', and at that point he called his primary researches into primitive sign language to a halt.[28]

But before long the government of the United States took up the burden. In 1877 a Colonel of the US Army named Garrick Mallery was transferred to the Bureau of Ethnology in Washington to co-ordinate research into the languages of American Indians. As a scientific anthropologist, Mallery regarded it as his duty to trace 'all forms of intellectual and social development' back to their original 'common source', and then work forwards again to reconstruct 'the march of mankind out of savagery'. In this perspective, he decided to focus attention on the Indian gesture-system, which, following Tylor, he took to be a 'vestige of the prehistoric epoch', and invaluable evidence of 'a stage of evolution once passed through by our own ancestors'.[29]

Mallery considered that Indian signs were essentially pantomimic – they were 'air-pictures', as he put it, 'of the most striking outline of an object'. And he was even more sanguine than Tylor – not to say credulous – about their power to unlock the secrets of cultural evolution as a whole.

> Gesture-language is, in fact, not only a picture language, but is actual writing, though dissolving and sympathetic, and neither alphabetic nor phonetic . . . This will be more apparent if the motions expressing the most prominent feature, attribute or function of an object are made, or supposed to be made, so as to leave a luminous track impressible to the eye, separate from the members producing it . . . A most interesting result has been obtained in the tentative comparison so far made between the gesture-signs of our Indians and some of the characters in the Chinese, Assyrian, Mexican and Runic alphabets or syllabaries, and also with Egyptian hieroglyphs.[30]

28 *Researches into the Early History of Mankind*, pp. 16, 22–3.
29 Garrick Mallery, *The Gesture Speech of Man*, Cincinnati, American Association for the Advancement of Science, 1881, pp. 3. 17.
30 Garrick Mallery, *Introduction to the Study of Sign Language among the North American Indians as illustrating the Gesture Speech of Mankind*, Washington, Government Printing Office, pp. 13, 14, 4–5. (Apparently Mallery was unaware of the phonetic interpretation of hieroglyphs, or at any rate unconvinced.)

In addition, Mallery confirmed a prediction of Tylor's by reporting that when savage Indians were brought East, to Washington or Pennsylvania, they had 'the greatest pleasure in meeting deaf-mutes', falling straight into eager gestural conversations with them, like compatriots in a foreign land.[31]

On the other hand, Mallery could not agree with Tylor's assumption that pure primitive sign systems are necessarily uniform: they did not constitute 'one language', he claimed, but only a family of overlapping dialects, some of which were mutually unintelligible. It was also possible, Mallery thought, that the same signs had different meanings for men and women: 'signs commonly used to men,' he said, 'are understood by women in a sense so different as to occasion embarrassment.' Gestural signs might in principle be capable of artificiality just as much as spoken words – indeed, he reasoned that since we have many limbs but only one voice, gestures could be a more expeditious means of formulating conventional expressions than speech itself. Thus it would be theoretically possible for gestural communication to acquire grammatical structure and become 'a cultivated art', suitable as a vehicle for abstract and subjective ideas. But – luckily for the scientific anthropologist in search of pure prehistoric cultures – neither the American aboriginals nor the deaf had yet made much progress in that direction.[32]

In short, Mallery said, gesture-language raised a series of profound issues in 'psychologic comparative philology', and progress in resolving them required the collection and collation of vast quantities of further factual information.[33] In the spring and summer of 1880, the Secretary of the Interior was persuaded to place more than one hundred Indians from numerous different tribes 'at the disposal' of Mallery's Bureau. Their speech was recorded phonetically by a team of Pitman-trained steno-phonographers, and their signs minutely described, sketched, and on occasion recorded in photographs. Mallery hurriedly published a 300-page draft report on his findings in the form of a *Collection of Gesture-Signs and Signals of the North American Indians*, covering

31 Garrick Mallery, *Introduction to the Study of Sign Language*, pp. 39–40; *The Gesture Speech of Man*, pp. 14, 22.
32 Garrick Mallery, *The Gesture Speech of Man*, pp. 16–17; *Introduction to the Study of Sign Language*, p. 4. Tylor's conciliatory response to Mallery's criticism is given in a manuscript note bound into the copy of *Introduction to the Study of Sign Language* in the Bodleian Library.
33 Garrick Mallery, *The Gesture Speech of Man*, p. 3.

more than a thousand English headwords, each followed by descriptions of the signs which corresponded to them amongst the Algonkian, Dakotan, Iroquoian, Kaiowan, Kutinean, Panian, Sahaptian, Shoshonian, Tinnean, Wichitan and Zuñian peoples. Where possible, these descriptions were supplemented by reports from investigators 'in the field', as well as accounts of 'deaf-mute natural sign' and 'Italian sign' taken from published sources. A total of nineteen signs are described as being equivalent to the word *man*, for example, including:

> Elevate the extended index before the right cheek, and throw the hand forward, keeping the palm towards the body. (*Dakota VI*)
>
> Place the extended index, pointing upward and forward, before the lower portion of the abdomen. (*Dakota VII*)
>
> *Deaf-mute natural signs.* Put the hands on the legs and draw the hands up, in imitation of the act of putting on a pair of pantaloons.

Or *love*:

> Pantomimic embrace. (*Arapaho I*)
>
> Hug both hands to the bosom as if clasping something affectionately. (*Wichita I*)
>
> *Deaf-mute natural signs.* Kiss your hand and point to the heart, with a happy smile.
>
> *Italian sign.* Place the open hand over the heart.[34]

Mallery's draft report on native American signs is an imposing monument to ethnographic industry, and will always remain the principal source of information on its subject, which was of course in the process of being destroyed faster than it could be recorded. But Mallery was not satisfied: there was an urgent need for further descriptions of these last remnants of primitive linguistic culture; and once all the information had been gathered in, he hoped to publish a 'final collation, in the form of a vocabulary, of all authentic signs, ancient and modern, found in any part of the world'.[35] This would allow the comparative linguists of the future to sit in their libraries and draw up

---

34 Garrick Mallery, *A Collection of Gesture-Signs and Signals of the North American Indians*, Washington, Government Printing Office, 1880, pp. 252–5.
35 *A Collection of Gesture-Signs and Signals*, pp. 7–8.

genealogies for gesture-language similar to those they had already devised for the speech-languages they called 'Indo-European'.

But the fieldwork must come first. Alongside the preliminary publication of his collection of signs, Mallery issued thousands of printed forms, to enable Army and Navy officers of all nations, and missionaries, travellers, and teachers of deaf-mutes, to contribute their observations of gestural signs to the collection at the Washington Bureau. (See Figures 30, 31 and 32.) Within a year Mallery was expressing delight at the scale of the response, and promising that the final compilation would soon be sent to the Government Printing Office. There was a difficult problem though. Reporters were not sending in the right information: their descriptions did not concentrate on pure primitive signs, on 'the radical or essential part as distinct from any individual flourish or mannerism on the one hand, and from a conventional or accidental abbreviation on the other'. They were attributing too much structure to primitive signs, forgetting that language must be 'studied historically' and that the users of signs, as 'living representatives of prehistoric man', were by definition incapable of the complex thoughts or organized sentences found in 'the languages of civilization'. A querulous tone troubles his customary robust mood as he begs his collaborators to concentrate, please, on 'genuine signs alone'.[36]

Colonel Mallery had indeed set himself a difficult task; and each new set of observations received through the post only made it harder. Like the earlier sign-language glossaries of de l'Épée, Sicard, de Gérando or de Jorio, Mallery's projected compilation was, in reality, more like a phrase book than a dictionary. It started with English headwords, that is to say, and then described the corresponding signs, rather than starting with the signs and then defining their meanings and grammatical functions. And the headwords were proliferating uncontrollably, together with the descriptions of signs that followed them. When Mallery was told of several different signs corresponding to the same word, he had to include them all, since he had no way of telling that they might really be different versions – variant pronunciations, so to speak – of what, to the signers, was one and the same sign.

36 Garrick Mallery, *Sign Language among North American Indians compared with that among other peoples and deaf-mutes*, in *First Annual Report of the Bureau of Ethnology, 1879–80*, Washington, Government Printing Office, 1881, pp. 263–552, pp. 269, 330–1, 359, 395, 637.

OUTLINES FOR ARM POSITIONS IN GESTURE-LANGUAGE.

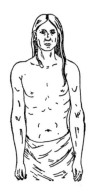
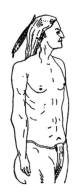

N. B.—The gestures, to be indicated by corrected positions of arms and by dotted lines showing the motion from the initial to the final positions (which are severally marked by an arrow-head and a cross—see sheet of EXAMPLES), will be always shown as they appear to an observer facing the gesturer, the front or side outline, or both, being used as most convenient. The special positions of hands and fingers will be designated by reference to the "TYPES OF HAND POSITIONS." For brevity in the written description, "hand" may be used for "right hand," when that one alone is employed in any particular gesture. In cases where the conception or origin of any sign is not obvious, if it can be ascertained or suggested, a note of that added to the description would be highly acceptable. Associated facial expression or bodily posture which may accentuate or qualify a gesture is necessarily left to the ingenuity of the contributor.

Word or Idea expressed by Sign:..

DESCRIPTION:

....

....

....

....

....

CONCEPTION OR ORIGIN:

....

Tribe:..

Locality:..

....
Observer.

FIG 30. Mallery's Proforma for reporting Primitive Gestural Signs, 1880

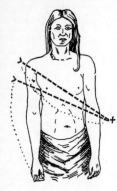

Word or idea expressed by sign: To cut, with an ax.

DESCRIPTION:

With the right hand flattened (X changed to right instead of left), palm upward, move it downward to the left side repeatedly from different elevations, ending each stroke at the same point.

Conception or origin: From the act of felling a tree.

Dotted lines indicate movements to place the hand and arm in position to commence the sign and not forming part of it.

>   Indicates commencement of movement in representing sign, or part of sign.

Dashes indicate the course of hand employed in the sign.

X   Represents the termination of movements.

Used in connection with dashes, shows the course of the latter when not otherwise clearly intelligible.

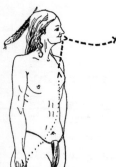

Word or idea expressed by sign: A lie.

DESCRIPTION:

Touch the left breast over the heart, and pass the hand forward from the mouth, the two first fingers only being extended and slightly separated (L, 1—with thumb resting on third finger).

Conception or origin: Double-tongued.

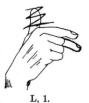

L, 1.

Dotted lines indicate movements to place the hand and arm in position to commence the sign and not forming part of it.

>   Indicates commencement of movement in representing sign, or part of sign.

Dashes indicate the course of hand employed in the sign.

X   Represents the termination of movements.

Used in connection with dashes, shows the course of the latter when not otherwise clearly intelligible.

FIG 31. TO CUT and A LIE from Mallery's field reports on Primiteive Gestures (1880).

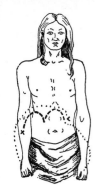

Word or idea expressed by sign: To ride.

DESCRIPTION:

Place the first two fingers of the right hand, thumb extended
(N, 1) downward, astraddle the first two joined and straight fingers of
the left (T, 1), sidewise, to the right, then make several short arched
movements forward with hands so joined.

Conception or origin: The horse mounted and in
motion.

N, 1.

T, 1.

Dotted lines indicate movements to place the hand and arm in position to commence
the sign and not forming part of it.

\> Indicates commencement of movement in representing sign, or part of sign.

Dashes indicate the course of hand employed in the sign.

X Represents the termination of movements.

Used in connection with dashes, shows the course of the latter when not otherwise
clearly intelligible.

FIG 32. TO RIDE from Mallery's field reports on Primitive Gestures (1880).

It was impossible, in short, for Mallery to create a systematic dictionary of signs out of the piles of verbal descriptions, photographs and
drawings sent in by his collaborators in the field. So, in the final phase
of his work, he turned his attention to American Indian paintings, in
the belief that these stylized pictures and designs functioned as a means
to 'fasten upon bark, skins or rocks the evanescent air-pictures of
signs' – in other words, that they might constitute a written notation
depicting gestures in the same way that alphabets depict speech.[37]

Colonel Mallery was mistaken of course: as the phonetic utopians
were discovering for themselves, the purpose of a writing system is
not to paint a portrait of a language, but to offer a theoretical analysis
of it.[38] Moreover the triumphant progress of Indo-European historical
linguistics was obviously based on a corpus of texts written in alphabetic scripts, rather than on impressionistic field-reports about how
people sounded when they spoke. Mallery died 'in harness' in 1893,
having just completed a vast and sumptuous report on Indian picto-

37 Garrick Mallery, *Picture-writing of the American Indians*, in *Tenth Annual Report of
the Bureau of Ethnology, 1888–9*, Washington, Government Printing Office, 1893, pp. 1–
822, p. 637.
38 See above, 269–70.

graphs. But despite all his efforts on behalf of a science of gestural language – and all those labours on classical rhetoric, pantomime, and ancient art, on hieroglyphs and Dactylological Prohellenic, on the signs used in the streets of Naples or in deaf schools round the world – he still lacked the one thing necessary: a method for writing gestures down.[39]

---

39 See D. Jean Umiker-Sebeok and Thomas A. Sebeok, *Aboriginal Sign Languages of the Americas and Australia*, 2 Vols, New York, Plenum Press, 1978, which reprints several doomed attempts to complete Mallery's work.

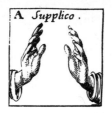

25

Writing signs

It had never been easy to see exactly what a writing system for gestural language was meant to achieve, or what obstacles might stand in its way. In the case of spoken language it had always seemed obvious that the problem was the passage from one sensory domain to another: that a writing system for speech had to transform a stream of audible sounds addressed to the ear into a row of visible marks addressed to the eye. But sign language is already composed of visible gestures, so it presented no such difficulty. Hence it was natural to assume that it could be recorded directly, in straightforward pictorial representations. The chirograms used by Bulwer in the seventeenth century might be too coarse-grained for modern scientific purposes, but two hundred years later they could be replaced by photographs and then, better still, by film. Technology seemed to have finally disposed of the problem of writing signs.

However, a comprehensive collection of photographs and films of gestural activities would not be much use without some method for detecting patterns in them. Rather like forensic scientists with their growing libraries of fingerprints, sign-language investigators felt the need for systems of optical classification which would abstract from the infinite visual variety of their materials and enable them to make the necessary judgements of similarity, difference and identity.

The natural place to seek a prototype for such a system was in

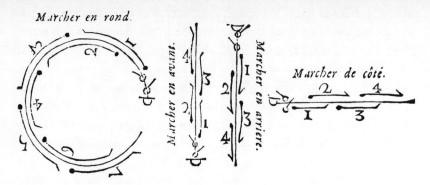

FIG 33. 'Walking by writing': simple steps in Feuillet's track-notation for dance

traditions of theatrical notation. The earliest graphic techniques for recording dance were based on the same principles as maps or architectural plans, providing a bird's-eye-view of a performing area, with an indication of the successive placements of each foot.[1] Raoul Auger Feuillet brought this system of 'track-diagrams' to a kind of perfection in 1700, using different symbols for each of five basic positions and five basic steps, and adding numbers to the diagram so that movements could be correlated with bar-lines in a musical score. (See Figure 33) The object was, as he said, to allow dances to be noted and decoded by dancers in just the same way that melodies were noted and decoded by musicians.[2] The new 'universal Character' for dance would, it was hoped, allow dance-compositions to be safely conserved in print, rather than entrusted to the precarious medium of memory.[3]

This early system of dance-writing did not specify movements of the arms and the rest of the body, however, and it had to be thoroughly reformed before it could be used to record the kind of theatrical dance that flourished in the nineteenth century. But the earliest attempt at a whole-body notation system was designed not for dance but for theatrical and rhetorical speaking. The 'chironomic' method published by Gilbert Austin in 1806 promised 'a language of symbols so simple

1 These 'track-drawings' appear to have been developed first as guides to the new art of 'dressing' horses in the seventeenth century: see William Cavendish, *Méthode et Invention Nouvelle de Dresser les Chevaux*, Antwerp, 1658.
2 Raoul Auger Feuillet, *Chorégraphie ou l'art de décrire la danse, par caractères, figures, et signes démonstratifs*, Paris, 1700, Preface.
3 See John Weaver, *Orchesography or The Art of Dancing by Characters and Demonstrative Figures* (translation of Feuillet, 1700), London, 1706, Dedication.

and so perfect as to . . . represent *every* action of an orator throughout his speech, or of an actor throughout the whole drama, and to record them for posterity, and for repetition and practice'.[4] Austin asked us to imagine a globe of gestural space surrounding the speaker, with letters referring to various points of longitude and latitude on its surface. (See Figure 34 overleaf.) The text of a speech could then be annotated by means of these letters, written either above the line for hands and arms, or below it for feet and legs, to offer a complete specification of all its gestural accompaniments.

But even the most sophisticated systems of notation for bodily movement were unlikely to be of much use in bringing order to the records of primitive gestural signs being amassed by Victorian anthropologists. And the hundreds of signs used by the deaf and their teachers, as described for example by Sicard and de Gérando, were even more intractable. The available notations were simply not schematic enough: they were too close to mere surface portraiture, and too distant from the severe but penetrating analytical abstractions of ordinary alphabetic writing. They would always specify the exact position of a gesturing hand, for example, even though it might be as irrelevant to the identification of a sign as the exact pitch of a voice is to the identification of a spoken word; and at the same time they might be incapable of representing certain small but vital differences that could totally alter a gesture's meaning. As Austin admitted, his notational method was appropriate for 'gesture suited to the illustration and enforcement of language', rather than 'gesture which supersedes its use'.[5] The writing of signs was a difficult matter; and, to make matters worse, it was difficult to see just what the difficulty was.

The young Joseph-Marie de Gérando had tried to dispose of the problem in his celebrated treatise on signs in 1800. His argument turned on the observation that in basic gestural communication 'everything is a painting, and each sign has to function as a picture'. This, he held, meant that the principles of sign language were fundamentally different from those of either speech or writing. In gestural language 'several signs are presented to our sight simultaneously', and this implied that

4 Gilbert Austin, *Chironomia; or a Treatise on Rhetorical Delivery*, London, 1806, pp. 274–5.
5 Gilbert Austin, *Chironomia*, p. 251.

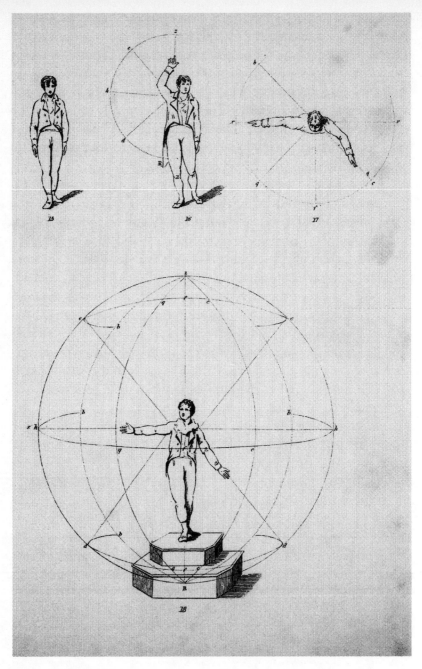

FIG 34. The 'Notation of Gestures' by Austin's Method (1806)

we could never 'stop and pause on any particular one'. Speech, by contrast, 'only ever displays its signs successively,' and 'writing, by giving its signs a lasting existence, allows us to unravel the ideas they represent with all the leisure we could wish.' The instantaneousness of gestural signs meant that there could never be a writing system for them, 'unless one chose to make drawings of gestures, which however would be far too difficult to execute, and take far too much time'.[6]

But this observation about the simultaneity of gestures as opposed to the successiveness of writing did not put an end to the quest for a script for writing signs. Indeed de Gérando himself, after a further quarter-century of experience with the Institution for Deaf Mutes in Paris, surmised that if the deaf were ever to 'unite and constitute themselves as a society' then they would have to devise 'a kind of alphabet' which would enable them to write directly in their own gestural language. However, since he regarded the idea of a 'deaf-mute people' as neither feasible nor desirable, and deprecated the extensive use of signs in the education of the deaf, he was happy to leave the details unexplored.[7]

The first investigator to make a committed assault on the problem of writing gestural signs was Roche-Ambroise Bébian, the embattled advocate of the purity and universality of sign language who had been driven from his post at the Institution in 1821 because of his intransigent opposition to the rising tide of oralism.[8] The essence of signs, according to Bébian, was their natural freedom. Since they were based entirely on innate gestural reactions like laughter and crying, they 'transmitted thought directly', he said, without reference to the kind of arbitrary 'fixed rules' that governed spoken languages. But their natural virtue was in constant danger: naughty deaf children could never resist the temptation of tampering with the perfection of their natural language; and most of the teachers who advocated the use of sign language, such as de l'Épée and Sicard, had inexcusably interfered with its lovely simplicity by subjecting it to alien and artificial grammatical principles drawn from Latin and French.[9]

6 De Gérando, *Des Signes*, Vol. 2, pp. 332, 339; Vol. 4, p. 477. See above, p. 185.
7 De Gérando, *De l'éducation des sourds-muets de naissance*, Vol. 1, pp. 266, 281; Vol. 2, p. 511.
8 See above, p. 204.
9 Roche-Ambroise Bébian, *Essai sur les sourds-muets et sur le langage naturel*, pp. 27, 23–5.

Bébian may have been an ultra-Rousseauist in his view of signs in the state of nature, but he did not subscribe to Rousseau's doctrine that writing was in itself dangerous and unnatural. On the contrary: he believed that the only way to save signs from degeneration was by devising a technique for writing them down. They could then be permanently preserved in print, safe from the corrupting influence of misguided teachers and irresponsible deaf children. Unlike his predecessors, however, Bébian was not attracted by the idea that gestural signs might be analogous to supposedly pictorial writing systems, such as the Egyptian or the Chinese. In any case, as he argued in 1817, the purpose of a script for signs was not to depict gestures in prolific living detail, but to 'classify them and fixate them for purposes of comparison'. The key to the writing of signs, Bébian continued, was to decompose them into combinations of elementary gestures, just as spoken words are analysed, in alphabetic writing, as sequences of elementary sounds. A writing system for signs, accordingly – or what he called a 'mimography' – depended on identifying the small collection of basic gestures which formed 'the material elements that constitute signs', allocating a separate character to each of them, and then writing the characters down 'in the same order as the gestures'. A small stock of mimographic characters should suffice to spell out 'all possible signs', just as the characters of the Latin alphabet could be used to spell out every possible spoken word.

And of course mimography would be an inestimable boon for the oppressed deaf-mute people. The correct form of natural mimic signs would be permanently conserved, and important messages, discourses and works of art in sign language would be preserved in print for future generations, just like the literatures of the other great languages of the world. Furthermore, mimography would enable the educated deaf to work entirely in their own language – to 'express their thoughts on paper immediately, just as clearly as in gestures, if not more so, and without having to translate them into a spoken language first, indeed without even having to know a single word of such a language'.[10]

Bébian's mimographic characters for manual signs fell into two classes, rather like the vowels and consonants of the alphabet. First of all, each

10 Bébian, *Essai*, pp. 27–8.

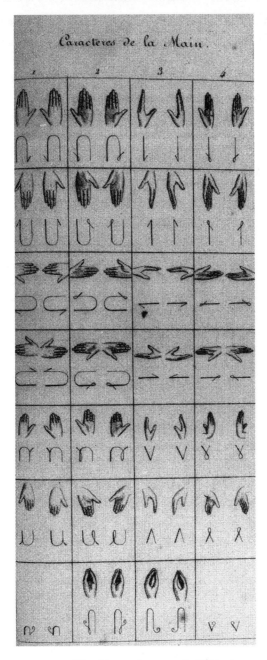

FIG 35. Handshape characters in Bébian's
Mimography, 1825 (Gallaudet University
Archives)

of the basic handshapes would have a character of its own, consisting of a severely stylized drawing. (See Figure 35.) But secondly there would be characters indicating how the hand should be moved: these would take the form of different segments of a circle with arrows indicating direction of movement (resembling a C and a reversed C, or a U and an inverted U), together with six different accents indicating whether the movement was slow or fast, long or short, successive or repetitive.[11] (See Figure 36.)

This was an excellent start; but the more Bébian developed his mimography, the further it diverged from its alphabetical model. The characters of a genuine alphabet are essentially simple, arbitrary, and mutually independent, whereas the arcs with arrows and accents which Bébian used for recording hand movements were descriptive and indeed imitative, more like dance notation than alphabetic writing. What is more, each character in an alphabetic text is meant to represent a temporal segment of the flow of speech, whereas it took a combination of several mimographs to depict a single momentary gesture. And as if that were not enough, Bébian felt obliged to extend the mimographic alphabet to other sites of gestural activity apart from hands and arms. In particular there were facial expressions, which he proposed to record by dividing the face into eight regions, and assigning a differently shaped curve to each. These facial characters would be written either above or below the line representing the sequence of manual gestures, to indicate upward and downward movements respectively, and they would also be associated with either one, two, or three dots to indicate the intensity of emotion they conveyed, whether mild, moderate or extreme.[12] (See Figure 37.)

But while this department of mimography provided a neat notation for 48 different facial expressions, it was not really alphabetic in its principles, so much as musical. And already the mimographic alphabet contained six times as many characters as the Roman alphabet. In 1825, when Bébian published a second account of the system, his invention was clearly beginning to fall apart: the supposed alphabet now designated eighty different shapes of the hand and other parts of the body, for instance. The august Baron de Gérando, while com-

11 Bébian, *Essai*, p. 29.
12 Bébian, *Essai*, p. 34.

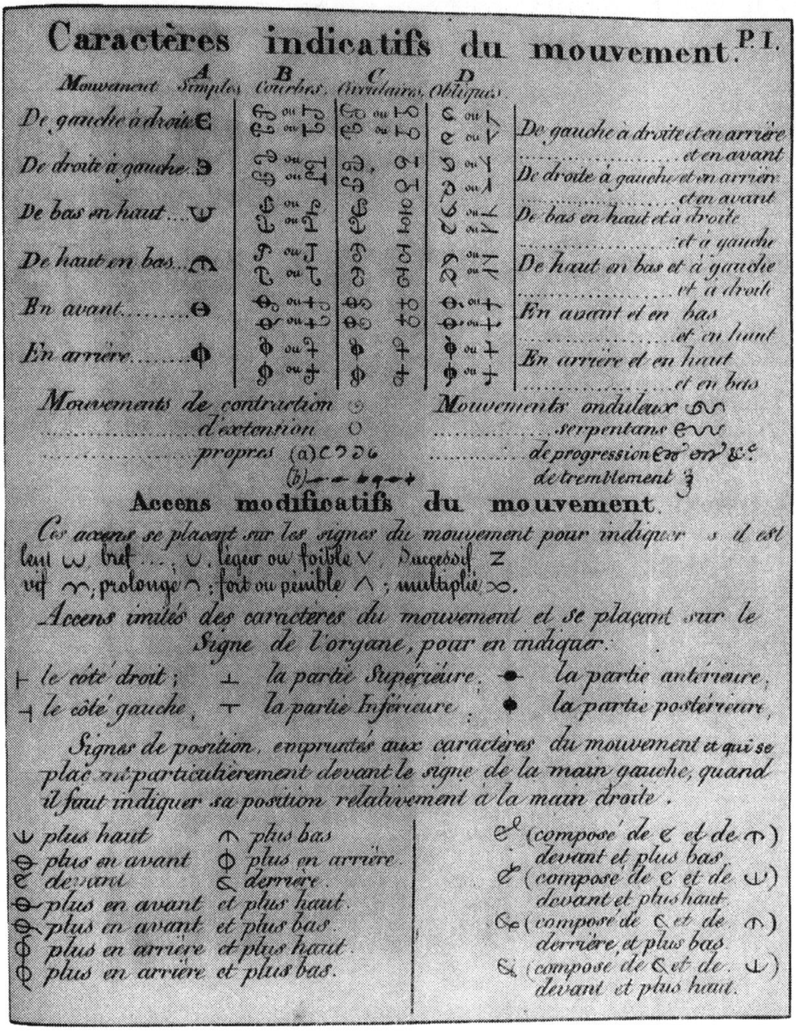

FIG 36. Movement characters in Bébian's
Mimography (Gallaudet University Archives)

mending Bébian's 'judiciousness', concluded that mimography was
really a form of 'drawing rather than writing'.[13] And Bébian's own claim
that the 150 characters of mimography could be mastered by a deaf
signer within 'eight or ten days' had a quality of crazed desperation,
as did his defiant citation of letters of recommendation from the Baron

13 De Gérando, *De l'éducation des sourds-muets de naissance*, Vol. 2, pp. 511, 264–8.

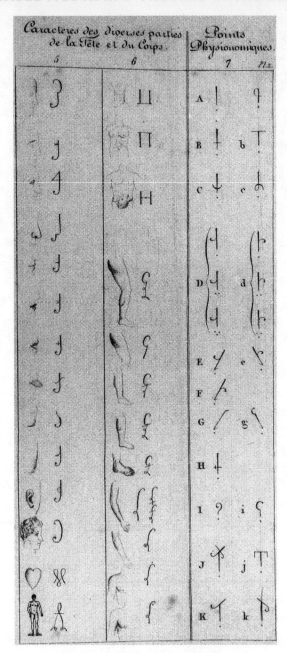

FIG 37. Head, body and face characters in
Bébian's Mimography (Gallaudet University
Archives)

de Gérando and the Institution Royale, from which he had been dismissed four years before.[14]

But although the adherents of the rising oralist orthodoxy were totally opposed to Bébian's practical advocacy of gestural signs, they were not entirely hostile to his theoretical perspectives on sign language. They were willing to agree that genuine mimic signs constituted a universal natural language, based in innate bodily gestures. And they also accepted that a huge gulf separated natural sign language from the artificial spoken languages of the civilized world – though of course they, unlike the growing band of deaf nationalists, concluded that signs are intellectually inferior to words. But even the most militant oralists might grant some place to natural gestural signs in the education of the deaf, at least for conveying a very preliminary outline of meanings to children who had not yet been introduced to a spoken language. And when they considered how signs should be used, they found themselves taking up again where the vanquished gesturalists had left off. Y.-L. Rémi Valade, for instance – an oralist professor at the Paris Institution in the 1850s – agreed with Bébian that sign language 'scorns all artifice, and is based in nature alone'.[15] It was able to 'depict nature directly, and independently of all convention, whereas artifice entered into speech almost at its origin, so that convention always intervenes between spoken words and their objects'.[16] Valade therefore supported Bébian when he criticized de l'Épée and Sicard for trying to turn sign language into 'an exact translation, sign for word, of spoken languages'. Sign language, rightly understood, had 'its own genius, its own laws, forms, and foibles': it had 'a life of its own', whose integrity ought to be respected and not interfered with. Despite his oralist convictions, therefore, Valade resolved to take over the project for a descriptive dictionary of natural sign language which Bébian had abandoned some twenty years before.[17]

Valade was magnanimous towards his predecessor, but confessed

14 Roche-Ambroise Bébian, *Mimographie ou essai d'écriture mimique propre à régulariser le langage des sourds-muets*, pp. 35, 40.
15 Y.-L. Rémi Valade, *Essai sur la grammaire du langage naturel des signes*, Paris, Roret, 1854, p. ix.
16 Y.-L. Rémi Valade, *Études sur la Lexicologie et la Grammaire du langage naturel des signes*, Paris, Ladrange, 1854, p. 64.
17 Valade, *Essai*, pp. vii–x.

that he found the idea of a mimographic script absurd. Bébian's notation was so cumbersome as to be almost unusable; but at the same
time it was not refined enough to distinguish between different signs.
Bébian's real achievement, in fact, was his unintentional demonstration
that mimography was an unrealizable dream, and that signs are not
susceptible to alphabetic analysis after all. The only puzzle was how
he could ever have 'deluded himself to the point of supposing that the
combinations of a small number of characters could ever be sufficient to
represent all possible signs'.[18] Valade's own dictionary of manual signs
(which in the event was never completed) would therefore consist of
a list of French headwords, each followed by a verbal description of the
corresponding natural gestural signs, supplemented where necessary by
'syrmographs', or stylized trace-drawings in which successive moments
in the execution of a sign were superimposed in a single image. Obviously this did not yield a special notation for sign language. But perhaps
no such thing was needed: according to Valade, the best way to record
gestural signs was by translating them and writing down their equivalents in French.

Valade had to acknowledge that sign discourses could never be
reconstructed from such transcriptions in the way that spoken discourses can be reconstituted from written records. But the imperfection was unavoidable, in Valade's opinion. It arose from a difficulty
of principle, which the unlucky Bébian had never anticipated: a problem not of 'nomenclature' (individual signs in isolation) but of 'syntax'
(techniques for linking them up to form statements, questions, or
commands). Now the most basic way of expressing syntactical relations
in spoken languages is, as Valade observed, by simple word order: 'cat
chases mouse' means one thing, 'mouse chases cat' something else.
In the course of the long evolution of civilized speech, however, simple
syntactical word order had almost disappeared owing to the proliferation of passive forms, inflections, and rampant rhetorical licence; and
that, as Valade recalled, was why Diderot had sought the advice of
uninstructed deaf mutes when trying to discover the structures of
original natural syntax.[19]

Valade agreed with Diderot that in a natural language 'ideas would

18 Valade, *Études*, p. 53.
19 See above, p. 135.

proceed in the same order as the facts that they depict': the cause would be mentioned first, then its activity, and then the object affected ('cat chases mouse' for example).[20] But then he noticed a prodigious syntactical divergence between signs and speech. In spoken languages, syntactic relations are expressed by word order, supplemented by inflections and grammatical particles. But sign language had an additional device at its disposal: it could exploit an 'order of disposition' in space as well as the 'order of emission' in time. It was not only that several different signs could be executed in a single instant, for example by using both hands at once, whereas words had to take their turn to be uttered, one after the other; that point was already familiar from the writings of Warburton, Rousseau and de Gérando. What Valade noticed was that the use of space in sign language could itself be extended in time. Meanings could be 'placed' in different locations or directions in an imaginary room or theatre, ready to be picked up again later. Signs could be used, as Valade put it, to 'circumscribe a region within whose limits an action is to be performed', and the significance of subsequent signs would depend on their 'localization' in the space so defined.[21]

According to Valade, the fact that sign syntax depended on spatial as well as temporal ordering – on the principle of the 'double construction' of sign language as he called it – was a necessary consequence of the fact that signs are exclusively visual. Vision, he argued, is essentially spatial and therefore plural: we can look at an animated scene, and see different processes all happening at the same time or moving between different positions within it. Sign language exploited the phenomenon of visible local simultaneity, and speech itself displayed the same features when observed by the eye rather than the ear: those who relied on 'lip reading' were obliged to follow the separate actions of throat, tongue, teeth and lips all at the same time in order to guess at what was being said. But when speech is perceived by the ears of those who can hear, then it takes the form of a single stream of sound which, though infinitely variable, remains 'simple in all its varieties'. The faculty of hearing spins its objects together into a single one-dimensional thread of sound, and it was the special privilege of speech

20 Valade, *Études*, pp. 63–4.
21 *Études*, pp. 127, 136.

to take advantage of this facility. Signs, on the other hand, could only generate a proliferating multitude of visual experiences, and never 'an impression of a different nature ... which could *summarize* them all, in the way that sound summarizes the combinations and the play of the organs of speech'.[22]

And that, according to Valade, was the basic flaw in Bébian's hope that the signing deaf might one day be able to write down their thoughts without first having to translate them into a language based in speech. A signer's gestures, like a speaker's facial movements, strike our eye with an irreducible simultaneous multiplicity; unlike the sounds of speech, they do not form a simple temporal line, which could then be expressed in a single spatial line of writing. Valade suggested that the syntax of signs might be partially represented by writing out words in the order of emission of the corresponding signs, and adding numerical superscripts to indicate their disposition in space: but of course this would only show that gestural signs, unlike spoken words, cannot be properly written down. 'In order for the resemblance to be as great as Bébian thought,' Valade said, 'each gesture or set of gestures would need to have a separate kind of effect on some sense other than vision: taste, for example, or smell.' In that case sign language would have been subjected to the discipline of linear or temporal syntax, and it would have been possible to record it in script. Unfortunately for Bébian, however, our sensory experience was not organized in that way; and the only human languages that could be written down were audible ones.[23]

Rémi Valade was not unaware of the paradoxes in this confrontation with the shade of Bébian. It was the anti-oralist Bébian, after all, who had believed most fervently in the qualitative difference between signs, which he took to be natural and lucid, and words, which he considered artificial and malign. It was Bébian who thought that the deaf were fortunate in being spared the mental deformities inflicted on the hearing by the rigid and unnatural conventions of civilized speech, and who had longed to restore the original natural language of signs. But Bébian's conviction that sign language could be rendered in linear

22 Valade, *Études*, pp. xv, 50.
23 *Études*, p. 50.

mimographic script implicitly slighted the peculiar excellences of signs, by reducing them to the compromises of conventional speech. If Valade had been more of a polemicist, indeed, he could have claimed that it was he and his fellow oralists who – by recognizing that signs are unwritable and 'far more recalcitrant to analysis than spoken words' – were acting in the best interests of natural sign language, and showing the greatest respect for its unique and indomitable spirit.[24]

The oralists might of course experience a twinge of theoretical regret at the thought that the necessities of nature had conspired to make mimographic writing systems impossible. But as de Gérando once observed, there would be little need to write signs down if, as he hoped, the deaf could be persuaded out of their gestures and into spoken languages instead.[25] And Valade went so far as to welcome Bébian's tragic failure. 'I am inclined to consider it a blessing,' he said: 'the deaf are already sufficiently attracted by their visual language, which they all learn without any effort; and if the convenience of writing were to be added to it as well, we would soon be confronted by the extraordinary phenomenon of a society of the dumb coming into existence in the midst of the society of the hearing.'[26]

In reality, of course, a 'society of the dumb' was already being nurtured within oralist schools, where deaf children were happily conversing with each other in signs despite the wrathful opposition of their teachers.[27] But the spontaneous growth of sign language within the newly formed deaf communities, though it appalled the oralists, was not enough to satisfy the deaf nationalists. The gestural systems that were now burgeoning amongst deaf children manifestly lacked the innocent pre-social naturalness imagined by Ferdinand Berthier or Roche-Ambroise Bébian: on the contrary, they flourished on artificial convention, much like the words of a spoken language, and they were teeming with exuberant and idiomatic poetic inventions. Nor were the deaf growing together into a single united nation thanks to the new-found strength of their language of signs. It was no longer plausible to refer to 'sign language' or 'the language of action' in the

24 Valade, *Études*, p. 51.
25 For de Gérando's balanced evaluation of mimography, see *De l'éducation des sourds-muets de naissance*, Vol. 2, p. 511.
26 Valade, *Études*, p. 168. (The term translated as 'visual language' is *langage imagé*.)
27 See above, p. 231.

singular. Gestural signs were evidently not a universal language of nature: sign languages were as arbitrary and diverse as spoken ones. Perhaps the deaf had not escaped the curse of Babel after all.

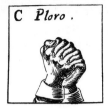

26

The science of Sign Languages

During the 1950s scientific linguists started to use the word 'natural' to distinguish traditional languages like French or Chinese from the 'artificial languages' of logic, mathematics, or computing. This meant that the diverse sign systems of the deaf, which could no longer be regarded as 'natural' in any Rousseauan, universal sense, could be classed as 'natural' in a modern linguistic sense instead. From now on, the primary natural sign languages of the deaf would be sharply separated from artificial 'signed' versions of spoken languages, such as de l'Épee's 'methodical signs', and also from 'secondary' signalling systems used as supplements to spoken languages, for example by Neapolitans or native Americans. Natural sign languages could be accorded the same psychological status as natural spoken languages, and investigated with the same theoretical instruments.

The new approach to sign languages was based on the argument advanced by Saussure fifty years before, that scientific linguistics must concentrate on formulating general principles operating across entire languages, rather than stockpiling miscellaneous historical information about the outward forms of words, meanings and writing systems.[1] It followed, as Saussure emphasized, that as far as linguistics was concerned 'the essence of language' had nothing to do with 'the phonic

1 See above, p. 267.

character of the linguistic sign'. The 'linguistic faculty as such' was indifferent to the 'material element' in which a language was expressed: linguistic systems of signs ranged from 'symbolic rituals' to 'forms of etiquette and military signals', and they could just as well be non-vocal as vocal, visible as audible.[2]

But despite this catholic theoretical programme, Saussure's own inquiries dealt exclusively with speech and alphabetic writing-systems. The only other sign systems he mentioned, in a passing reference, were the handshapes of the 'deaf-mute alphabet'.[3]

This was a massively obtuse suggestion. Saussure must have known that manual spelling is not a separate linguistic system, but only an alternative way of representing the letters of an alphabet. He must have been aware, too, that the deaf were widely credited with a distinct form of communication, consisting of gestures that had nothing to do with spoken or written words; but for some reason he chose to ignore gestural signs completely. Having made the concept of 'signs' the cornerstone of his science of language, Saussure contrived to neglect the language of signs.

The idea that the sign systems of the deaf might be languages in a broadly Saussurean sense was not taken up and carried forward till 1957, when a young hearing teacher at Gallaudet College in Washington began to consider applying the conceptual framework of spoken-language linguistics to the signs used by his deaf students and colleagues.[4] William C. Stokoe's essay on *Sign Language Structure*, which appeared in 1960, proposed a system of 'cherology' that would do for manual signs what phonology had done for spoken words. Stokoe shadowed the phonological distinction between *phonemes* and *allophones* with a cherological distinction between *cheremes* and *allochers*: aspects of an utterance that are linguistically significant as opposed to

---

2 See Ferdinand de Saussure *Cours de linguistique générale*, pp. 21, 164, 26–7, 33.
3 *Cours de linguistique générale*, p. 33.
4 Leonard Bloomfield's influential textbook of 1933 grouped 'deaf-and-dumb language' with the gestures of 'lower-class Neapolitans . . . Trappist monks [and] . . . the Indians of our Western plains', describing them all as either 'derivatives of language', or else mere substitutes for it. (*Language*, pp. 144, 39–40.) Chomsky, too, defined languages as systems of 'sound-meaning correspondences' until his attention was drawn to the problem of sign language in 1967, whereupon he substituted 'signal' for 'sound'. See Noam Chomsky, 'The General Properties of Language', in F. Darley, ed., *Brain Mechanisms Underlying Speech and Language*, New York, Grune and Stratton, 1967, pp. 73–88, p. 85.

those that can vary according to individual whim without affecting its meaning. He then analysed sign languages as devices which artificially select a finite number of 'cheremic' elements from the continuous spectrum of gestural movements, just as spoken languages make their selection of phonemic elements from the infinite array of vocal sounds. The other aspects of signed utterances could then be deemed 'allocheric': of no linguistic consequence, as far as that language was concerned. (In particular, Stokoe and his followers regarded facial expressions as optional or allocheric variations with no linguistic significance.)

Stokoe identified three kinds of chereme: hand positions (the tabula or *tab*), handshapes (the designator or *dez*), and hand movements (the signation or *sig*). All the signs of a gestural language, he argued, could be analysed as various combinations or permutations of these three classes of chereme.[5] From observing the signing of the deaf students and staff around him in Washington, Stokoe concluded that their sign system comprised a total of 55 cheremes. There were twelve *tab* cheremes (positions), nineteen *dez* cheremes (handshapes), and twenty-four *sig* cheremes (movements): 'just fifty-five things visibly unlike all the rest,' he said. He only needed to assign a character to each chereme, and he would have created a writing system for signs. 'The language has never before been written,' as Stokoe put it in the introduction to his *Dictionary of American sign language on Linguistic Principles*, published in 1965; but 'it is written here and can be written because of what we know of its structure'. Any simple sign would be notated by spelling out its *tab*, *dez* and *sig*; complex signs involving combined or successive movements were specified by two *sigs* either in parallel or in series; and those involving two hands, by a *double-dez*. Sign language had become writable at last, and Stokoe's revolutionary dictionary could be seen as the final fulfilment, thanks to de Courtenay and Saussure, of Bébian's dream.[6]

5 William C. Stokoe, *Sign Language Structure: An Outline of the Visual Communication Systems of the American Deaf* (*Studies in Linquistics*, Occasional Paper 8), Buffalo, 1960, pp. 30, 39–40.
6 William C. Stokoe, Dorothy C. Casterline and Carl G. Croneberg, *A Dictionary of American sign language on Linguistic Principles*, Washington, Gallaudet College Press, 1965; second edition, Silver Spring MD., Linstok Press, 1976, pp. vii-x. The magnificent *Dictionary of British Sign Language/English* (edited by David Brien, with an introduction by Mary Brennan, London, Faber and Faber, 1992) is a long-matured tribute to Stokoe's work.

The system of manual signs described and notated by Stokoe was found to be in use thoughout most of the United States and parts of Canada, and in about 1970 it began to be dignified with a fully capitalized name: American Sign Language, or ASL for short. During the following twenty years, investigators using some version of Stokoe's notation identified more than seventy other Sign Languages, from Adomorobe, Algerian, and American, through British, Chinese, Costa Rican and Czech, to Venezuelan and Yugoslavian.[7]

It was now clear that if signing had indeed been linguistically crude in the past, that was only because the deaf had never been given the opportunity to develop it. Most signers would have made their first furtive encounter with their gestural system when they were already past the normal age of first-language learning, and it may be doubted whether a spoken language could have survived at all under such unfavourable conditions. After Stokoe, however, Sign Languages began to lose their stigma, and many more infants were exposed to them from birth, learning to sign in just the same effortless way that children surrounded by speech will learn to talk. Very young signers may in fact be more advanced than very young talkers, since infants can control the movements of their hands more accurately than the sounds of their voices. In any case both groups will pass through the same psycho-linguistic learning stages, in the same order, and at about the same age: even their exploratory games of pre-linguistic echoing and babbling have been shown to be exactly similar in the manual and the vocal modes.[8]

But the attempt to vindicate the primary sign systems of the deaf as natural languages comparable to speech ran into severe opposition; indeed the descendants of Alexander Graham Bell registered their objections to Stokoe's work almost before it had begun.[9] Sign Languages could never be the equal of speech, according to the oralists, not just because of their form and structure, but because of their

7 See Adam Kendon, 'Sign Language, an Overview', in William Bright, ed., *An International Encyclopedia of Linguistics*, New York, Oxford University Press, 1992, Vol. 3, pp. 432–5.
8 See Laura Ann Petitto and Paula F. Marentette, 'Babbling in the Manual Mode: Evidence for the Ontogeny of Language', *Science*, Vol. 251, 22 March 1991, pp. 1493–6.
9 See William C. Stokoe, 'Editorial', in *Sign Language Studies*, Vol. 71, Summer 1991, pp. 99–106.

history. Spoken languages were, amongst other things, treasuries of the thoughts and expressions of the past, and bulwarks of cultural continuity; indeed they might even be regarded as the substance of tradition as such, the basic means by which speaking adults recruit the young into their collective culture. When children acquire Sign Languages, however, they typically learn them from other children, so they cannot be imbibing the distilled wisdom of past generations, matured in a national collective memory. Sign Languages, it seemed, could not commemorate anything except the eternal childishness of the deaf.

Indignant Deaf nationalists, encouraged by the linguistic respectability newly conferred upon signs by the Stokoe notation, retaliated by claiming that Sign Languages too have long and venerable pedigrees: for example, that modern French Sign Language is the same as the system which Bébian took to be the true language of nature, or that the gestures used by the Gostwicke brothers or Lord Downing's servant are direct ancestors of British Sign Language.[10] But such claims are unsustainable and inherently improbable. The linguistic history of signing before the first signed films is so obscure as to be beyond conjecture. Like spoken languages that have become extinct without being written down or mechanically recorded, the gestural systems casually observed by Plato, Montaigne, Descartes, Wallis, Diderot or Dickens are now irretrievably lost. The rare descriptions of signs left by investigators like de Gérando, Bébian or Valade, or by the deaf in their own publications, are sketchy at best, and such evidence as they provide concerns the form of a few hundred isolated individual signs, frozen in a moment of time, and gives no guidance at all to their systematic linguistic function.

The only useful evidence about the history of Sign Languages is indirect. For instance there are numerous similarities between modern French and American Sign Languages, which perhaps go back to Laurent Clerc's journey from Paris to Hartford in 1816; and some of the shared features – for example, aspects of their tense or gender systems – may possibly be due to artificial conventions introduced by the Abbé

10 Harlan Lane, for example, gives the misleading impression that Bébian's concept of 'free natural signs' refers to ASL or French Sign Language (*The Wild Boy of Aveyron*, p. 220); and Peter W. Jackson considers that 'BSL was in common usage . . . by the 1630s' (*Britain's Deaf Heritage*, p. 3).

de l'Épée and derived from the grammar of Latin and French. On the other hand, if it is really true that Clerc was able to communicate in Sign Language with English boys at Dr Watson's asylum in 1815, then they cannot have been using French and British Sign Language respectively, since the two modern systems are unrelated and mutually unintelligible. Asian sign languages are even more mysterious: European philosophers used to imagine that signing would be encouraged in the East, because of its supposed similarity to non-alphabetic scripts, but it would seem that there are no records of indigenous Eastern signing systems, and modern Chinese Sign Language appears to have originated in schools set up by Western missionaries.[11] A historian who wants to investigate the linguistic pedigrees of Sign Languages before the twentieth century is staring into a black hole.

But the problem is not just that Sign Languages have left very little trace of themselves on the historical record. Given the instabilities and discontinuities which afflicted the collective life of the deaf before the creation of permanent institutions of deaf education, and the lack of any workable system of notation for signs before 1960, no Sign Languages were likely to survive more than one or two generations. Indeed children in deaf schools have been observed to invent a completely new Sign Language for themselves in the space of a few years, without any tradition to build on or any assistance from outside.[12] The deaf may indeed have grounds for linguistic pride, but it should be based on the tireless poetic imagination with which they have kept creating new languages out of nothing, rather than on speculative projections of modern Sign Languages on to an unknown linguistic past.

11 See Yau Shun-Chiu, 'Sign Languages in Asia', in R. E. Aster, ed., *The Encyclopedia of Language and Linguistics*, Oxford, Pergamon, 1994, Vol. 7, p. 3921.
12 In the 1980s, the Sandinista government created the first deaf schools in Nicaragua. They were oral institutions, but the pupils quickly improvised an elementary sign system. The language was learned by younger children who joined the school later, and they adapted the language and made it so much more compact that its original inventors could no longer follow it. Thus a handful of children created a Sign Language for themselves, and then transformed it into another, within the space of less than ten years. These findings, reported by J. Kegl, G. A. Iwata and A. M. H. Lopez in 1989–90, are described in Stephen Pinker, *The Language Instinct: the New Science of Language and Mind*, London, Allen Lane, 1994, pp. 36–7. See also Rolf Kuschel, 'The Silent Inventor: the creation of a sign language by the only deaf-mute on a Polynesian island', *Sign Language Studies* 3, October 1973, pp. 1–27.

When Stokoe embarked on his researches into the structures of American Sign Language, many of his signing deaf students and colleagues at Gallaudet College refused to co-operate. They were convinced that their signs signified not as part of a Saussurean linguistic system, but directly, naturally and automatically, in terms of how the gestures 'felt' and what 'picture' they made. They were affronted by Stokoe's presumption that their unique system of communication might yield to the same kind of scientific analysis as conventional spoken language, or that it might ever be stilled by the dead hand of a written script.[13]

But then all of us are inclined to be churlish when linguistic theories are applied to our own knowledge of language. We find it hard to credit the amount of information we had to take in when we learned our first language: whether signers or speakers, we tend to assume that our linguistic knowledge must be very simple, because its acquisition cost us no pains. Speakers are unlikely ever to realize their mistake unless they are exposed to other languages, or to foreigners speaking their own – an experience which has not been available to most signers, since they have typically been confined to one signing community. Moreover they have been constantly encouraged to underestimate their linguistic knowledge by the confident patronage of speakers, who are always impressed by the range of signs (for eating or drinking, for example) whose form gives an unmistakable clue to their meaning. Indeed, speakers often imagine that they need only do a bit of pointing and mimicry in order to become members of a Sign Language community themselves. And before the rise of Sign Language linguistics, signers often accepted this condescension uncomplainingly, agreeing that they should be ashamed of using any gestures that could not be seen as self-explanatory pantomimes.

The iconicity of certain signs may be the first thing that strikes outsiders, but it is a misleading starting point for theoretical inquiries. The signs for 'tree' in American, Chinese and Danish Sign Language all have a manifestly tree-like look to them, for instance; but the signs do not resemble each other much – particularly in the eyes of signers, who pay no more attention to the shapes of their signs than speakers do to the sounds of their words.[14] Even infant signers are unaware of

13 See Carol Padden and Tom Humphries, *Deaf in America*, p. 80.
14 Edward S. Klima and Ursula Bellugi, *The Signs of Language*, Cambridge, Harvard University Press, 1979, p. 21.

the iconic origins of their gestures when they use them as signs. No gesture, for example, could be more obvious and universal than pointing inwards to indicate yourself, and pointing outwards to indicate others. It is hardly surprising, therefore, that the signs for 'me' and 'you' in American Sign Language are based on forms of these pointing gestures. To a signer in ASL, however, their linguistic meaning completely masks their iconic origin. At about twenty-four months, an English-speaking child, having been referred to as 'you', will sometimes over-generalize its limited grammatical knowledge, mistake the pronoun for its own personal name, and call itself 'you' as well. And ASL-signing children of the same age will make exactly the same grammatical mistake, pointing outwards towards their partners when they mean to refer to themselves.[15] The iconic pantomimes of a Sign Language, it seems, exist only in the eye of those who do not understand it.

But scientific research has not entirely supported the view that Sign Languages are structurally exactly similar to spoken ones. In particular some of its findings have confirmed Rémi Valade's opinion that gestural systems are unique in the way they exploit the visible disposition of signs in space. Stokoe himself agreed with Valade in claiming that whereas words are sequences of successive linguistic features, signs involve the production of several different features simultaneously. In his notation, the cheremes of a given sign are always written in the sequence *tab*, *dez* and *sig*, but this does not imply that the signer first indicates a position, then makes a handshape, and finally executes a movement. Unlike phonemes, cheremes do not have to succeed each other in time. In the 1980s, the parallel was partially restored when some of Stokoe's followers – so-called 'Sign Language phonologists' – demonstrated that many signs do in fact comprise successive segments, just like spoken words, even if signers tend to think of them as instantaneous unities rather than articulated sequences.[16]

15 Laura Ann Petitto, ' "Language" in the prelinguistic child', in Frank S. Kessel, ed., *The development of language and of language researchers*, Hillsdale, Erlbaum, 1988, pp. 187–221, pp. 193–4.
16 See Scott K. Liddell, 'Think and Believe: Sequentiality in American Sign Language', *Language* 60, 2, June 1984, pp. 372–99; the argument is taken further in C. A. Padden and D. M. Perlmutter, 'American Sign Language and the Architecture of Phonological Theory', *Natural Language and Linguistic Theory* 5, August 1987, pp. 335–75. See also Edwin G. Pulleyblank, 'The Meaning of Duality of Patterning and its importance in language evolution', *Sign Language Studies* 51, Summer 1986, pp. 101–20.

The problem of assimilating Sign Languages to the temporal formats of speech is even harder in the field of syntax. As Valade had postulated in his doctrine of 'double construction', certain elements of sign syntax are expressed 'in space' rather than 'in time'. Instead of using pronouns like 'he', 'she' or 'it', for instance, or 'the former' and 'the latter', signers can invoke a kind of imaginary table-top spread out in front of them, assign various objects and characters to different locations on it, and re-identify them by indicating those locations once again; or, still more compendiously, they can specify the subject and object of a verb by moving their signing hand between one location and another.[17]

The spatial syntax of Sign Languages is not only a barrier to a fully unified theory of spoken and gestural communication; it is also a grave setback for Bébian's hope that signers may one day have a writing system of their own, comparable to the alphabetic scripts used for speech. The mere fact that signers can make different linguistic signs simultaneously with each hand, and possibly with other parts of the body as well, means that any Sign Language script will have to be written in more than one string of characters – more like polyphony than a single vocal line.[18] Of course signers could adapt their linguistic behaviour, just as speakers sometimes do, to make it more convenient to write down; and they may eventually develop flourishing written traditions of Sign Language poetry, theatre and narrative fiction; but the prospects of establishing an adequate way of writing signs that would be sufficiently simple to enter into general daily use have receded as the science of Sign Language has advanced.

17 The same applies to morphology: 'The modality in which the language develops appears to make a crucial difference in the form of its inflectional patterning: ASL signs undergo simultaneous multidimensional changes, resulting in complex spatial-temporal forms' (Klima and Bellugi, *The Signs of Language*, p. 314). For an excellent survey see Ursula Bellugi, 'The Acquisition of a Spatial Language', in Kessell, *The development of language and of language researchers*, pp. 153–85. See also Elisabeth Engberg-Pedersen, *Space in Danish Sign Language*, Hamburg, Signum, 1993, which includes discussion of the effect of this method of indexing on direct and indirect 'speech' in sign language.
18 In a note to their ambitious revision of Stokoe notation, Liddell and Johnson remark that 'discourse strings must be represented as several simultaneous strings: one for each hand, since each produces segments, and one for each linguistically independent complex of torso, head, and facial behaviours.' See Scott K. Liddell and Robert E. Johnson, 'American Sign Language: the Phonological Base', in *Sign Language Studies* 64, Fall 1989, pp. 195–277, p. 210.

There were further grounds for doubts about Stokoe's revolution. Non-linguistic gesticulations play an obvious role in the communicative behaviour of both speakers and signers. They are used not only for emphasis and rhythm or mimicry and pantomime, but to convey information that cannot easily be put into words – the size of a fish, the shape of a window-frame, or the best method of chopping an onion, for example. But whilst spoken words are easily separated from the gesticulations that accompany them, gestural signs are not. When you make the sign for KISS in ASL, it will be impossible to avoid suggesting what kind of kiss you have in mind, through the location of your sign; when you mention a STREET, the movements and positions of your hands will simultaneously indicate whether it is meant to be straight or twisted, narrow or broad; when you say that something has IMPROVED, you will inevitably imply some particular degree of improvement through the point of contact of your sign.[19] The gestures of Sign Language, it seems, cannot be detached from their articulatory background as easily as spoken words.

In the 1990s this kind of consideration led to an attempted counter-revolution against formal Sign Language linguistics as a whole; and its leader was none other than the original revolutionary, William Stokoe: a fugitive from the camp of victory, a Valade to his own Bébian. Thirty years of scientific collaboration based on his paradigm had convinced him that cherological or phonological analysis was applicable only to languages which exploit the single temporal dimension peculiar to the experience of hearing sounds.[20] 'Visible signs' were 'essentially different from audible signs,' he now said, and therefore incapable in principle of being represented in any kind of script. The idealized and artificial notation that he himself had developed should be discarded, he argued, and replaced by physiological and kinetic descriptions based in video-recordings of real gestures.[21]

The basis of Stokoe's counter-revolution was general and metaphysical rather than scientific and particular. He and his collaborators now objected to 'structural/formalist linguistics' as a whole, especially to

19 See Elizabeth Macken, John Perry, Cathy Haas, 'Richly Grounding Symbols in ASL', *Sign Language Studies* 81, Winter 1993, pp. 375–94, p. 386.
20 William C. Stokoe, 'Semantic Phonology', *Sign Language Studies* 71, Summer 1991, pp. 107–14, p. 113.
21 William C. Stokoe, 'Dictionary Making, Then and Now', *Sign Language Studies* 79, Summer 1993, pp. 128–42, pp. 136, 138–9, 142.

Saussure's conception of languages as systems of 'abstract linguistic units'. Even in its application to spoken languages, Stokoe pointed out, Saussurean formalism presupposed a 'dualistic separation' between linguistic codes on the one hand and bodily activities on the other; and this 'dualism' was not only biologically unjustified, but incompatible with the general facts of evolution.[22]

In a very general way Stokoe may have been right to reject 'dualism'. It is clearly preposterous to expect the world to divide into separate segments, like the two halves of a walnut, just because scientists choose to draw an abstract theoretical line across it. It is undoubtedly artificial to distinguish between words and the vocal sounds of which they are composed, or signs and the gesticulations that make them up. Experience certainly discloses no clear and absolute rift between what is linguistically coded in our communicative activity, and what is merely naturally expressive.

But perhaps Stokoe's doubts about the 'dualism' between abstract linguistic structures and concrete natural expressions were not aimed in quite the right direction. For one thing, they count against attempts to isolate the structures of spoken language as much as those of gestural ones. In any case, the attempt to disentangle artificial linguistic conventions from the expressive wilderness of natural bodily reactions is not the brainchild of 'formalistic' zealots following in the wake of Saussure. It is built into the institution of language itself. Any community which makes use of a system of communicative conventions must ceaselessly try to differentiate between abstract, repeatable linguistic features and their variable concrete forms: a spoken word, for instance, and the innumerable ways it can be pronounced, or a gestural sign and the different styles in which it can be performed. Of course our decisions as to where to draw the line on any particular occasion are based on theoretical judgements, and we are always at risk of getting them wrong: what we take to be an idiosyncratic mannerism of speech or gesture might really indicate a distinct word or sign. But it is a risk we cannot avoid, unless we choose to opt out of linguistic activity altogether. We always have to make a separation between non-language and language, continuum and code, reaction and repetition.

22 David F. Armstrong, William C. Stokoe and Sherman E. Wilcox, *Gesture and the Nature of Language*, Cambridge, Cambridge University Press, 1995, pp. 71, 8, 36.

We have no choice but to be theoretical dualists in our own linguistic practice.[23]

One of Saussure's greatest achievements was the realization that our decisions about where to draw this linguistic line are closely connected with the nature of writing. Every spoken language divides the stream of vocal sounds into a finite number of repeatable elements (phonemes), out of which all its messages will be composed. And writing systems, ideally, supply symbols for each of these elements, or for certain combinations of them, and permit their various possible permutations to be represented in a script. They are neither portraits of the speaking voice, nor arbitrary grids imposed on it from outside; they are attempts to reproduce or anticipate the discriminations that we already have to make in order to pick out a definite linguistic message from a stream of vocal sound. (That is why we often feel insecure about pronouncing an unfamiliar word until we know how it is written, as we can expect the spelling to identify linguistically the essential core of its sound.) Of course, a writing system is never better than a well-founded conjecture as to the elements of the language to which it is applied, and it may always need to be revised; but still the kinds of abstractions it encodes are inherent in linguistic understanding itself: everything that is linguistic must in principle be writable as well.

But Saussure's insight into the connection between language and writing is closely associated with a strange obfuscation. It was 'the central principle of all useful reflections on words', he wrote, that 'the elements which form a word follow one another'.[24] Every element of language was 'auditory in character', and therefore 'unfolds in time alone'. Hence it must represent a one-dimensional extension: in short, 'it is a line'. It was linguistically impossible to 'pronounce two different

---

23 Cf. Kenneth Pike's distinction (derived from the terms *phonemic* and *phonetic*) between 'emic' analyses, which cleave to the distinctions which are significant to 'native participants', and 'etic' or 'physical' analyses, which 'deal only with continua of various kinds without reference to the fact that natives . . . react to that behavior as if it were comprised of discrete particles'. See Kenneth L. Pike, 'Towards a theory of the structure of human behavior' (1956), in *Selected Writings*, edited by Ruth M. Brend, The Hague, Mouton, 1972, pp. 106–16, p. 108.

24 The comment comes from Saussure's notes on anagrams of 1906–9. See Jean Starobinski, *Les mots sous les mots, les anagrammes de Saussure*, Paris, Gallimard, 1971, p. 46, translated by Olivia Emmet as *Words upon Words*, New Haven, Yale University Press, 1979, p. 30.

elements at the same time', Saussure claimed, because words 'are always confined to the line of time; their elements present themselves one by one; they form a chain'.[25]

Saussure regarded the doctrine of the unilinear temporality of language as a 'simple' and 'obvious' truth with 'incalculable implications' for linguistic science; but subsequent developments have shown it to be thoroughly paradoxical and contradictory. In the first place, his insistence on the essential role of temporal succession in language is flatly incompatible with his plea for a science of language that would embrace other systems of signs apart from speech – for example, codes of etiquette and military signalling, both of which make use of simultaneous signs. Secondly, the principle of linearity does not even apply satisfactorily to the sounds of speech.[26] Saussure might be able to analyse spoken messages as temporal sequences of phonemes; but the phonemes can in turn be broken down – as Roman Jakobson demonstrated in detail in the 1940s – into smaller co-occurring types of sound, or 'simultaneous bundles of distinctive features'.[27] An instantaneous slice of spoken sound can contain linguistically significant structure, and – as Jakobson put it – Saussure was clearly mistaken in subscribing to 'the traditional belief in the linear character of language'.[28] There is nothing in the nature of speech to support the idea that language extends itself only along the line of time.

Following Jakobson, Jacques Derrida made the notorious allegation that Saussure's comments on the line of time and the sequentiality of language stem from 'a metaphysical presupposition about the relationship between speech and writing', a 'traditional belief' in the virtuous innocence of time, vocality, and the sense of hearing as contrasted with the menacing threat posed by space, writing, and the sense of sight. Like Rousseau before him, Saussure believed – or so Derrida

25 *Cours de linguistique générale*, pp. 170, 103.
26 Saussure himself acknowledged, however inconsistently, that the successive segments of a word need to be understood partly in terms of their simultaneous 'associative relations'. See *Cours de linguistique générale*, p. 171; see also David Holdcroft, *Saussure: Signs, System and Arbitrariness*, Cambridge, Cambridge University Press, 1991, pp. 56–61.
27 Roman Jakobson, 'On the Relation between Visual and Auditory Signs' (1964, 1973), in *Language in Literature*, pp. 466–73, p. 469. The 'distinctive feature' theory was first proposed in 1942, and published in Roman Jakobson and Morris Halle, *Fundamentals of Language*, The Hague, Mouton, 1956.
28 Roman Jakobson, 'Two Aspects of Language and Two Types of Aphasic Disturbances' (1956), in *Language in Literature*, pp. 95–114, p. 99.

alleged – that writing systems debauch the healthy relationship between the audible voice and subjective meaning by making an obscene visible spectacle of it: writing was an insult to the metaphysical purity of language, 'worse than a theoretical error, worse than a moral fault: a kind of pollution and above all a sin'.[29]

But there are no grounds whatsoever for attributing this fantastic hatred of writing to Saussure. Both in theory and in practice, Saussure's linguistics concentrated – excessively, some would say – on written examples. Of course he would sometimes warn his students against making uncritical use of written texts as evidence about spoken languages, reminding them of two important historical truths: that literacy is usually the monopoly of a social elite, whose biases will affect the kinds of speech that get to be preserved in writing; and that changes in spelling tend to lag behind changes in pronunciation.[30] But these warnings were appeals for caution in the interpretation of documents, not expressions of any irrational prejudice against writing.

If Saussurean linguistics really is deformed by a concealed 'metaphysical presupposition', then the prejudice in question is almost the opposite of what Derrida alleged. For Saussure regarded the principle of linguistic linearity as a matter of ocular not aural proof: it was demonstrated, as he put it, when words 'are represented in writing, with a spatial line of written signs substituted for sequence in time',[31] and this suggests that for Saussure the principle of one-dimensional linearity applies to visible writing more directly than to audible speech. So if Saussure was the victim of a metaphysical prepossession, it was not in favour of speech, still less of temporality, or of sound and the sense of hearing: on the contrary, it was – despite Derrida – on behalf of scripts and the visible linearity of alphabetic writing. And if he was guilty of gratuitous intolerance towards certain forms of communication, it was not directed at writing, or visible or spatial signs in general, but languages which had not yet been reduced to writing: in particular, against the one kind of language which Saussure – together with Derrida, and all the other philosophers of language of the twen-

29 See Jacques Derrida, *De la grammatologie*, Paris, Minuit, 1967, pp. 44, 52–3; English translation by Gayatri Chakravorty Spivak, *Of Grammatology*, Baltimore, Johns Hopkins University Press, 1976, pp. 28, 34–5.
30 Saussure, *Cours de linguistique générale*, pp. 44–54.
31 *Cours de linguistique générale*, p. 103.

tieth century – managed never to acknowledge at all, namely the Sign
Languages of the deaf.

Ironically, the recognition that the gestural communication systems
of the deaf are natural languages with broadly the same structural and
psychological characteristics as any others can itself be traced back to
Saussure's argument that the physical nature of signs has no bearing
on their systematic functioning within a language. After that it slowly
became clear that the pioneers of deaf education – gesturalists as much
as oralists, nationalists as much as integrationists, deaf as much as
hearing – had always been hung up on a metaphysical folly: eternally
returning to a few persistent old assumptions embedded in the folk
metaphysics of the voice, and taking it for granted that the differences
between gestural languages and spoken ones can be deduced from the
difference between vision and hearing, and that they must be somehow
connected to the relationships between writing and speech, space and
time, and simultaneity and succession.

The flaws in all these assumptions should perhaps have been obvious
from ordinary unsystematic observation all along. Signers have always
been able to communicate in the dark by lightly touching each other's
hands, so their comprehension of signs was never exclusively 'visual'.
And the hard-of-hearing have always watched a speaker's face for clues
as to what words are being spoken, so their understanding of speech
was not purely 'auditory'. And words can always be spelled out in an
audible or tangible alphabet instead of a visible one, so writing itself
cannot be essentially a visual medium. The sense of hearing, moreover,
has never been confined to sequences of simple sensations strung out
one after another along the 'line of time'. As every child knows, and
every musician too, the ear can perceive thousands of different sounds
at the same time: vision is not the only sense that is responsive to
simultaneous complexity. Nor does it have a monopoly in spatial apprehension: distances are perceived by touch as well as vision, and they
can also be explored by the sense of hearing. And finally, the distinction
between succession and simultaneity does not correspond to the difference between time and space; nor can either of them be mapped on
to the distinction between hearing and vision, or speech and writing,
or vocal language and the language of signs. The idea that there is a
metaphysical gulf dividing communication by visible gestures from

communication by audible words, in short, is a fantasy without foundation, a hallucination rather than a theory. But still it is sufficiently
convincing to have caused countless generations of deaf people to be
condemned to lives of pointless suffering, at least until it was eventually
dispelled – if it has been – by the hesitant and wavering progress of
twentieth-century linguistics.

It is always hard, looking back, to understand how the journey that
led to what we presently regard as the commanding heights of scientific
knowledge could have been so tortuous and perplexing, and why it
took so long. But the obstacles that blocked the way to an adequate
theory of the linguistic capacities of the deaf were not just a few
scattered errors that could be quickly identified and then cleared away.
They belong not only to the history of science, but also to the history
of metaphysics on the one hand, and the history of philosophy on the
other. Our attitudes to Sign Languages have been constructed out of
commonsense interpretations of experience and the five senses; and
when our delusions are part of our habitual interpretation of ourselves,
we can become as attached to them as to our finest truths.

THREE

THE SENSES AND THE SELF

A history of philosophy

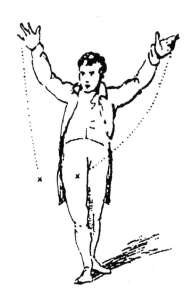

We can never escape our own metaphysical imaginations. On the other hand, the story of the deaf and their relationship to speech and writing has thoroughly discredited our folk metaphysical doctrines about the voice, the five senses, and space and time: experience refuting our metaphysics, and history teaching us philosophy by examples.

The tale of the scientific vindication of sign languages is echoed in the development of philosophy itself. The History of Philosophy suggests, indeed, that the theory of the five senses – or 'aesthetic theory' in the general sense of the phrase – has always been the main issue preoccupying and dividing the philosophers. From Plato and Aristotle on, it seems, they have all been trying to work out the nature of sensory experience (or *aisthêsis*), its relation to the 'inner' faculties of reason, memory and imagination, and its place in human knowledge.

The aesthetic theory of knowledge attempts to trace all the contents of our experience to sources in our separate senses, especially touch, sight and hearing; but the project collapses because it is unable to reconstruct the unity of our world out of disparate sensory impressions.

Thanks to the theoretical revolutions wrought by Descartes, Kant and Husserl, the philosophical question of knowledge and experience has been progressively clarified, and the old model of five 'outer' senses supplemented by several inner faculties has been completely abandoned within philosophy. In the same way that linguistics slowly learned that languages are essentially systems of abstract elements, rather than collections of concrete sounds and sights, so philosophy gradually discovered that some grasp of the world in general must precede our apprehension of particular sensory qualities within it. Our primary sense organ is not our eyes or ears or fingers or nose or tongue: it is our body as a whole. Experience, like language, is nothing if not systematic.

The aesthetic theory of knowledge had to go the same way as the commonsense theory of language – the aesthetic theory of language as it might be called. But before aesthetic theory was finally discarded, it colonized the field of the arts, reducing them too to classifications and theorizations based on the doctrine of the five senses, with 'visual' arts assigned to two or three dimensions of space, and 'auditory' arts to the single dimension of time.

But the aesthetic theory of the arts proved as unworkable as aesthetic theories of knowledge and language, and for much the same reasons: the arts cannot be reduced to compendia of sensory impressions, since they too presuppose an experience of the world as a whole, a systematic experience which cannot be built up from the separate inputs of the five senses.

Contrary to aesthetic theory, works of art are not objects of experience, so much as ways of putting it into question – means of inciting us to attend to discrepancies between particulars and totalities, contents and forms, facts and schemes, objectivities and subjectivities. Works of art are invitations to notice the complexity, multiplicity and precariousness of our ordinary perception of the world. They succeed in their work when they bring it home to us that the identities and continuities that confront us in the world are our inventions as well as our discoveries – including the identities and continuities of language, selfhood and the human voice.

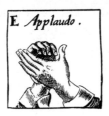

27

The five senses and
the history of philosophy

The History of Philosophy – the discipline which tries to fit the classic texts of Western philosophy into a comprehensive scheme divided into periods and sects and governed by an overall sense of chronological direction – came of age in the last quarter of the eighteeenth century, thanks mainly to Immanuel Kant. It was not just that Kant's 'Critical Philosophy' offered a new vantage point for looking back on philosophy's past. It was also that Kantian Criticism was internally preoccupied with the question of its own place in history. Kant regarded himself as an intellectual revolutionary, and hoped he would be remembered as the philosopher who had confronted the debilitating quarrelsomeness of previous philosophizing, traced it back to its underlying cause, and found a definitive cure. He presumed that future historians would regard him as having inaugurated a new epoch, and this anticipated retrospect on himself was an integral part of his thinking.

The main disputes in all previous philosophy, Kant thought, were aspects of a single fundamental dilemma concerning the source of our knowledge. If knowledge came from the intellect, as 'rationalist' philosophers like Plato, Leibniz and Wolff supposed, then it was impossible to see why we need wait for sensory experience to provide us with information about the world; but if it came from the senses, as 'empiricists' such as Epicurus, Aristotle and Locke maintained, then it was impossible to account for the certainty of our knowledge of universal truths in logic, mathematics and natural science.[1]

Kant thought he had resolved this dilemma through a revolutionary reformulation of the relationship between necessity and experience – a revolution which he compared to Copernicus's reinterpretation of the relationship between cosmological truth and astronomical observation. Up to the sixteenth century, Kant pointed out, most astronomers tried to explain the pattern of observable movements of heavenly bodies 'on the supposition that they all revolved round the spectator', as if the earth were the centre of the cosmos. Copernicus, however, asked 'whether he might not have greater success if he made the spectator to revolve and the stars to remain at rest'. If the earth itself was a wandering star, then the old insoluble difficulties immediately became tractable. The anomalies that had always been observable in the movements of the heavenly bodies were not real after all: they were simply the effects of our own movements as observers stationed on the earth, which we had then projected onto the extra-terrestrial world and mistaken for real objective facts.

In the same way, Kant argued, the great intractable problems of metaphysics – concerning the nature of God, freedom and the soul, for example – arose from our own eccentric ways of thinking, rather than the objective nature of things themselves. He was therefore going to abandon the traditional assumption that 'our knowledge must conform to objects' and replace it with a 'new point of view', the hypothesis that 'objects must conform to our knowledge'. Experience was a collaborative enterprise: our senses delivered information to us, but it would never become objective knowledge until it had been subjectively organized and unified by our understanding or intellect. 'The intellect can sense nothing, the senses can think nothing; only through their union can knowledge arise,' Kant wrote. This implied that the overall shape of the knowable world was framed in advance by the intellect. Our intellectual knowledge of universal truths was due not to some miraculous pre-established harmony between the ways of the world and the ways of our minds; it arose simply from what 'we ourselves

1 Immanuel Kant, 'The History of Pure Reason', *Critique of Pure Reason* (1781, 1787), A 852–6, B 880–4, translated by Norman Kemp Smith, London, Macmillan, 1933, pp. 666–9.

put into' the structure of our world.[2] That was the programme of Kant's philosophical revolution: the Critical Philosophy was the solution to the riddle of the History of Philosophy, and it knew itself to be the solution.

According to Kant, it was not just our intellect which gave order to experience. In their own way our senses did the same, because they constrained us to interpret the world in terms of time and space. Just like the categories supplied by our intellect or understanding, the spatial and temporal 'forms' were always apt to be mistaken by us for inherent attributes of things in themselves, though in fact they were only the subjective scaffolding of our knowledge; and geometry and arithmetic were merely descriptions of how we organize our experience in terms of space and time. 'If the subject, or even only the subjective constitution of the senses in general, be removed,' Kant wrote, 'the whole constitution and all the relations of objects in space and time, nay space and time themselves, would vanish.'[3]

But there was an essential difference between space and time, and this difference would prove to be the basis for a profound distinction between two different kinds of experience. On the one hand, all experience whatsoever was inescapably temporal. The parts of our experience were 'always successive', and anything that affected our senses had to impinge on them at some particular time: 'all objects of the senses are in time, and necessarily stand in time-relations.' On the other hand, an important sector of our experience was differentiated from the rest by being assigned to space as well as time. 'Outer appearances' belonged distinctively to the world of space, whereas our 'inner state' – comprising the private emotions and desires revealed to 'inner sense' – was governed by temporality alone.[4] Our experience was objective only to the extent that it was imprinted with the form of space.

Kant's suggestion that inner experience is essentially temporal, and that outer experience distinguishes itself by being spatial as well, was indeed revolutionary. Ever since Aristotle had propounded the doc-

---

2 Kant, *Critique of Pure Reason*, Preface to Second Edition, B xvi, p. 22, and Introduction to Transcendental Logic, A 51, B 75, p. 93 (translation amended, substituting 'intellect' for 'understanding' as the equivalent of *Verstand*).
3 *Critique of Pure Reason*, Transcendental Aesthetic, A 42, B 59, p. 82.
4 *Critique of Pure Reason*, Transcendental Aesthetic, A 33–4, B 49–51, p. 77.

trine that our knowledge and understanding of the world depend on sensory perception (*aisthêsis*), philosophers had habitually treated experience as a complex additive process in which the distinct senses of sight, hearing, taste, smell and touch all flowed into a common pool, like five separate rivers converging from different directions on the great reservoir of human knowledge.[5] But Aristotle himself had noted a difficulty in this simple 'aesthetic' theory of experience, pointing out that whilst we can tell whiteness from blackness by using our eyes, or sweetness from bitterness by using our tongue, neither tongue nor eyes can distinguish whiteness from sweetness: such discriminations, it would seem, presuppose a further faculty that somehow co-ordinates or supervises the separate deliverances of our five senses.[6] In addition, Aristotle observed that many of the most important objects of sensation – items like movement, shape, size and number – are not 'special to any one sense, but common to all'.[7] It would clearly be a mistake to postulate an additional sense-organ to perceive these *koina aisthêta*, or 'common sensibles'. (That would lead to an infinite regress: you would need another sense-organ to perceive what it shared with the other five.) So Aristotle described the common sensibles as objects of a 'common sense' (*koine aisthêsis* in Greek, and *sensus communis* or *sensorium* in Latin translation) which was conceived as the governing organization of our sensibility, a bit like a sixth sense, but somehow distributed amongst the usual five.[8]

Aristotle's idea of the five senses as sources of all our knowledge became a first principle of medieval philosophy: **nihil est in intellectu quod non prius fuerit in sensu** ('there is nothing in the intellect that was not first in sensation'). And the supplementary concept of a 'common sense' was expanded too, the eleventh-century Muslim thinker Ibn Sina elaborating it into an array of five 'inner senses', a kind of internal counterpart to sight, hearing, taste, smell and touch. The first and most significant of these inner senses was the Aristotelian *sensus communis*, and then there were formative imagination, comparative imagination, cogitation (*vis aestimationis*), and memory.[9] Aquinas

---

5 Aristotle, *De Anima* III 9, 432a 6; III 1, 424b 22.
6 *De Anima* III 2, 436b 9–30.
7 *De Anima* II 6, 418a 18.
8 *De Anima* III 1, 425a 15, 27.
9 Avicenna, *Liber de Anima, seu Sextus de Naturalibus*, edited by S. Van Riet, Louvain, Peeters, 1972, Vol. 1, pp. 87–8.

broadly accepted this list,[10] and the idea of the *sensus communis* and the five inner senses (or 'five wits'), was to remain one of the staples of philosophizing throughout the Middle Ages and the Renaissance.[11]

But – as Aristotle could have foreseen – the postulation of several inner senses only prolonged the difficulty: surely we would need a sixth inner sense to collate the deliverances of the first five? No doubt this was one of the considerations which, in the 1630s, led Descartes to sweep away the whole cumbersome apparatus of distinct 'senses' as separate sources of knowledge. In the first place, he offered a purely physiological account of sense perception, and of the *sensus communis* as an organ of the brain on which the sensory nerves were supposed to converge.[12] He then put forward an austere general concept of mental contents ('ideas' as he called them), designed to cover the entire field of experience, both intellectual and sensory, both inner and outer. For Descartes, the senses depended on the intellect as much as the intellect on the senses: there was no dichotomy between sensory and intellectual knowledge, only various degrees of clarity and distinctness amongst our ideas.[13] Leibniz, following Descartes, was thus able to add an amendment to the old Aristotelian commonplace: *nihil est in intellectu quod non prius fuerit in sensu*, no doubt: *Excipe: nisi ipse intellectus* – except, that is, for the innate contents of the intellect itself.[14]

This new analysis of experience left most philosophers puzzled and unsatisfied. Descartes's attempt to blur the old distinction between intellect and senses by means of an amphibious concept of 'ideas' seemed not so much a solution as an evasion; and in particular it appeared to take no account of the natural or physical peculiarities of our sense organs and therefore our sensory worlds. Half a century later, John Locke – though wholeheartedly adopting the new usage of the word 'idea' – sought to correct Descartes's deficiency by insisting on plain answers to the question how the ideas which furnish 'the

10 Aquinas's doctrine of the inner senses did, however, discard Avicenna's concept of a formative imagination. See *Summa Theologiae*, Prima Pars, Qu. 78, 4.

11 See C. S. Lewis, *Studies in Words*, Cambridge, Cambridge University Press, 1967, pp. 146–8.

12 Descartes, *Discours de la méthode* (1637), Part Five, *Œuvres*, Vol. 6, p. 55.

13 Descartes, *Second Meditation*, in *Meditationes de prima philosophia* (1641), II, *Œuvres*, Vol. 7, p. 32.

14 G. W. F. Leibniz, *Nouveaux Essais sur l'Entendement Humain* (1703–5, published 1765), in *Philosophische Schriften*, Vol. 6, Berlin, Akademie-Verlag, 1990, pp. 110–1.

Materials of all our Knowledge' are able to 'come into the Mind' in the first place.[15] In his *Essay concerning Human Understanding* (first published, after long gestation, in 1689), he affirmed that there are only two 'Fountains of Knowledge', namely Sensation and Reflection. Reflection was the source of the mind's ideas about its own operations ('*Believing, Reasoning, Knowing, Willing*' for instance), and hence 'might properly enough be call'd internal Sense'. And Sensation was the source of those ideas which the ordinary five external senses 'convey into the mind' ('*White, Heat, Cold, Soft, Hard, Bitter*').[16]

Locke then attempted to compile a systematic inventory of different kinds of ideas, ordered according to their respective sources in Sensation and Reflection. In addition to the obvious ones '*which have admittance only through one Sense*', he noted a special group of ideas 'suggested to the mind *by all the ways of Sensation and Reflection*' ('*Pleasure, Pain, Power, Existence, Unity* and *Succession*') and a further set 'that convey themselves into the mind *by more senses than one*', notably '*Space*, or *Extension, Figure, Rest*, and *Motion*' which are received 'both by seeing and feeling'.[17] Once ideas of these various kinds had been garnered into the mind's storehouse, they could be endlessly repeated and recombined to create complex new ideas; but it was impossible, Locke argued, to extend our basic stock of simple ideas except by exposing ourselves to further new experiences. It was 'not in the Power of the most exalted Wit, or enlarged Understanding, by any quickness or variety of thought, to *invent or frame one new simple* Idea in the mind'. Whether we liked it or not, we had to make do with ideas 'received in by [our] Senses, from external Objects; or by reflection from the Operations of [our] own mind about them.'[18]

Over in Dublin, the first edition of Locke's *Essay* was read attentively by a philosophizing lawyer called William Molyneux. Molyneux approved of Locke's attempt to parcel out the materials of knowledge according to their various sensory 'inlets', but he noticed that it had some rather strange implications, and in 1693 he wrote to Locke asking his opinion on a hypothetical hard case.

15 John Locke, *An Essay concerning Human Understanding* (1689), Book I, Chapter II, §2, p. 119; Chapter I, §8, p. 48.
16 *Essay*, Book II, Chapter I, §§3–4, p. 105.
17 *Essay*, Book II, Chapter III, §1, p. 121; Chapter VII, §§1, 9, pp. 128, 131; Chapter IV, p. 127.
18 *Essay*, Book II, Chapter II, §2, pp. 119–20.

Suppose a Man born blind, and now adult, and taught by his touch to distinguish between a Cube, and a Sphere of the same metal, and nighly of the same bigness, so as to tell, when he felt one and t'other, which is the Cube, which the Sphere. Suppose then the Cube and Sphere placed on a Table, and the Blind Man to be made to see. Quaere, Whether by his sight, before he touch'd them, he could now distinguish, and tell, which is the Globe, which the Cube.

Molyneux reported that nearly all those he asked began by presuming that the blind man would be able to see the difference between the globe and the cube immediately his sight was restored. But Molyneux would then convince them they were making a mistake, reasoning on Lockean principles as follows:

For though he [the blind man] has obtain'd the experience of, how a Globe, how a Cube affects his touch; yet he has not yet attained the Experience, that what affects his touch so or so, must affect his sight so or so; Or that a protuberant angle in the Cube, that pressed his hand unequally, shall appear to his eye, as it does in the Cube.

If it is accepted that different senses give rise to different ideas, then Molyneux's conclusion is indeed unavoidable, and in the second edition of the *Essay*, Locke cited Molyneux with the comment: 'I agree with this thinking Gent., whom I am proud to call my friend.'[19]

But it was a seriously damaging concession. Locke had originally maintained that certain ideas were common to several sources, and in particular that ideas of shape and size were shared by the senses of sight and touch. And with very good reason, too: otherwise there would be no greater connection between visible and tangible shapes than there is between, say, colours and temperatures, or flavours and sounds. If Molyneux was right in thinking that a cured blind man would not immediately receive the same ideas of shapes from his eyes as he was accustomed to getting from his fingers, then the whole Lockean fabric of experience was doomed to unravel. Indeed, the unlucky man's difficulty with the relationship between the shapes he had always been able to recognize by touch and the shapes he could

19 *Essay*, Book II, Chapter IX, §8, p. 146.

now see would be absolutely insuperable. Of course he might eventually learn from experience to associate the feel of a cube with the look of a cube, and similarly for other shapes; but he would never be able to identify shapes felt with shapes seen in general, nor even to perceive any systematic and necessary connection between them. They would be as separate from each other as the feel of apples and their smell, or the smell of a fire and its sound. Indeed none of us, however perfect our sensory equipment, could even dream of matching the deliverances of one sense with those of another. Sight, touch, smell, taste and hearing would open on to separate and uncommunicating worlds, like the rooms in Bluebeard's castle. Our experience would be so radically disorganized that it could scarcely be described as experience at all.

Back in Dublin, in 1709, George Berkeley seized on Locke's answer to Molyneux's question, and gleefully endorsed the inference that visible and tangible shapes have nothing whatever in common. Indeed it was a pure play on words, in Berkeley's opinion, to use the same term to describe the objects of different senses. For example shapes, properly speaking, were invisible: they belonged exclusively to the province of touch, and vision had no claim on them, being confined to the fleeting amorphous world of coloured points. And formal geometry, Berkeley argued, was essentially a tactile science, having no necessary connection with the visible world.[20]

Berkeley's arguments, though intended to turn back the rising tide of Newtonian science, received influential support in the lovable person of Nicholas Saunderson, Lucasian Professor of Mathematics at Cambridge and Fellow of the Royal Society from 1719 to his death in 1739. Saunderson was renowned for his brilliant lectures on the principles of Newtonian mathematics and optics. He had exceptionally clear and penetrating ideas of geometrical form, in short; but – tragically – he had been totally blind since infancy. His ideas must therefore have been derived, as his admiring colleagues observed, not from vision but from touch. Of course the range of our ordinary passive tactile experiences of space and number is quite limited, but Saunderson ingeniously augmented his by designing small wooden boards drilled with a regular pattern of holes, and then using pegs to record numerals,

20 George Berkeley, *An Essay towards a New Theory of Vision* (1709), §§ 132–7, 150–9.

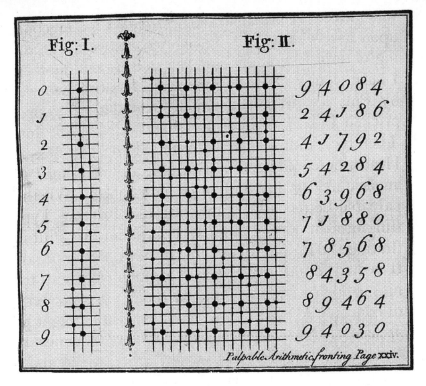

FIG 38. Saunderson's Palpable Arithmetic, 1740
(The large peg is a cipher representing zero; replacing a small peg, it stands for
the number 1; 2–9 are presented by a small peg inserted in a hole adjacent to the
large one, starting with 2 immediately above and then moving clockwise.)

and joining them with silk thread to construct 'palpable or tangible
Symbols . . . to convey those ideas to his Understanding, which were
denied entrance through his Eyes'. (See Figure 38.) By this means, it
was said, Saunderson 'could perform any Arithmetical Operations, by
the Sense of Feeling only; which therefore may be called his *Palpable
Arithmetic*'.[21]

Further empirical confirmation of Berkeley's disaggregated view of
sensory experience was provided in 1728, when the oculist William
Cheselden described restoring the sight of a young gentleman by
removing cataracts from his eyes:

21 See 'Memoirs of the Life and Character of Dr Nicholas Saunderson' and 'Palpable
Arithmetic', in Nicholas Saunderson, *The Elements of Algebra*, Cambridge, 1740, Vol. 1,
pp. i–xxvi, pp. x–xii, xx, xxv.

> When he first saw, he was so far from making any Judgement
> about Distances, that he thought all Objects whatever touch'd
> his Eyes, (as he express'd it) as what he felt, did his Skin . . .
> He knew not the Shape of any Thing, nor any one Thing from
> another, however different in Shape, or Magnitude.

Even familiar objects gave him difficulties, and he had to take particular
pains to imprint their visible aspect on his memory:

> Having often forgot which was the Cat, and which the Dog,
> he was asham'd to ask; but catching the Cat (which he knew
> by feeling) he was observ'd to look at her stedfastly, and then
> setting her down, said, So puss! I shall know you another time.

The young man was puzzled by pictures too:

> We thought he soon knew what Pictures represented, which
> were shew'd to him, but we found afterwards we were mis-
> taken, for about two Months after he was couch'd, he dis-
> covered at once, they represented solid Bodies; when to that
> Time he consider'd them only as Party-colour'd Planes, or
> surfaces diversified with Variety of Paint, but even then he was
> no less surpriz'd, and was amaz'd when he found those Parts,
> which by their Light and Shadow appear'd now round and
> uneven, felt only flat like the rest; and ask'd which was the
> lying sense, Feeling or Seeing?[22]

In 1738, Voltaire picked up the arguments and anecdotes of Molyneux, Locke, Berkeley, Saunderson and Cheselden and broadcast them
all over Europe.[23] The 'English' practice of tracing every idea back to
its separate origin in one of the five senses should act as a corrective,
Voltaire thought, to the typically Gallic precipitation of Descartes, who
was 'possessed by the urge to establish a system' and never paused to
examine the nature and limitations of sensory knowledge. Natural
scientists needed to emulate the caution of Locke and Berkeley, rather
than assuming, like Descartes, that experience automatically provides

22 William Cheselden, 'An account of some observations made by a young gentleman,
who was born blind, or lost his sight so early, that he had no remembrance of ever
having seen, and was couch'd between 13 and 14 years of age', *Philosophical Transactions
of the Royal Society*, Vol. 35, No 402, April–June 1728, pp. 447–50.
23 See Michael J. Morgan, *Molyneux's Question: Vision, Touch and the Philosophy of
Perception*, Cambridge, Cambridge University Press, 1977.

us with a more or less distinct representation of a unified natural world. Voltaire drove home his point with an example.

> First I hear the noise of a carriage from my room; then I open the window and see it; and then I go down and get into it. But the carriage that I heard, the carriage that I saw, and the carriage that I touched are three absolutely separate objects of three of my senses, and between them there is no immediate relationship whatsoever.[24]

But once experience had been broken up into its sensory parts, how could it ever be put back together again? That was the challenge which, through Voltaire, Molyneux issued to all the great spirits of the European Enlightenment.[25]

In his exuberant *Letter on the Blind* of 1749, Diderot took over Locke's basic assumption that our imagination or 'inner sense' is confined to the recollection and recombination of ideas received from the external senses. He then carelessly inferred, as Locke had not, that even our most elevated moral and metaphysical ideas must be involuntary – an impiety which earned him three months of incarceration in Vincennes. He was also fascinated by the apparent implication that we have an inherent tendency to carry our language rather further than the ideas that are supposed to support it. His anonymous 'blind man of Puiseaux', for example, would speak plausibly about vision and mirrors, so that his hearers might almost forget that he 'could not have attached any idea to the terms he was using' – a lesson which, Diderot suggests, we would do well to apply to all the other glib gabblers who can discourse endlessly about matters they do not remotely understand.

But Diderot thought that his friend's blindness also made him acutely aware of perceptual discrepancies and linguistic niceties that

---

24 Voltaire, *Élémens de la philosophie de Newton, mis à la portée de tout le monde*, Amsterdam, Desbordes, 1738, pp. 16, 78.
25 See for example Julien Offray de La Mettrie, *Histoire naturelle de l'âme*, Paris, 1747, pp. 302–6; Etienne Bonnot de Condillac, *Essai sur l'origine des connoissances humaines*, Amsterdam, Mortier, 1746, Vol. 1, pp. 238–65. These works, like Condillac's later *Traité des Sensations* (1754), owe a debt not only to Molyneux but to Descartes's *Traité de l'homme* (written before 1633, published posthumously in 1664), which imagined constructing a human body as if it were 'a statue or an earthy machine', successively equipping it with the 'five external senses' of touch, taste, smell, hearing, and – last but not least – vision. See *Traité de l'homme, Œuvres*, Vol. 11, pp. 120, 141–63.

the rest of us, in the hasty laziness of daily life, are liable to pass over. Why was it, for example, that a mirror should reflect a visible replica of us but not a tangible one?

> Look, said the blind man, at how these two senses [vision and touch] are set in contradiction with each other by your little machine. Perhaps a better machine would bring them into agreement – though still without rendering the objects in its reflections any more real. And perhaps an even more perfect machine, and a less perfidious one, would make the objects disappear completely, and so make us aware of our mistake.[26]

It seemed, therefore, that the only thing we could reliably learn from our senses is that they do not always agree. Like witnesses in a contentious court case, they give conflicting evidence and point off in different directions. Like restless adventurers, they constantly strayed into each other's territories, bent on mischief and destruction. Our sensory ideas were too mobile and erratic ever to furnish us with a durable and coherent representation of the world. Our knowledge was founded on nothing but ideas derived from the senses, no doubt; but it was built not on solid rock but on shifting sands.

That, according to Diderot, explains the austere intelligence of the blind. Shortage of ideas concentrates their minds. The imagination of those of us who can see is filled with throngs of 'visible or coloured points', whereas the imagination of the blind is free to concentrate on 'sensations of touch' and elaborate them to infinity. 'It follows,' Diderot wrote, 'that those who were born blind perceive things in a far more abstract manner than we do,' and this truth was borne out, Diderot thought, by the case of Nicholas Saunderson and the 'palpable arithmetic' with which the blind Newtonian had elucidated the nature of light and colours.[27]

Sensory destitution could also be a spur to imaginative fertility. As well as being steeped in classical poetry, Saunderson was celebrated for his verbal inventiveness – a natural effect, according to Diderot, of being deprived of visual ideas. He resembled those who have only a rudimentary knowledge of a foreign language: 'word-famine' compels

---

26 Diderot, *Lettre sur les aveugles, à l'usage de ceux qui voient* (1749), in *Œuvres Philosophiques*, pp. 96, 84–5.
27 *Lettre sur les aveugles*, pp. 95, 98, 111.

them 'to say everything using a very small number of terms, which sometimes leads them to employ their words very felicitously'. In the same way, Saunderson's blindness meant that 'he only half understood what he was saying, since he was unaware of half the ideas that are attached to the terms he was using'. He would make use of expressions which, for him, referred literally to ideas derived from the sense of touch. Unknown to him, however, his expressions were 'metaphorical in relation to another sense, for example the eyes; which provided a double illumination for the person spoken to: the true and literal light of the expression itself, and also the reflected light of metaphor.'[28]

A serious historian of philosophy is bound to point out that Diderot could hardly have stayed loyal to the Lockean tradition if he had not had a relish for reducing solemn philosophizing to picaresque tail-chasing. Other philosophers, however, were not amused. Kant referred in some exasperation to Cheselden's bewildered patient, citing his pathetic question, when confronted by a deceptively realistic picture, as to 'which was the lying sense, Feeling or Seeing?' The supposed quarrel between the tangible and the visible was, according to Kant, factitious and tedious; indeed it was no more than an expression of the equally illusory conflict between 'rationalists' and 'empiricists'. In Kant's opinion, 'empiricism is based on a felt necessity, rationalism on a visible one'; but of course for Kant the true necessities of our experience were due not to the peculiarities of the different sense organs, but to the transcendental mathematical forms of space and time.[29]

This could have been expected to put an abrupt end to the century-old Lockean habit of harping on the sensory provenances and pedigrees of our ideas. Readers of the *Critique of Pure Reason* were invited to think in terms of a single faculty of outer sense, in place of Locke's old tour round the five external senses; and instead of his impossibly versatile and protean 'Reflection', there was now the monolithic faculty of inner sense. Moreover, both inner and outer experience now had their own proper fields – time and space respectively – each rigorously

28 *Lettre sur les aveugles*, pp. 110–11.
29 'Was betrügt mich, das Gesicht oder Gefühl? (Denn der Empirismus gründet sich auf einer gefühlten, der Rationalismus aber auf einer eingesehenen Notwendigkeit.)' See Immanuel Kant, *Kritik der Praktischen Vernunft* (1797), edited by Karl Vorländer, Hamburg, Meiner, 1929, Preface, p. 14; *Critique of Practical Reason*, translated by Lewis White Beck, New York, Macmillan, 1993, p. 14.

unified by its own mathematical laws. The architecture of our 'inner state' was essentially temporal, and since time is inherently one-dimensional (like 'a line progressing to infinity'), our inner experiences had to occur one after another in time, in accordance with the principles of simple arithmetic.[30] Outer experience, however, was constituted by the laws of three-dimensional geometry as well, which ordained that all its objects must lie 'side by side in space'.[31] Thus Kant's revolution restored and reinforced the unity and orderliness of experience that Locke, Berkeley and their French followers had all but destroyed. As Hegel was to comment with some complacency (and exaggeration too), the old slogan could now be entirely reversed: *Nihil est in sensu, quod non fuerit in intellectu* – there was nothing in our senses, that had not been in our intellect all along.[32]

Twentieth-century philosophy began with a further Copernican revolution in the theory of sensory experience, a revolution which can be seen as completing those of Descartes and Kant. The phenomenology of Edmund Husserl was explicitly designed to redraw both the Kantian boundary between 'sensibility' and 'intellect' (or 'understanding') and the Lockean boundary between 'sensation' and 'reflection' (or 'inner sense'). Husserl suggested that a far more fundamental distinction was required, dividing our mental life into two kinds of acts – 'sensuous' and 'categorial'. Sensuous acts were aimed at objects (whether 'inner' or 'outer') that we take to be 'real' in the sense of having a depth of existence that will never be fully revealed in our apprehension of them; and categorial ones (such as those involving 'being' or 'time') are not directed towards any 'objective correlative' at all, but have their 'fulfilment' within the sphere of thinking itself.[33]

This new approach implied that sensory perception is always directed (whether successfully or not) towards real objects. Contrary to Kant, our experience did not consist of mental contents which start off purely

30 *Critique of Pure Reason*, Transcendental Aesthetic, A 33, B 49–50, p. 77.
31 *Critique of Pure Reason*, Transcendental Aesthetic, A 27, B 43, p. 72.
32 Hegel, *Logic* (Encyclopedia), Introduction, §8, translated by William Wallace, Oxford, Oxford University Press, 1892, p. 15.
33 'kein mögliches *objectives Korrelat*'. See Edmund Husserl, *Logical Investigations* (1900–1901), Chapter 6, §43, translated by J. N. Findlay, London, Routledge and Kegan Paul, 1970, Vol. 2, p. 781.

subjective, to be synthesized subsequently into representations of 'real things'. As Husserl observed in 1901,

> We may handle the thing from all sides in a *continuous perceptual series*, feeling it over as it were with our senses. But each single perception [*Wahrnehmung*] in this series is already a perception of the thing. Whether I look at this book from above or below, from inside or outside, I always see *this book*. It is always one and the same thing, not merely in some purely physical sense, but in the view of our perceptions themselves.[34]

Our perceptions must be anchored from the outset in objective reality, therefore – otherwise the very idea of objectivity could have no meaning for us – and they can never be separated from the world of real things.

From the point of view of the History of Philosophy, Husserl's phenomenology could be described as uniting the two great tendencies in philosophy since Descartes: on the one hand, the loving attention to contingent and perhaps chaotic perceptual detail characteristic of Locke, Berkeley and Diderot, and on the other, the rigorous explication of orderly transcendental forms characteristic of Kant. And historians may also present phenomenology as a belated return to plain healthy common sense, in the non-technical meaning of that word. Husserl, as Sartre put it, liberated us from the stuffy old philosophy of the 'inner life'. We were finally out in the open air and philosophy could breathe again. 'At last, everything is outside; everything, including ourselves, is outside, in the world, amongst others.'[35] The pre-phenomenological philosophers had tried to persuade us that our experience is fundamentally subjective; but they were ignoring the irrepressible objective worldly reference of all our perceptions. The world is not a kind of afterthought, a quality we tentatively infer from regular correlations amongst our sensory ideas. Nor is it a subjective three-dimensional geometrical form that we clamp on to certain ideas in order to differentiate them from the inner experiences which take

34 'nach der Meinung der Wahrnehmung selbst'. *Logical Investigations*, Chapter 6, §47, p. 789 (translation modified).
35 Jean-Paul Sartre, 'Une idée fondamentale de la phénoménologie de Husserl: l'intentionnalité' (1939), in *Situations I*, Paris, Gallimard, 1947, pp. 29–32, p. 32, translated in *Journal of the British Society for Phenomenology*, 1, May 1970, pp. 4–5.

place only in the single dimension of time. Despite the ingenuity of the old subjectivist philosophers, the world is always with us, whether we know it or not.

When you come to consider it, you may suspect that the truths of phenomenology have been familiar to you all along, if only obscurely. You have never really supposed that the content of your experience is defined primarily by the sensory channel through which it reaches you. You perceive people, animals, plants and inanimate things before you perceive colours, shapes, smells, flavours and sounds. You can be aware of comfort or danger without being conscious of any particular sensory ideas. You have a sense of orientation amongst the things that surround you before you have any knowledge of the mathematics of space and time. In addition, you will respond to stories and events without having to react to the specific sensory medium by which they are conveyed. If you catch an unexpected glimpse of someone you adore, your inner commotion is a matter of love rather than optics. You understand the words or signs of a familiar language without needing to notice the exact sounds or gestures of which they are composed. If you are distraught on hearing of the death of a friend, what you suffer is not auditory distress. Even our dreams are not reducible to subjective sensory imagination: you can dream of your mother, for example, through a dream-image which bears no visible resemblance to her, or through no image at all. Your experience always contains people and stories, words and things, signs and meanings, rather than metaphysical abstractions such as space and time, or the deliverances of the five senses. And that is why phenomenology can easily sound like a belated reawakening of solid common sense.

But Husserl did not present himself as a philosophical friend of the people. He described phenomenology as a corrective to the doctrines of sensation and reflection that had been 'universally put about since the time of Locke', but he did not claim to be repairing the damage suffered by ordinary worldly common sense at the hands of theory-intoxicated Lockeans and Kantians. Locke's views were indeed 'quite misguided', according to Husserl, but at the same time they were both 'natural' and 'obvious'.[36] Philosophical errors, in other words, were no less firmly anchored in experience than philosophical truths: indeed

---

36 'naheliegend'. *Logical Investigations*, Chapter 6, §44, p. 782.

the origins of Locke's misinterpretations lay, as Husserl put it, 'in the naive metaphysics and anthropology of everyday life'.[37]

The strife between different conceptualizations of experience, in short, was not an idle squabble between leisured philosophers, conducted over the heads of everyone else. The misunderstandings articulated in traditional philosophy were woven into experience itself, not projected on to it from outside. It did not take Locke to make us suppose, however obscurely, that our experience is pieced together from the separate subjective deliverances of the five senses. Nor did it take Kant to lead us to connect the outer world with space and the inner world with time. Neither did we need Diderot to suggest that our senses may never quite match up with each other. Nor, indeed, did we have to wait for Husserl to tell us that anything we can count as a perceptual experience must contain the possibility of being interpreted and misinterpreted in the ways made explicit by Locke, Diderot, or Kant. Infants playing with their own bodies, or children experimenting with echoes and shadows and reflections and refractions, are already embarked on the same folk-metaphysical excursions: behind the grand procession of great dead philosophers, the permanent puzzlements of ordinary human experience.

37 'Die veraltete Rede von äusseren und inneren Sinnen, die den Ursprung aus dem Alltagsleben mit seiner naiven Metaphysik und Anthropologie nicht verleugnet . . .' *Logical Investigations*, Chapter 6, p. 786.

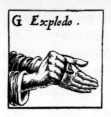

28

Space, time and the aesthetic theory of art

The first part of the *Critique of Pure Reason* – where Kant tried to sweep away the quaint old philosophies of knowledge based on the different qualities revealed to us by our five outer senses and a rather uncertain number of inner ones – is called 'Transcendental Aesthetic'. Kant's doctrine of outer and inner sensibility as having strictly organized fields, thoroughly unified by the mathematical structures of space and time, was *transcendental* because it was concerned with the forms of experience, rather than its externally given content. And it was *aesthetic* in the classical meaning of the term: it was concerned with sense perception or *aisthêsis*, as opposed to intellectual knowledge or *noêsis*.

In a footnote in the first edition, published in 1781, Kant admitted that this use of the word 'aesthetic' might strike readers as perverse and old-fashioned. It was nearly fifty years since Alexander Baumgarten had adopted the term and applied it to the theory of art, in an attempt – as Kant interpreted it – to 'bring the critical treatment of the beautiful under rational principles, and so to raise its rules to the rank of a science'. But although Kant respected Baumgarten – indeed he used his textbook on metaphysics in his own lecture courses – he was convinced that this idea of philosophical aesthetics was 'fruitless' and incoherent. It was our taste that determined the rules of artistic value, he thought, and not the other way round. Hence 'aesthetic' should be retained as the title for the general philosophy of sensory perception, leaving 'critique of taste' as the name for the theory of art.[1]

Perhaps Kant had a point. But his readers may have wondered why such a fastidious thinker should have found the concept of artistic 'taste' any clearer than Baumgarten's proposed 'aesthetics'. And then, what ground could he have for presuming that the various fine arts have enough in common to make them objects of a unified theory at all?

The philosophical tradition certainly gave little enough authority for such assumptions. If its founders discussed art at all, they treated it from the point of view of the *poiêtês* or 'maker', rather than the critic, observer or dilettante. In the *Republic*, for instance, Plato merely said that children should be trained in dramatic recitation and lyrical singing, so as to give 'rhythm and harmony' to their souls, and in the *Laws* he emphasized the political benefits of organized choral singing and dancing.[2] Similarly, Aristotle's *Poetics* concentrated on tragic drama, and the *Politics* recommended musical education for the 'formation of character'.[3] Painting and sculpture did not figure much in these classical discussions, however, and poetry, music and dance were presented as methods of political and personal training, rather than valuable or praiseworthy activities in themselves.

Although the classical philosophers did not have any general concept of 'art', let alone a theory of artistic value, they always recognized the idea of beauty as a central philosophical question. But beauty belonged to nature as well as art: it included anything that could be a source of pleasure or gratification. As Plato recognized, it was popularly associated with the five senses – especially vision and hearing, he thought – and thus with the body; but he held that true beauty was non-sensory, and accessible only to the philosophically purified intellect.[4] Aristotle, too, was disquieted by the connection between beauty and sensual gratification, even lasciviousness.[5] But he noted that the pleasures of the three nobler senses – vision, hearing and (he said) smell – were relatively safe: even if you doted excessively on sights, sounds or per-

1 Immanuel Kant, *Critique of Pure Reason*, A21, B35–6, fn., pp. 66–7.
2 Plato, *Republic* 40ld, *Laws* 654b–665a.
3 Aristotle, *Politics* 1340b11–15.
4 *Republic* 475b–476c.
5 Aristotle, *Problems* X, 52, 896b10–29.

fumes you would not necessarily sink into profligacy as a result, provided your enjoyment remained contemplative and free of any urge to consume or possess the objects of your delectation. The other two senses however – touch and taste – were always fraught with ethical danger: they were directly associated with brutal bodily appetites, and appeasing them could lead directly to drunkenness, gluttony, and lechery.[6] The pursuit of beauty needed to be subjected to critical judgements; but these judgements, for the classical philosophers, belonged more to ethics than to art. Nor were judgements of beauty classically connected with a special faculty of 'taste'. In medieval philosophy, the concept of taste was still taken literally, and the scholastic slogan *de gustibus et coloribus non est disputandum* simply meant that it was pointless to argue about what colours we see or what flavours we taste. It was not till after the Renaissance that 'taste' became an emblem of all that was personal, idiosyncratic and aristocratic in artistic judgement.[7] '*De gustibus non est disputandum*; – that is, there is no disputing against HOBBY HORSES,' as Sterne interprets the old principle in *Tristram Shandy*.[8]

The eighteenth-century idea of taste also required a general category of 'art' as distinct from mere manual craft. Painting, sculpture and architecture had begun to claim the status of 'fine arts' during the Italian Renaissance (perhaps with the publication of Vasari's *Lives of the Most Eminent Architects, Painters and Sculptors* in 1550). But it was not till Diderot's *Encyclopédie* in the 1750s that the standard modern list of five *beaux arts* was established: architecture, sculpture, painting, music and poetry would now be regarded as forming a single field, in which connoisseurs or virtuosos could cultivate and exercise their good taste.[9]

And many of these persons of taste began to think that they could look to philosophy for guidance, and indeed that philosophy ought to culminate in an aesthetic theory of art. But Kant, in 1781, was

---

6 Aristotle, *Eudemian Ethics* III, 2, 1230b21–1231a26; cf. *Nicomachean Ethics* VII, 7, 1150Ia8–15.

7 On the origins of the eighteenth-century idea of 'good taste' see Benedetto Croce, *Aesthetic as Science of Expression and General Linguistic* (1901), translated by Douglas Ainslie, London, Peter Owen, 1922, pp. 191–3.

8 Laurence Sterne, *The Life and Opinions of Tristram Shandy* (1759–67), edited by Ian Campbell Ross, Oxford, Oxford University Press, 1983, p. 12.

9 See Paul Oskar Kristeller, 'The Modern System of the Arts' (1951), in *Renaissance Thought II*, New York, Harper and Row, 1965, pp. 163–227, esp. pp. 182, 165, 202.

determined to take exception to the idea, on the grounds that to subject taste to philosophy would be to deny the autonomy of artistic judgement. That is why he objected to Baumgarten, and proposed to confine the word 'aesthetic' to the theory of sensory knowledge in general, with no special reference to art.[10]

Kant was not quite fair to his predecessor, however. For Baumgarten's idea of aesthetics was also rooted in the classical distinction between sensibility and intellect, experience and logic, *aisthêsis* and *noêsis*. In his *Reflections on Poetry*, published in 1735, Baumgarten had merely raised a question concerning the literary forms appropriate to these two different kinds of knowledge. Logic, he found, was already so rigorously systematic that its truths could be propounded 'just as they are thought', without any need for artistic embellishment or rhetorical skill. Logic was a complete guide to its own presentation, and when it had to be cast into a literary or discursive form, Baumgarten said, there were 'no special rules of arrangement to be observed'.[11]

But the exposition of 'sensory' or 'aesthetic' matters – the contingencies of history, nature, politics, law or sentiment, as opposed to the necessities of reason – could not be expected to take care of itself in the same way. And the ancient disciplines of rhetoric failed to provide the necessary guidance, because they were more concerned with winning over an audience than with clearly expounding the truth. Therefore, according to Baumgarten, there was need for a new kind of 'general poetics', stationed midway between rhetoric and logic: like rhetoric, it would teach techniques for discoursing on sensory topics; but like logic, it would seek to do full justice to its materials. Its output would be 'perfect discourse about sensory matters' (*oratio perfecta sensitiva*), that is to say poetry, correctly defined: language so well chosen and aptly arranged that, even when expressing tedious or distasteful subjects, it would remain vivid and lively and 'pleasing to the ear'.[12]

---

10 Kant proposed 'to give up using the name in this sense of critique of taste, and to reserve it for that doctrine of sensibility which is true science, thus approximating to the language and sense of the ancients, in their far-famed division of knowledge into *aisthêta kai noêta*'. Kant *Critique of Pure Reason*, A21, fn., pp. 66–7.
11 Alexander Baumgarten, *Meditationes Philosophicae de nonnullis ad poema pertinentibus*, Magdeburg, 1735, §117, pp. 39–40. The text is reproduced with an English translation as *Reflections on Poetry*, translated by Karl Aschenbrenner and William B. Holther, Berkeley, University of California Press, 1954; see p. 78.
12 Baumgarten, *Meditationes Philosophicae*, §§117, 95–6, pp. 39–40, 32–3; *Reflections on Poetry*, pp. 78, 70.

Baumgarten's later works were devoted to promoting his conception of poetics as a kind of medium between logic and rhetoric, under the influential title of *Aesthetica*. But although he added some hints towards a general doctrine of 'cogitating beautifully', and suggestions about poetics as a guide in 'all the liberal arts',[13] he never regarded 'aesthetics' as a universal guide to artistic judgement. The only subject to which Baumgarten ventured to suggest that the new discipline might be applied, beyond rhetoric and poetry, was music, insofar as it was a representation of various types of human character.[14] The idea that Baumgarten had proposed a rationalistic deduction of the principles of 'aesthetic pleasure' in general was, it would seem, a figment of Kant's antagonistic imagination.[15]

And not only Kant. Lessing too – in his *Laokoön*, published in 1766 – criticized Baumgarten for failing to offer a general 'aesthetic' theory of the fine arts, and especially for neglecting what Lessing called the 'visual' or 'plastic' arts (*bildende Künste*), or simply 'art' without qualification.[16] Irritated by poets who engaged in 'scene-painting' as opposed to story-telling – a practice which he condemned for confounding the aims of two distinct forms of fine art – Lessing took over the idea of 'aesthetics', but sent it off in a direction never envisaged by Baumgarten. He was concerned not with the proper representation of 'sensory' as opposed to 'intellectual' topics, but with the appeal made to the different senses by the various fine arts. Whereas Baumgarten defined the arts by their sensory subject-matter, Lessing defined them by their sensory medium, and the five fine arts were now to be differentiated according to how they addressed the five external senses.

Eyesight, according to Lessing, was the only sense that could perceive many different realities in 'one instant of vision' or 'a single moment of time'.[17] The other senses, in contrast – the 'dark senses', as Lessing called them – could only present us with a succession of

---

13 Alexander Baumgarten, *Aesthetica* (1750, 1758), Bari, Laterza, 1936, §§1, 69, 71, pp. 55, 76.
14 Aristotle, *Politics* 1340a19-b6.
15 As Croce concludes (*Aesthetic as Science of Expression and General Linguistic*, pp. 218–19): 'the new name is devoid of new matter.'
16 Gotthold Ephraim Lessing, *Laokoön: an essay on the limits of paintings and poetry* (1766), translated by Edward Allen McCormick, Baltimore, Johns Hopkins University Press, 1984, Preface, p. 5.
17 'der einzige Augenblick' – see *Laokoön*, Chapter 3, p. 19.

qualities, one by one. That was why objects like putrefying wounds, which would make us retch and vomit if they were presented to the senses of taste or smell or touch, could be contemplated calmly by our eyes: the dark senses could not mitigate our disgust, whereas sight would dilute it by presenting many other objects to our sensibility at the same time. 'Our sense of sight perceives in them and with them a number of other realities,' as Lessing put it: 'realities whose pleasant images weaken and obscure the unpleasant ones to the point where they can have no noticeable influence on our body.'[18]

But taste, smell and touch, though unrivalled as potential sources of disgust, were the 'lower senses', and had no great significance for the fine arts. The only worthy counterparts to the arts that appealed to vision were those that addressed the ear – especially the arts of poetry, or literature in general. Poetry and painting were thus the two principal 'kinds of imitation', according to Lessing, and their true nature or vocation was to be inferred from the simple truism that 'colours are not sounds and ears are not eyes'.[19] Paintings consisted of 'figures and colours in space', whereas poems comprised 'signs that follow one another', or 'articulated sounds in time'. Painting was a spatial art whose task was to delight the eye by depicting 'objects whose wholes or parts coexist', whilst poetry was a temporal art, which gave pleasure to the ear by representing 'actions', or 'objects whose wholes or parts are consecutive'.[20] Once this had been made clear, Lessing thought, the two leading art forms could be properly separated at last, and they need never trespass on each other's territories again.

There is a certain plausibility to Lessing's argument. A painting can only represent a single frozen moment, whereas poetry can show a whole series of events taking place at different times. On the other hand, that scarcely means that vision is essentially spatial and instantaneous, and hearing essentially temporal and successive. If Lessing had paused to consider the arts of drama, opera, or especially dance, he would have had to admit that they propose temporal patternings to our eyes, just as much as poetry does to our ears. And if he had attended to the music of, say, Rameau, Bach, Handel, Scarlatti, Gluck

18 *Laokoön*, Chapter 25, p. 131.
19 *Laokoön*, Chapters 11, 15, pp. 62, 76.
20 *Laokoön*, Chapter 16, p. 78.

or Haydn, he could hardly have failed to notice that it consists of several different streams of sound, playing concertedly, rather than a sequence of simple tones, one after the other; in fact he need only have glanced at an orchestral score in order to grasp the point. Furthermore, even the simplest musical line cannot be understood unless its successive moments are attended to simultaneously, held together in memory and anticipation: otherwise you would never notice the patterns of repetition and return, invocation and echo, that make a coherent melody of it. Even poetry – Lessing's paradigm of auditory art – does not conform to his principle of successivity: if you heard a portion of language as a set of separate sounds passing through your consciousness one by one, like sheep jumping over a stile, you would not even be able to recognize words in it, let alone grasp their meaning and syntactical relations, or appreciate their tunes and rhythmic patterns. Hearing is no more specifically temporal than seeing is specifically spatial, and the only puzzle, it would seem, is that such notions could ever have been considered a plausible basis for a theory of art.

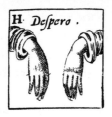

29

Art against aesthetics

Kant could not possibly accept Lessing's analysis of sensory experience. According to the Kantian transcendental aesthetic, space was the form of external sensibility as a whole – of touch, taste, smell and hearing, that is to say, as well as vision and the visual arts. And time was the form of inner sensibility in general, and therefore by extension of all experience whatsoever, so it had no special connection with hearing or the auditory arts.

But Lessing's attempt to classify and unify the five fine arts on the basis of a theory of space, time and the senses fascinated Kant nevertheless. In 1787 he swallowed his disdain and began work on his own theory of 'the foundations of the Critique of Taste', so that the first half of his *Critique of Judgement*, published in 1790, was given over to 'aesthetics' in the very sense he had deprecated in the *Critique of Pure Reason* less than ten years before.[1]

Of course, Kant was never tempted to reduce the operation of the fine arts to a mere 'organic sensation' of sensory pleasure. He argued, on the contrary, that true art excited a purely 'reflective' enjoyment, arising not from a passive physical response but from the active exercise of our faculty of judgement.[2] This activity not only enhanced our

---

1 See Ernst Cassirer, *Kant's Life and Thought* (1918), translated by James Haden, Yale University Press, 1981, p. 271.
2 Immanuel Kant, *Critique of Judgement* (1790), translated by James Creed Meredith, Oxford, Oxford University Press, 1952, §44, p. 166.

'feeling of life', but also improved us mentally and socially: although our aesthetic judgements were purely personal, we might nevertheless be expected to adjust or defend them in the light of the judgements of others – and this, as Kant remarked, would have the effect of cultivating our minds 'in the interests of social communication', thus promoting the 'urbanity' of our cognitive powers.[3] (Kant took pleasure in describing the 'large banquets' and 'dinner parties' where aesthetic taste might be exhibited and improved through the 'free flow of conversation between guest and guest'.) The benefits of cultivating good taste, it seems, were sedentary successors to the character-forming powers attributed to dance and song by Plato and Aristotle.[4]

Aesthetic taste, for Kant, was concerned not with the content of sensory experience but with its form. Hence the classification of the arts had to start from the distinction between the two basic mathematical forms of experience, namely three-dimensional space and one-dimensional time.[5] Space was the medium used by the 'formative' arts (*bildende Künste* – painting, sculpture, architecture and landscape gardening). On the other hand, the arts of the 'beautiful play of sensations' – especially music – occupied the medium of time. Then, somewhat inconsistently, Kant attempted to share out these two forms of art between the different senses: the spatial arts, according to him, belonged not only to the eye, as Lessing had thought, but to touch as well; and the temporal arts could be addressed to the eye as well as the ear – for Kant believed that in addition to sound-music there could in principle be colour-music as well, based in our unconscious appreciation of the mathematics of harmonious vibration in light of different colours.[6]

Like Lessing, Kant regarded artistic activities that straddled the terms of his classification as impure and therefore regrettable. Theatre or dance, for example, or pantomime and opera, were freakish hybrids,

---

3 Kant, *Critique of Judgement*, §28, p. 110, §20, p. 82, §1, p. 42, §40, p. 151, §44, p. 166, §53, p. 195.
4 On the agreeable pleasures of the refined dinner party see *Critique of Judgement*, §44, pp. 165–6.
5 *Critique of Judgement*, §19, pp. 67–8.
6 Unlike Lessing, Kant did not think of music in terms of temporal patterning. He concerned himself not with melody, but only harmony – 'the numerical relation of the vibrations in the air in the same time, so far as there is combination of the tones simultaneously or in succession.' He also permitted himself to doubt whether anyone could judge such relations clearly enough to derive truly aesthetic pleasure from them. See *Critique of Judgement*, §53, p. 194, see also §51, pp. 186, 189–90.

each of them a 'combination of fine arts' rather than a true art form in its own right.[7] But there was another field that Kant found difficult to accommodate in his aesthetic classification, namely the not insignificant 'arts of speech' (*redende Künste*) – by which he meant rhetoric or literature, especially poetry.[8] And Kant really loved poetry: he loved it, he said, because it was not only prodigally suggestive but also sincere and direct, and because it never attempted to 'ensnare the understanding with a sensuous presentation', or so he thought. But it was difficult to fit it into an aesthetic theory of art: despite Lessing, it could not be attributed either to the sense of hearing or to the medium of time. All the same, 'I must confess,' Kant wrote, 'to the pure delight I have ever been afforded by a beautiful poem.'[9] So although it made fair nonsense of his system of classification, Kant gallantly placed poetry in 'the first rank among all the arts'.[10]

A generation later, Hegel returned to Kant's system of the fine arts and tried to restore it to good order and bring it back into harmony with Lessing. The ultimate aim of all human activities, Hegel thought, was to lead us ever upwards to a realm of higher spiritual truth. But the distinctive speciality of the fine arts – as he explained in his *Lectures on Aesthetics*, first delivered in Berlin in 1823 – was that they were rooted in our sensory experience. The starting point for the theory of art must therefore be the 'specific characterization of the senses'. Like his predecessors, Hegel was quick to exclude touch, smell, and taste for being attuned to sensory plea-sure rather than artistic beauty. ('The fondling [*Herumtatscheln*] of the voluptuous parts of marble statues of female goddesses,' he gravely informed his audience, 'has nothing to do with the contemplation or enjoyment of art.')[11] That left eyes and ears as the only senses with any relevance to the fine arts, and Hegel was happy to restore Lessing's simple equivalences: 'just as sight relates to light or physicalised space,' he wrote, 'so hearing relates to sound or physicalised time.'[12]

In Hegel's classification, space and the eyes were less spiritual than

---

7 *Critique of Judgement*, §52, p. 190, §14, p. 68.
8 *Critique of Judgement*, §51, p. 184.
9 *Critique of Judgement*, §53, p. 193 and fn.
10 *Critique of Judgement*, §53, p. 191.
11 G. W. F. Hegel, *Aesthetics: Lectures on Fine Art*, pp. 621, 39, 621.
12 Hegel, *Philosophy of Mind*, §401; see *Hegel's Philosophy of Subjective Spirit*, translated by M. J. Petry, Vol. 2, p. 171.

time and the ears, and the three 'visual arts' were inferior to the 'art of sound'. Architecture obviously lay at the bottom of the pyramid, being weighted down with heavy matter in three dimensions. Next came sculpture, which was somewhat lighter because it represented the human body. Then there was painting, which was clearly less materialistic than either architecture or sculpture, since it had only two dimensions. But it was still dependent on physical colours lying inertly on a solid surface, and therefore ranked below music ('the art of sound'), sounds being essentially weightless and evanescent, and hence more 'adequate to spirit' than colours. But whilst music could give perfect expression to 'essentially shapeless feeling', the specificity of 'spiritual meanings' was expressible only in language. And that was why – as Kant had realized, though without quite knowing his reasons – the highest of the arts was 'the art of speech' (*die Kunst der Rede*), in other words poetry. Poetry, for Hegel as for Kant, topped off the pyramid of the arts: it was 'total art', Hegel said, and 'the absolute and true art of the spirit'.[13]

But if the fine arts were all concerned with the senses, and poetry was the finest art of all, then which of the senses was poetry addressed to? The question had defeated Kant, but Hegel was able to suggest an adroitly dialectical answer. He realized that we do not hear speech by simply listening to it. Even our own mother tongue remains inexplicable to us unless we know how to look at it, in other words how to recognize and analyse it through the medium of alphabetic writing. In some ways, Hegel said, writing is inferior to speech, offering us only a 'roundabout way to ideas'. But, he continued, we have to be able to represent speech to ourselves in written form in order to grasp what it essentially is – namely a finite set of arbitrary 'simple elements', rather than a limitless array of particular sounds. Thus the contradiction between the two aspects of language – language as sound, spoken 'in time' to the ear, and language as script, written 'in space' for the eye – served to raise our consciousness towards 'the more formal nature of the sounding word and its abstract elements' – a transfiguration which was 'essential in order to establish and purify the basis of inwardness within the subject'.[14]

13 Hegel, *Aesthetics*, pp. 622–6.
14 Hegel, *Philosophy of Mind*, §459; see *Hegel's Philosophy of Subjective Spirit*, Vol. 3, pp. 187–91.

Thus poetry in its essence was neither audible nor visible. It was composed of language itself, which was not a material substance but a spiritual one. The physical sound of poetry, at least genuine poetry, did not have 'a value on its own account', and that accounted for poetry's superiority over music.[15] The contradictory relations of speech to visible space and audible time raised the arts of language like an angel above the sensory forms of all the other arts, and justified poetry's place at their head.

But Hegel's neat attempt to reconcile Lessing with Kant and refurbish the aesthetic system of the five fine arts did not dispose of those art forms which appeared as curious and derivative confections in which one art was messily mixed up with another. Dancing, for example: Kant had already objected to its promiscuous way of trying to appeal to more than one sense at the same time,[16] and Hegel took it as a paradigm of 'imperfect art'. While conceding that it might contain 'much that is enjoyable, graceful and meritorious', he was in no doubt that it was essentially a 'hybrid' or an 'amphibian', flouting 'essential differences grounded in the thing itself', and thus giving expression not to spiritual freedom but to sheer 'impotence'.[17] He was not surprised to find that contemporary admirers of dance were incapable of approaching it in a properly aesthetic manner, that is to say as a purely visual experience of space, detached and disinterested: 'those who know about these things are captivated by the extraordinarily developed bravura and suppleness of the legs,' Hegel complained, 'and this always plays the chief part in dancing nowadays.'[18]

The intertwining of the athletic with the aesthetic in the appreciation of a dancer's legs had long been a sore point in philosophy. Locke, for example, held that a good training in dance came second only to books and study in the education of a gentleman, since it imparted a 'perfect graceful carriage' and 'manliness and a becoming confidence'. However, he maintained that a badly conducted dance lesson was worse than none at all. Children should never be permitted to get engrossed by 'the jigging part, and the figures of dances', and it would

---

15 Hegel, *Aesthetics*, p. 627.
16 Kant, *Critique of Judgement*, §52, p. 190.
17 *Aesthetics*, pp. 627–8.
18 *Aesthetics*, p. 1192.

be better to remain forever in 'natural unfashionableness', Locke wrote, and 'put off the hat, and make a leg, like an honest country gentleman', than to adopt 'apish, affected postures . . . like an ill-fashioned dancing master'.[19]

It is not entirely surprising, of course, that the arts of dance have occasioned philosophical misgivings. You would have to be a very abstracted aesthetic philosopher to imagine that the experience of watching a dance, let alone performing one, could ever be quite so exclusively 'visual' and 'painterly' as Kant desired.[20] In an impudent passage of the *Critique of Judgement*, Kant imagined 'playing a trick' on lovers of natural beauty. He wanted to catch any of us who might be pretending to enjoy an aesthetic experience of nature, when in fact we were simply indulging dozily in the sensuous or sentimental pleasures of a fragrant summer afternoon in the garden. His suggested stratagem was to stick artificial flowers in the ground, and suspend painted carvings of birds in the trees. If our pleasure in these objects vanished when we discovered the deception, then we would be exposed as aesthetic hypocrites – interested not in a high-minded experience of beauty, but in something rather more coarsely material that might lie behind it.[21]

Kant could have proposed a parallel experiment with the dance. He might have arranged for us to witness a glorious and moving performance, with the most rhythmical steps, the most breath-taking leaps, and the most graceful pirouettes, the most responsive partnering – except that he was deceiving us by an optical trick, or presenting us with featherweight mechanical dolls, not real human dancers. If our enjoyment disappeared when the trick was revealed, then our appreciation could not have been truly aesthetic, since it would have been dependent on the existence of its objects rather than the form of our experience.

It is hard to believe, however, that anyone would ever bother with dancing if obliged to consider it in Kantian terms. You watch a dance not simply with the eyes, nor with the mind, but with a kind of muscular sympathy, a projective identification with the bodies of dan-

19 John Locke, *Some Thoughts concerning Education* (1690), §196, *Works*, 1824, Vol. 9, pp. 190–1.
20 Kant's word is '*malerisch*': see *Critique of Judgement*, §52, p. 190.
21 *Critique of Judgement*, §42, p. 158.

cers. What you see is not a general visual impression, but a particular body: 'this dancer who is now this moment under your eyes,' as George Balanchine put it.[22] From the point of view of aesthetics, the dancer's physical body may be an impurity; but take it away, and the art of dance vanishes with it.

The same applies to singing as well. Hegel regarded the human voice as the 'most perfect' of musical instruments: it expressed the essence of music by uniting the virtues of the wind instruments with those of the strings.[23] But he was of course referring to pure vocalizing, to songs without words; like Kant, he was uneasy about mixing music with poetry and asking the singer to utter not only a musical line but also 'words which give us the idea of a specific subject-matter'.[24]

And those are not the only defects of singing from an aesthetic point of view. Singers have to breathe, for instance, their range is limited to three octaves at most, and a woman's voice sounds different from a man's, a child's from an adult's. But it would hardly be an artistic improvement if grainy, idiosyncratic human voices were replaced with pingingly accurate and absolutely indistinguishable voice machines capable of holding their perfect notes indefinitely. Nor would it help if singers stripped their songs of their texts. The task of speaking words meaningfully may conflict with that of singing tunes musically; but the strife between the two is the very substance of singing, not its unlucky affliction. Singing involves a combination of elements that can never be perfectly combined.[25] That may make it extravagant and unnatural from the point of view of philosophical aesthetics; but nothing comes to children more instinctively than the chanting of words, except dancing perhaps. All of us must have sung and danced, or tried to, at least when young; and the memories, however deeply

22 George Balanchine, quoted by Francis Sparshott in his invaluable *Off the Ground, First Steps to a Philosophical Consideration of the Dance*, Princeton, Princeton University Press, 1988, p. 232.
23 Hegel, *Aesthetics*, p. 922.
24 *Aesthetics*, pp. 909, 934; see also Kant, *Critique of Judgement*, §52, p. 190. Hegel's discussion of music as 'accompaniment' to words (*Aesthetics*, pp. 937–51) treats it only as a step towards 'independent music' which he says (p. 953) 'cannot be vocal'.
25 As Verdi wrote to Antonio Ghislanzoni, librettist of *Aida*, in 1870: 'It is sometimes necessary in the theatre for poets and composers to have the talent not to write either poetry or music.' See Charles Osborne, *Verdi: A Life in the Theatre* (1987), London, Michael O'Mara Books, 1990, p. 215.

sedimented, still guide us when we try to follow the singing and dancing of others, even within the limits of fine art.

Kant and Hegel would perhaps have admitted that the significance of singing and dancing is inseparable from imperfection and individual bodily existence, and even from half-buried memories of childhood. But it would not have worried them much, since – unlike Plato and Aristotle – they regarded song and dance as subsidiary and dispensable art forms: what really mattered to them were the aesthetically pure arts – painting, abstract music, and of course the sublime art of poetry.

However, it may be hard to prevent the same line of thought, once admitted for the lowly arts of singing and dancing, from spreading to loftier realms – as in Nietzsche's raucous physiological aesthetics, where all kinds of art were called upon to 'act through suggestion on the muscles and the senses', even poetry. 'We always hear with our muscles,' Nietzsche says; indeed 'we even read with our muscles.'[26]

That may seem to dig a deep pit beneath Hegel's aesthetic hierarchy of the fine arts, paradoxically culminating by the art whose medium was intelligible rather than visible or audible, namely poetry. And yet Hegel's emphasis on the universality or generality of works of art was not entirely misconceived. If a poem is to do its work, it must act as more than an instantaneous muscular tonic. The experience of reading or hearing a poem is not confined to its fleeting moment of actuality: to treat a set of words as poetry is to regard them as constituting a work that may be returned to – recollected in different circumstances, with new significances, and performed with endless variations of stress, pronunciation, tempo and vocal style. In poetry, as in language in general, to exist is to be repeatable. If there is something universal about poetry, it is not because it floats above the regular structures of our experience of language, but because it plays repeatedly through them all.[27]

Poetry, Paul Valéry once said, is a kind of 'verbal materialism'. It is interested in nothing but words, in words as words. But even in their

26 Friedrich Nietzsche, *The Will to Power*, §809; *Der Wille zur Macht*, edited by Peter Gast (1906), Leipzig, Alfred Kröner Verlag, 1959, pp. 543–4.
27 As Gaston Bachelard remarked, even silent poetic reading institutes a 'primitive economy of breathing', perhaps even affirming implicitly 'the primacy of vocality over hearing'. See 'La déclamation muette', in *L'air et les songes: Essai sur l'imagination du mouvement*, Paris, José Corti, 1943, pp. 271–80, pp. 272, 279.

most ponderous materiality, words are not supine and inert and isolated: they activate and catalyse and resonate. '*Hearing?* But it is the same as *speaking*. You cannot understand what you have heard unless you can also say it yourself for other purposes.'[28] A poem, as Valéry put it, 'entails a continuous linkage between the *voice that is*, the *voice that impends*, and the *voice that is to come*.'[29]

Of all the joys of the anticipated voice that are treasured by Valéry's verbal materialists, none will be more highly prized than its infinite capacity for rhythm – for the patterns of stress and timing that are characteristic of any given language, but which also serve to individualize its different speakers, and differentiate its places and occasions.[30] Linguistic rhythm is amongst our earliest social experiences, the immediate content of our babbling, echoing, and unselfconscious song and dance. And poetry, as an art which specializes in rhythm, stays close to these forgotten layers of linguistic experience: to the infantile linguality, as it might be called, that is carried as a kind of ballast by all our vocal experience.[31]

But that is not how Hegel interpreted poetry's universality. For him, poetry was the 'universal teacher of humanity', furnishing us with an understanding of 'the powers governing spiritual life' in general.[32] And poetic rhythm was 'essentially external' – poets imposed 'regularity and symmetry' on language as a kind of alien chronometrical pattern,[33] rather like gardeners clipping their shrubs into identical regular shapes, or sergeants drilling their new recruits to march like rigid machines run by clockwork.

No doubt it is true, in a sense, that to experience a poem is to subject oneself to someone else's control: as Valéry put it, we make

28 Paul Valéry, 'Calepin d'un poète' (1928), *Œuvres*, edited by Jean Hytier, Paris, Gallimard, 1957, Vol. 1, pp. 1447–63, 1456, 1448.
29 Valéry, 'Première Leçon du Cours de Poétique' (1937), *Œuvres*, Vol. 1, pp. 1340–58, p. 1349.
30 See Émile Benveniste, 'La notion de "rythme" dans son expression linguistique' (1951), *Problèmes de linguistique générale*, Paris, Gallimard, 1966, pp. 327–35.
31 This line of argument can be traced in Julia Kristeva, 'Rythmes phoniques et sémantiques', in *La Révolution du langage poétique*, Paris, Seuil, 1974, pp. 209–63, and 'Contraintes rythmiques et langage poétique' (1974), in *Polylogue*, Paris, Seuil, 1977, pp. 437–66; Henri Meschonnic, *Critique du rythme: anthropologie historique du langage*, Paris, Verdier, 1982; and Ivan Fónagy, *La vive voix: Essais de psycho-phonétique*, Paris, Payot, 1983.
32 Hegel, *Aesthetics*, p. 972.
33 *Aesthetics*, pp. 249–50.

ourselves into 'the instrument of what has been written, so that our voice, our intelligence, and the entire range of our sensibility' are bent to the task of realizing the poem's power.[34] But when we allow it to take us over and 'act on our muscular organization through its rhythms', we are not – despite Hegel – subordinating ourselves to an external force. The language of the poem was already ours before we read it: it belongs to us as much as to our poet, and the poem will work for us only if it can inhabit our own linguistic world.[35]

Following Nietzsche, Valéry totally inverted Hegel's aesthetic interpretation of poetry's universality. Poetry, as he pointed out, need not be regarded as the antithesis or antipodes of the dance. Prose is like walking somewhere you need to get to: it is of no interest apart from its destination. Poetry, on the other hand, is an invitation to linger, so that 'starting to speak a poem is like entering into a verbal dance'.[36] The whole point of dancing is that it 'makes use of the *very same* limbs, organs, bones, muscles and nerves as walking'.[37] In just the same way, poetry uses the same grammar, rhythms, sounds, meanings, and spellings as the language of the rest of our lives: only it probes them, stretches them, discusses them, and tests them to their limits. Poetry, one might say, is a way of being philosophical about language. Indeed it is in itself a kind of philosophy of language; but instead of marching briskly over a Hegelian horizon, hoping to look back eventually and see language as a distant object of sublime knowledge, it is content to stay where it is, and dance.

The aesthetic theorists of art were correct, no doubt, in thinking that art is concerned with sensory experience. They were right, too, to insist that the function of art is not confined to the fleeting subjective instant. But they had the misfortune to inherit a theory of perception – an aesthetic or pre-phenomenological theory of the five senses, as it might be described by a historian of philosophy – which assumes that the mind is a private place where isolated perceptions, each closed in upon itself, are matched up and pieced together into a conjectural representation of an external reality.

34 Valéry, 'Questions de poésie' (1935), Œuvres, Vol. 1, pp. 1280–94, p. 1289.
35 Valéry, 'Propos sur la poésie' (1927), Œuvres, Vol. 1, pp. 1361–78, pp. 1374–5.
36 Valéry, 'Philosophie de la danse' (1936), Œuvres, Vol. 1, pp. 1390–403, p. 1400.
37 Valéry, 'Propos sur la poésie', p. 1371 (emphasis added).

If we look at something, though – a mountain, for instance – we are not gathering up a collection of subjective sensations, comparing them, and then venturing the hypothesis that a mountain is facing us, or that we are facing a mountain. When we look at the mountain, we are already planted there in the landscape, ourselves and our futures and our pasts, together with everything that makes up our sense of town and country, of history and nature, of walking and running, murmuring and shouting, of earth and water and wind and sun, of the colours of the heather or the seasons of the year. And a successful painting will not be an account of how the mountain happens to look to us subjectively; nor will it be about how the mountain is in itself objectively. The painting will discuss how the mountain manages to be as it looks to us, and how it manages to look to us as it is in itself. It will investigate, in other words, how it is constituted as a reality in our experience. The painting puts questions to the mountain: as Maurice Merleau-Ponty said, it 'asks it to reveal the means . . . by which it comes to be a mountain before our eyes'.[38]

The painting reveals a truth, but not the kind of truth that would contribute to the solution of a scientific problem. Despite the self-conscious 'modernities', 'movements' and 'avant-gardes' that have been inspired by the aesthetic theory of art, there is no reason to believe that art, in its work as art, makes any progress from one epoch to the next, or indeed that the period-concepts of the History of Art have anything to say about works of art and how they work. For their work starts afresh with every new life that begins, and with every day that dawns. 'Even if the world lasted for millions of years, it would still need to be painted, and the task would never be completed,' as Merleau-Ponty puts it.[39] The discussion of ourselves, our perceptions, and our world that art draws us into – and philosophy as well – is always going to be incomplete: not imperfect, just perfectly incomplete.

38 Maurice Merleau-Ponty, *L'Œil et l'Esprit*, Paris, Gallimard, 1964, pp. 28–9.
39 *L'Œil et l'Esprit*, p. 90.

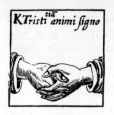

30

A voice of your own?

Aesthetic theories of art would seem to be following aesthetic theories of language and knowledge into what a historian of philosophy might regard as a metaphysical limbo, a scrapyard for obsolete theories. But the five-sided template of taste, smell, touch, hearing and vision is not about to sink into oblivion. The folk metaphysics of the five senses endures, with all its insights, contradictions, ambiguities and oversights; and it is still the first device we turn to when we try to make sense of the world and how we experience it.

We will never quite manage to prevent ourselves from assuming that our grasp of our situation in the world has been pieced together like a mosaic out of many separate sensations, conveyed to us through the separate channels of our senses. The very earliest games we played with our bodies – shutting our eyes and trying to think what it would be like to be blind, or stopping our ears and imagining ourselves deprived of hearing – will have suggested that our senses are just so many gateways through which flavours and fragrances, textures, colours or sounds gain admission to our consciousness, where we link them up to form our picture of the world. After all, if we can analyse our experience by subtracting our senses one by one in our imagination, then elementary arithmetic seems to imply that it can be reconstructed by adding them all up again. The commonsense metaphysics of the senses is, it would seem, an unavoidable part of our interpretations of the world, of other people and of ourselves.

Interpreting ourselves involves trying to understand our interpretations: our experiences, our responses, and above all what we and others have to say. *Saying* can of course take many forms – gesturing and writing as well as speech, for example – but it always involves uttering some semblance of coherent sense. You cannot say anything without saying *something*.

But the notion of saying something can be treacherous.

It is obvious that the meaning of any message depends on the relations amongst the signs by which it is expressed. But that implies that before you can understand any message, you have to make at least a preliminary judgement as to which signs belong with each other in the same group, and in what order. When you look through a newspaper, you could always choose to pursue a horizontal row of type from one column to the next, thus stringing together sentence-fragments from several different articles. But even if you could make sense of the resulting collections of words, it would be no way of finding out what the paper had to say. In the same way, if several people are speaking to you simultaneously, you may be able to pick up one word from each of them in turn, and perhaps make them add up to a perfectly good sentence: but still you will not have understood what any of them was saying.

One of the recurrent obsessions of aesthetic theories of language – one which even Saussure was unable to escape – is the supposition that the coherence of a group of signs must either be conveyed to the eye, preferably as a spatial sequence of letters in a single line of script, or to the ear, as a temporal sequence of sounds in a single line of speech.[1] But as Saussure ought to have known – and perhaps he did know it some of the time – the insistent old issues about time as against space, succession in contrast with simultaneity, or hearing as opposed to seeing, have absolutely nothing to do with the question of linguistic organization: a sequence can be coded any way we like, and all that is linguistically necessary is that we should be able to identify it as a

---

1 On Saussure's attempts to explain the linearity of language, see above, pp. 320–2.

structured set of signs, and experience it as a single *line of language*, as it might be called.

However it is not always easy to identify and disentangle different lines of language. You may be able to trace a set of words back to the mouths that physically spoke them, or the hands that physically wrote. But what if the words are being copied or quoted? What happens when people are uttering another person's words and not their own? Or what if someone is talking directly to you at the same time as conducting a separate conversation on the telephone? And what of the celebrated virtuosity of Julius Caesar dictating several letters simultaneously, to a circle of laborious scribes? How can you extricate several different lines of language issuing from a single physical source?

And the difficulties may go far deeper. Consciously or unconsciously, people often fail to say what they mean, or mean what they say. A single phrase may carry a double message, deliberately or not – words of comfort and reassurance perhaps, but spoken in a tone of menace or sarcasm, or an offensive remark which may have been meant as a friendly joke, or ironies which seem to say one thing but, to the initiated, mean something very different.

When we try to unscramble even such simple layerings of meaning, we will always be tempted to think in terms of a kind of subjective inner world – a private space enclosed in the breast or the head – which is the seat of a self or a soul, or perhaps of a constellation of selves or souls, each responsible for different strands of meaning and different lines of language. This habit of inward projection can either be a device of blame ('Lay not that flattering unction to your soul, That not your trespass but my madness speaks,' as Hamlet upbraids his mother) or of exculpation ('If Hamlet from himself be ta'en away,' as he says of his own crime, then 'Hamlet does it not, Hamlet denies it: Who does it then? – His madness.').[2]

Stern philosophers may warn us against postulating such inner *personae*: we are simply getting carried away, they will say, by our over-weening wish to keep different lines of language separate, and to discover a unified message in every collection of signs. After all, what is the idea of an inner spirit except a vague metaphorical sublimation of the breath that carries the human voice – a *persona*, in fact, in the

2 Shakespeare, *Hamlet*, III.iv.147–8; V.ii.230–4.

etymological sense of the word: a theatrical mask through which a voice sounds out?

But the idea that there must be a voice behind every message – the voice of a mother, perhaps, or a master's voice or the voice of conscience or of God – may be hard to shake off. Even when we are silently reading – looking through a century-old anonymous report, say, or a letter from someone we do not know, or an error message on a computer screen – we will often find ourselves conjuring up a mocking or friendly voice – male or female, young or old, attractive or ugly – calling rudely or wanly to us from between the lines. Some of us in fact find it hard to read anything at all without imagining it being spoken in a specific voice out loud: we treat books as texts for performance – as if they were musical scores – and when we do not know how to pronounce a word or a symbol, we will make a guess or imagine a name rather than treat it as a purely visible mark to be passed over in silence. We can get quite hoarse after a solitary evening absorbed in a book.

Still, the habit of listening for the voice behind a text has never had the approval of philosophical theorists. Hegel thought that anyone who 'reads out loud in order to catch the meaning in the sound' must be sadly under-educated: reading is essentially a 'hieroglyphic' activity, he said: purely spatial and visual, and utterly abstracted from the voice. We westerners would do well to forget that our writing system was originally a representation of sounds; we should learn to become like the Chinese mandarins – 'dumb' in our writing, according to Hegel, and 'deaf' in our reading.[3]

Nearly all the theoretical leaders of twentieth-century literary avant-gardes were good Hegelians too, doing their bit, in the cause of artistic progress, to expel the ghost of the living voice from the machinic structures of modernist writing. References to vocal experience were spurned on suspicion of being infected by romantic notions of a sovereign subjectivity, cosy, self-enclosed and smugly unified. In the 1920s, for instance, Ezra Pound sought to revolutionize European poetry by reminding it of the principles of Chinese script – principles which, according to him, were based on sight rather than sound, and for that

---

3 Hegel, 'Ein taubes Lesen und ein stummes Schreiben': see *Philosophy of Mind*, §459; see *Hegel's Philosophy of Subjective Spirit*, Vol. 3, p. 189.

reason had always been 'unrecognised in the West'.[4] And in the 1940s, Joseph Frank inverted and twisted the terms of Lessing's distinction between the poetic and the pictorial, by arguing that the whole essence of literary modernism resides in the promotion of visibility and 'spatial form', and the abandonment of temporality and the ear.[5] Wellek and Warren's pioneering work in literary theory also insisted that readers do not pronounce words to themselves, not even silently, unless they are 'almost illiterate'.[6] In the sixties, Roland Barthes argued that the essence of Eastern writing systems was their 'emptiness of speech'.[7] And then Derrida went so far as to link the task of disarming European metaphysics to the necessity of protecting the art of writing from what he called 'phonocentrism', meaning our supposed fascination with the authoritative power of the voice, conceived as the source of all meaning and value.[8] Even in the 1980s, progressive poets and critics were still getting angry at the 'pusillanimous' way in which their more conventional colleagues wanted literature to be 'grounded in the presence of a legitimating voice'.[9]

Why did they all get so upset? What made them suppose that every reference to the speaking voice must be mendacious and coercive? The metaphysical notion of fixed subjective identities may well deserve its philosophical disrepute, but why should it be associated with the experience of the human voice? The still-inarticulate cries of an infant are hardly the expression of a readymade original unity, after all; and the semi-speech of a child learning its first language is audibly a kind

---

4 Pound was basing himself on the shaky authority of Ernest Fenollosa: see his introduction to 'The Chinese Written Character' in *Instigations of Ezra Pound*, New York, Boni and Liveright, 1920, pp. 357–88; and his notes to Fenollosa's *The Chinese Written Character as a Medium for Poetry*, London, Stanley Nott, 1936. See also *ABC of Reading* (1934), London, Faber and Faber, 1961, pp. 20–1.
5 Joseph Frank, 'Spatial Form in Modern Literature' (1945), reprinted with additional materials in his *The Idea of Spatial Form*, New Brunswick, Rutgers University Press, 1991.
6 René Wellek and Austin Warren, *Theory of Literature* (1949), Harmondsworth, Penguin, 1963, p. 144.
7 See Roland Barthes, *L'empire des signes* (1970), Paris, Flammarion, 1984, p. 10.
8 For Derrida the critique of phonocentrism was also a generalization of the Heideggerian critique of Western philosophy as a whole: 'We already have a foreboding that phonocentrism merges with the historical determination of the meaning of being in general as presence.' See Jacques Derrida, *Of Grammatology*, p. 12.
9 See Crozier's introduction to Andrew Crozier and Tim Longville, eds, *A Various Art*, Manchester, Carcanet, 1987, p. 12.

of crossroads, a market-place where fragments of words and phrases, tunes, tones, rhythms and accents are passed around and traded back and forth, or returned inquiringly to their original utterers, and chanted and echoed till any hint of originality has been beaten out of them. It is hard to hear any peremptory claim to authority in these vocalizations, and impossible to decompose their fluid intermingling into a definite number of separate 'voices'. And the same applies to adult vocalization too: it is only on the most artificial and solemn occasions – speaking under oath, reading out a sacred text or prayer, or perhaps recording a message on an answering machine – that you will try to make your voice express a rigidly consistent personality; and even then the result is likely to sound ludicrously artificial and unlike you, not reassuringly natural and authentic. Relaxed conversational intimacy is characterized by exchanges that are unfathomably various and often silly, rather than by monotonous self-centred uniformity.

And then consider oral story-telling: not just the self-conscious artistry of traditional tellers or professional performers, but also the spontaneous circulation of gossip and anecdotes which forms a large part of ordinary human sociability. Listen to the way the narrator's voice moulds itself to its theme: the plight of the injured bird evoked in a hurried whisper, the cruelty of the cat with a tone of screech and snarl. Furthermore, many narratives include word-for-word repetitions of things said by characters within a story, and oral story-tellers will often mimic a character's phrases or vocal style without distinguishing them sharply from those of the teller. None of us speaks with just one voice, in short: not because we have a choice of two or three or ten, but because our voice does not contain any stable unities that can be counted on at all. No doubt that is why bureaucrats, and perhaps literary modernizers too, have always preferred to say things in writing.

When a spoken story comes to be written down, most of the vocal variety is bound to get stripped out: the most we can hope for, very often, is a bare record identifying which words were uttered and in what order. This was indeed how early writing systems worked, as they possessed no devices for indicating diversity or discontinuity in the linguistic line. Ancient Greek and Roman texts consisted of unbroken rows of letters, gaps being left only to indicate paragraphs or chapters. At the end of the fourth century, Saint Jerome initiated the useful practice of starting each new unit of sense or 'sentence' on a new line, and scribes working in Ireland in the seventh century began to leave spaces between words as well.[10] The 'diple' – a sort of arrow (>) pointing in from the margin – was sometimes used to pick out citations from the Bible, and then a range of 'points' was invented to indicate whether a sentence had a rising, a falling, or an undulating tune – not so much a guide to sense, more a help for those reading aloud in acts of worship.[11] In addition, scribes could use different varieties of ink, and different styles and sizes of lettering, to distinguish different categories of text on the same page.

But such textual practices could not be standardized before the spread of printing in the sixteenth century. And of all the many transformations in literary technique that came about as a result, none was more fateful than the invention of methods for setting off certain passages in a text from the rest in order to indicate that they belonged to different lines of language – that they were citations, or 'quotations' as they were called in English on account of the numerals which identified the authority referred to. Some early printers set citations in italic type, but in France the diple was reintroduced in the form of a pair of semicircular marks printed at the beginning of each cited line (») – a device known as the *guillemet* after its supposed inventor, a printer named Guillaume. From the beginning of the seventeenth century British printers imitated the effect by using commas raised to the top of the line of print, and these 'inverted commas', as they came to be called, became their favoured form of quotation mark.

The punctuation practices associated with printed books allowed more flexibility than one might expect for writers wanting to capture the versatility of oral story-telling, and as early as the 1570s quotation marks were being used to distinguish a character's words from those of the narrator in narrative fiction.[12] But the marking of quotations could also be an annoyance, since it forced writers to give a definite attribution to each word in their story: if it was in quotation marks,

10 See M. B. Parkes, *Pause and Effect: An Introduction to the History of Punctuation in the West*, p. 24.
11 M. B. Parkes, 'Punctuation, or Pause and Effect', in James J. Murphy, ed., *Medieval Eloquence: Studies in the Theory and Practice of Medieval Rhetoric*, Berkeley, University of California Press, 1978, pp. 127–42, pp. 139–40; see also Parkes, *Pause and Effect*, pp. 35–7. See also above, p. 247.
12 Parkes, *Pause and Effect*, pp. 58–61.

it belonged to a character, otherwise it belonged to the narrator, and the indeterminate middle ground occupied by oral story-tellers was thus ruled out of bounds. It was like a literary counterpart to the enclosure of common lands.[13] Writers trying to reclaim some of the freedom of the oral teller (chiefly by using the grammatical techniques sometimes theorized as 'Free Indirect Speech') have often been quite baffled about what to do with their quotation marks: Jane Austen, for instance, famously resorted to putting quotation marks round passages expressing a character's point of view, even though, grammatically speaking, the words could not belong to anyone but her narrator.[14]

But it is possible to regard almost any book as a kind of script for vocal performance. Søren Kierkegaard's incomparably fluent philosophical prose was practised vocally before being committed to the page: 'most of what I have written was spoken aloud many, many times,' he wrote. 'I have been able to sit for hours at a time, like a flautist entertaining himself with his flute.'[15] And according to Charles Dickens, 'every writer of fiction, though he may not adopt the dramatic form, writes in effect for the stage.'[16] His own writing room was equipped with a mirror so that – like a composer at the piano – he could try out different effects while he was writing, and Thomas Carlyle said that one could have 'no conception before hearing Dickens read, of what capacities lie in the human face and voice'.[17] In the later part of his life, in fact, Dickens made public recitals into a second career, reading from specially marked-up texts and using a kind of conductor's baton to emphasize his rhythms.[18] (See Figure 39.)

13 It also has an effect on a narrator's use of tags: see C. E. Montague, ' "Sez 'e" or "Thinks 'e",' in *A Writer's Notes on His Trade*, London, Chatto and Windus, 1930, pp. 39–50.
14 'She found herself accosted by Captain Wentworth, in a reserved yet hurried sort of farewell. "He must wish her goodnight. He was going – he should get home as fast as he could." ' See Jane Austen, *Persuasion* (1818), edited by D. W. Harding, Harmondsworth, Penguin, 1965, pp. 198–9. A more orthodox case of 'Free Indirect Speech' is to be found in her preceding paragraph. See also Dorrit Cohn, *Transparent Minds: Narrative Modes for Presenting Consciousness in Fiction*, Princeton, Princeton University Press, 1978.
15 Søren Kierkegaard, *Journals* (1854), translated by Alastair Hannay in *Journals and Papers*, p. 588.
16 See *The Speeches of Charles Dickens*, edited by K. J. Fielding, Oxford, Oxford University Press, 1960, p. 262.
17 Cited in *Charles Dickens, Sikes and Nancy and other Public Readings*, edited by Phillip Collins, Oxford, Oxford University Press, 1983, p. xvi.
18 See Hesketh Pearson, *Dickens*, London, Methuen, 1949, pp. 307–8, and Peter Ackroyd, *Dickens*, London, Sinclair-Stevenson, 1990, p. 561.

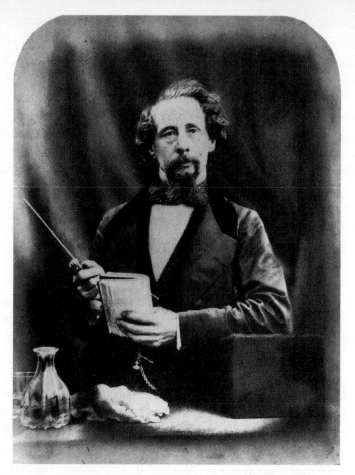

FIG 38. Reading with a baton: Charles Dickens in 1854

Although quotation marks might seem out of place in texts written for performance, Dickens exploited them with rare exuberance. For instance he would close them temporarily in order to interrupt his characters in mid-phrase, as if to remind them who was in charge.[19] ('"Do you suppose," Mr Lorry went on, with a laughing twinkle in his bright eye, as it looked kindly at her, "that Doctor Manette has any theory of his own. . . ?"')[20] But Dickens was also prepared to abandon

19 See Mark Lambert, *Dickens and the Suspended Quotation*, New Haven, Yale University Press, 1981.
20 Charles Dickens, *A Tale of Two Cities* (1859), edited by George Woodcock, Harmondsworth, Penguin, 1970, p. 127.

quotation marks completely, letting a dialogue run on undisturbed, almost as if the narrator had lost interest in it. ('Ever been in prison? Certainly not. Never in a debtor's prison? Didn't see what that had to do with it. Never in a debtor's prison? – Come, once again. Never? Yes. How many times? Two or three times. Not five or six? Perhaps.)'[21]

A few years later, in *Our Mutual Friend*, Dickens attempted some further small rebellions against the conventions of narrative notation, using a long bracket at the edge of the text to indicate that several characters are speaking their lines at the same time, as in vocal ensembles in opera or oratorio.[22] In the same book he depicted a kind of slow-witted representative of his own theatrical self in the love-child Sloppy, who delights his doting minder by reading aloud from court reports in the newspaper: 'And I do love a newspaper. You mightn't think it, but Sloppy is a beautiful reader of a newspaper. He does the Police in different voices.'[23] Shy pretty little Bella, however, has no need to be so vocal: she can punctuate her speech with an inaudible smile, isolating chosen phrases not with inverted commas but 'with a look as if she italicised the word by putting one of her dimples under it'.[24]

After Dickens, however, novelists began to find quotation marks increasingly irksome. French authors managed to get away with a sparing use of dashes, but printers in the English-speaking world were reluctant to give their authors such freedoms. Virginia Woolf and Samuel Beckett both rebelled against the requirement that they always divide up their narrative into separate linguistic parcels, and James Joyce railed against his printers for taking out his French-style dashes and italics and replacing them with 'perverted commas', as he called them: they 'are most unsightly and give an impression of unreality', as he said.[25]

Writers of factual and theoretical prose, in contrast, were developing a galloping appetite for quotation marks. They used them not only

21 *A Tale of Two Cities*, p. 97.
22 Charles Dickens, *Our Mutual Friend* (1865), Oxford, Oxford University Press, 1952, pp. 12, 410.
23 *Our Mutual Friend*, p. 198; see also p. 785.
24 *Our Mutual Friend*, p. 519.
25 See Robert E. Scholes, 'Some Observations on the Text of *Dubliners*: "The Dead",' *Studies in Bibliography*, Vol. 15. 1962, pp. 191–205, p. 200 n. 14. See also Scholes's note in his edition of James Joyce, *Dubliners*, London, Jonathan Cape, 1967.

for identifying material cited from other writers, but also for wrapping up any words for which they wanted to signal their disdain, without having to give up using them. The use of 'scare quotes' even spread from the printed page to the spoken word, and one of the most curious developments in twentieth-century speech was the rise of what may be called *punctuation pronunciations* – ways of speaking which express the punctuation that would be required if the words were to be written down, a comma here, a semicolon there, and the occasional flourish of a full stop and new paragraph. And the flow of speech even came to be broken up with quotation marks – sometimes spoken ('quote . . . unquote') or gesticulated (hands fluttering in the air), and sometimes implied by the adoption of a voice intended to be heard as not being truly one's own: in short, a 'funny voice'.[26]

Proust had occasion to comment on the practice early in the century, when he referred to Swann's dismissive way of talking about 'la "*hiér-archie!*" des arts':

> whenever he used an expression which seemed to imply a definite opinion upon some important subject, he would take care to isolate it in a special intonation, mechanical and ironic, as though he had put it in quotation marks [*entre guillemets*] and was anxious to disclaim any personal responsibility for it . . . But then, if it was so absurd, why did he use the word? . . . I found it all contradictory. What other life did he set apart for saying in all seriousness what he thought about things, for formulating judgements which he need not put between quotation marks . . . ?[27]

The implicit metaphysics of the quotation mark is indeed quite deliri-ous: if you really wanted to mark out every word that is not wholly your own with inverted commas or a funny voice, then – like a modern sorcerer's apprentice – you would hardly know how to bring the pro-cess to a halt. For what you say and how you say it are always going to form part of patterns that spread much wider than your individual

26 See Jonathan Rée, 'Funny Voices: Stories, Punctuation, and Personal Identity', *New Literary History*, Vol. 21, No. 4, Autumn 1990, pp. 1039–58, and 'Les mots des autres', in Henri Meschonnic, ed., *Le langage comme défi*, Paris, Presses Universitaires de Vincennes, 1991.
27 Marcel Proust, *Du Côté de chez Swann* (1913), *A la recherche du temps perdu*, Vol. 1, p. 98; *Swann's Way, Remembrance of Things Past*, Vol. 1, 105–6.

existence, far beyond the limits of what you can know or even imagine.

We are none of us linguistic islands, after all; more like lost swimmers out at sea, buffeted by waves and dragged by currents that have no regard for our carefully groomed individualities. And our interpretations of ourselves will never become the serene sky-borne perspectives we might like them to be. They are just our wary thoughts about the changeable weather of our existence: not objective sciences gone wrong, but anxious glances at the fragile techniques with which we try to keep ourselves and our objectivities afloat. Strictly speaking, we have no such thing as a voice of our own.

AFTERWORD

Afterword

Once, you could have expected all aspiring philosophers to produce a philosophical system of their own – a treatise, perhaps unfinished, or a sequence of volumes, probably incomplete, promising a comprehensive personal overview of knowledge, existence and the meaning of life as a whole. Since the beginning of the twentieth century, however, such synoptic ambitions have come in for suspicion, and the great systematic philosophers of the past, from Plato and Aristotle to Hegel and Schopenhauer, have been reduced to objects of pity or mere antiquarian curiosity: sterile daydreamers who, in less enlightened times, mistook their private intellectual caprices for transcendent truths, and somehow persuaded others to do so as well.

Nowadays, if 'theories of everything' have any credibility at all, they are a province of natural science, not philosophy. In fact it is widely supposed that the only positive result of two thousand years of formal philosophical inquiry is a confirmation of what everyone should always have known – that knowledge comes from experience, application and the scientific method, not head-in-air speculation. Which leaves us philosophers looking like forlorn remnants of a discredited sect, perpetuating our obsolete texts and empty rites merely because we cannot imagine anything else to do.

And yet philosophy has survived; and it may even have profited from the collapse of its public prestige and learned a belated lesson about its own intellectual limitations. Philosophers have at least managed to differentiate philosophy from mere 'metaphysics' – the more or less unconscious myths, maxims and metaphors we live by – and even to transform their discipline, to the satisfaction of some, into a field of 'research' in the shrunken modern sense of the word: a domain for specialists only, rather than an active part of some larger intellectual culture. Just like natural scientists, philosophers have learned to concentrate on well-defined problems that can be tackled in accordance with professionally agreed protocols so as to produce measurable increments in the stock of human knowledge. The achievements may not be large, and they may be of little interest to anyone outside the profession, but at least they promise to be more durable than the inflated conceits of the philosophical system-builders of the past.

But it is not so easy to eradicate the urge to think connectedly about our knowledge and feelings, our experience of the world and of ourselves. It is still rather tempting to try and revive the soaring ambitions of traditional philosophy, perhaps temper them with some modern good sense, and work out a hard-headed and clear-sighted philosophical system suited to our sceptical and post-philosophical age.

There are obstacles to such a scheme, however. Philosophical enlightenment, as has often been remarked, arises from particular details sharply observed, not looming shapes suggestively sketched: it is to be sought in the fine textures of our concepts, practices and theories, rather than in some overall general tendency that we may be inclined to impute to things in general. But when we try to bring the disparate fragments of experience together we are liable to find that we cannot fit them all into each other with self-evident exactness. Experience is not a jigsaw puzzle, waiting to be assembled into a pre-ordained pattern, with no odd pieces left over.

We live in a world revealed to us by our bodily senses; we also live in our passions, hopes and anxieties, and in societies, languages and religions, and in traditions of science, technology and art. But when we compare our experiences in these different domains we keep confronting systematic discrepancies amongst them, not to say disharmonies, incoherences, even conflicts. If your parents die, for instance, then it is a banal biological event, entirely unremarkable, and an ordinary social fact; but it also marks an epoch in your life: it may clarify your sense of yourself or bewilder you completely, change your interests, ambitions and tastes, relieve you of anxiety or lead to emotional calamity. Perhaps each of these items can be analysed separately and given a satisfying philosophical gloss; but that does not mean they can all be collated or added up and subjected to a common measure. The mere fact that they have cohabited in the stream of your experience does not make them parts of a cohesive totality. Your experiences may all share certain characteristics, defined by your body, your memories and your expectations, but such unity as they have will always be more like a provisional conjectural summation than a final incontrovertible settlement. And the discrepancies are not accidental distortions, to be discounted or silently corrected for the sake of a comprehensive theoretical reckoning: if you ignored the elements that do not fit, you might be missing the most essential parts.

There will always be something that eludes the quest for philosophical self-knowledge. You can never observe the point of view from which you are watching yourself: the eye is its own blind spot, and you cannot jump out of your skin. The only way you can catch yourself in the act of reflecting on yourself is by becoming another self – a self which, when it looks down on your reflecting self, will not be included in the reflection. If you want to understand yourself better, you always have to keep on the move.

If philosophy is to win back some of its old cultural dignity, it will therefore have to approach the task of systematic self-understanding with a bit more caution and circumspection, a bit more agility, and more sensitivity to its own situation. Instead of pretending that it can station itself at an infinite distance from the fractured contingencies of our individual existences, it should learn to study them close up, and to recognize itself in them. Instead of trying to abstract from the thousands of little threads – linguistic, practical and conceptual – that connect it to its local habitation, it should focus on them consciously. Our thoughts are woven into webs with an infinitely complex past, and so are our thoughts about our thoughts. If we are to improve our philosophical self-understanding, therefore, we must get serious about history: about the history that leads up to us, the history we contribute to, and the history that we are. Our philosophical arguments, even our philosophical systems, need to be constantly reinvented as philosophical histories.

Philosophical history, as I understand it, is a discipline that may not yet exist (despite some prototypes by Foucault and Deleuze), but whose arrival is long overdue. Negatively, philosophical history can be defined as a reaction against the unfettered speculativeness that philosophical inquiry is always prone to – its preference for general explanations over exact descriptions, and its weakness for analysing and criticizing extreme metaphysical follies that have never existed outside the imagination of the philosopher who wants to triumph over them. Philosophical history will therefore devote itself to metaphysical notions that have infiltrated ordinary common sense and become real forces in the world, guiding our individual choices and even determining the destiny of whole groups or classes: for example the ideas about the five senses and the human voice which, till recently, ensured a miserable fate for most of those born deaf.

Philosophical history is not the same as History of Philosophy though; in fact in some ways the two are thoroughly opposed. History of Philosophy is the curiously ritualized discipline that has managed to dominate academic philosophy ever since the eighteenth century, busying itself with canonical texts from the ancient Greeks to the present, and forcing them into a narrative pattern with a beginning, a middle and an end. In the History of Philosophy, as Søren Kierkegaard once wrote in his Journal, 'a professor commands the whole range of thinkers from Greece to modern times,' and it 'looks as if the professor stood over them all'. The professor traces their filiations and disagreements, their borrowings and derivations, and offers commentaries and value-judgements on the issues that are supposed to divide them. But his self-righteous serenity is quite incompatible with the infinite intellectual diffidence that Kierkegaard saw as the supreme philosophical virtue. 'Well, thanks,' as Kierkegaard says to his professor.[1]

Nevertheless the History of Philosophy persists in presenting itself as the key to all the philosophies – simultaneously the gateway, the foundation and the pinnacle of philosophy as a professional discipline. Sometimes, historians of philosophy will be found setting their philosophers against each other, like children playing with toy soldiers; sometimes they scold, cajole and correct them, like old-fashioned teachers returning faulty work to apprehensive pupils. Or they may seek to assign each philosopher to a unique place in a perfect table of classification, like botanists or bibliomaniacs; or attempt to conciliate

---

1 Søren Kierkegaard, *Papers and Journals* X 1 A 609, 1849, translated and edited by Alastair Hannay, Harmondsworth, Penguin, 1996, p. 406.

the irreconcilable, like gullible international peacemakers. In any case they always remain in thrall to the same old sad conceit, as they try to hoist themselves above the dialectical fray and put every past philosophy in its place, dividing and interpreting all that they survey, and permanently exempting themselves from the belittling comparisons they apply to everything else.

Another damaging effect of the History of Philosophy is that it scants the peculiar ordinariness of philosophical inquiry. It is so preoccupied with comparing its classical texts with each other that it forgets to listen for what they may have to say about the rest of the world. Philosophy has always been a sophisticated form of thinking, no doubt, and heavily dependent on inherited traditions; it is even, in its way, a highly specialized art form. But like the other arts it is far more than the sum of its classics. Its raw material, and perhaps its touchstone too, is found on the rough pathways of everyday thoughtful reflection, not the far reaches of high theory. There was philosophical experience long before there were philosophers or philosophical books; for philosophy is what happens whenever people allow themselves to be surprised, perhaps taken aback, by the habits of thinking they usually take for granted – by the folk metaphysics of their everyday life. The historical development of philosophy will never make much sense if it is treated as a bloodless struggle between great books, with all the local flavours, fragrances, noises, temperatures, and colours of ordinary experience left out.

And finally, the History of Philosophy suffers from its rigid sense of historical rhythm. There is, we may assume, an unchanging basic programme of philosophical problems that never changes much: death and finitude, say, or love and duty, injustice and happiness, or the scope of knowledge, rationality and justice – an agenda which imposes itself wherever philosophy is practised, in other words whenever our thoughts are carefully thought through. But the range and multiplicity of the responses these questions have provoked cannot be comprehended within a historian's doctrine of epochs: a sequence of discrete historical periods, that is to say, from the pre-Socratics through the Enlightenment to Postmodernism, with all their mutual differences and individual identities proceeding nose-to-tail through time. For philosophical experience is not a succession of separate episodes, first one thing, then another; it is more like a tangled heap of co-existences,

each pulsing to a tempo of its own. They play across each other, some
with a rapidity that makes them blur, others with a trans-epochal
slowness in which no movement is perceptible at all – though it is
worth remembering that even the oldest of philosophical tales can be
shockingly new to whoever hears it for the first time. The rhythms of
philosophical experience are no respecters of the metronomical divisions decreed by the History of Philosophy.[2]

More positively, a philosophical history will have to be mobile, complicated, stratified, and detailed. It will cut cinematically between close
and distant perspectives, making use of the rememorative methods of
autobiography and the evocative polyphonies of fiction, as well as the
exacting crafts of historical research and philosophical criticism. Like
any other fundamental intellectual inquiry, its results may not lend
themselves to abstract summary. It will always be taking us on journeys
whose purpose and pay-off may not be apparent till we reach the end,
or even later; down paths which, instead of leading us somewhere new,
simply help us understand, for the first time, where we have been all
along.

But you may already have convinced yourself that a historical study
of the byways of philosophical experience is going to be a waste of
effort: would it not be better, you might ask, to take a direct route to
the summit, and describe the objective facts of nature and society in
terms of the best scientific concepts now available, working at the
cutting edge of tomorrow's world instead of tarrying with mere old-
fashioned folklore, obsolete technology and fatuous antique metaphysics – with discarded superstitions and unhinged metaphors, all
contradicting each other, all equally undisciplined, all utterly jejune?
Why not try to be a bit more up to date? Ought we not to forget
about metaphysics altogether, and philosophy too, and stick to the
tried and tested methods of modern science?

Perhaps we ought; but on the other hand perhaps we have no choice.
There is a risk that our ideas of objectivity, method and science, and
indeed of being 'up to date', will introduce distortions of their own.
They have their own peculiar histories after all, and they too can carry

2 See Jonathan Rée, 'The Vanity of Historicism', *New Literary History* Vol. 22, No 4,
Autumn 1991, pp. 961–83.

unsuspected biases. That is why there is a standing cultural necessity for philosophy – for philosophy as a critique of metaphysics (though not necessarily distinct from it), and for philosophy as distinct from science (but not necessarily opposed to it): in short, for philosophy in the form which has slowly become explicit since the beginning of the twentieth century under the broad rubric of phenomenology. The purpose of phenomenology is to enable us to describe the world of our experience without forcing preconceived ideas on to it. In particular, it helps us resist the easy assumption that we can know in advance how to disentangle some unbiddable nature-given objective content of truth from the idiosyncratic and history-bound forms through which we perceive and evaluate it. Phenomenology constantly challenges us to undertake the humble but endlessly complex task of describing the world in terms of what it can mean to us, to each of us, in whatever specific situation we happen to find ourselves.

Through the teachings of (most notably) Husserl, Heidegger, Sartre and Merleau-Ponty, phenomenology has sought to free us from the mesmerizing choice between the objective theoretical sciences on the one hand, and the subjective irrational arts on the other. It offers the philosopher in each of us a chance to turn away from the newsy world of controversies and conferences, opinions, interventions and debates, and face up to the large structures of experience and self-interpretation without which nothing at all – neither personal subjectivity nor objective science – could ever have sense or value for us in the first place.

In a way, these contingent structures of meaning are obvious, if not trivial. The fact that we experience ourselves as living continuous lives in the midst of material objects that we perceive with our senses, for example, and as having bodies that are part of the ordinary physical world – a world we share with others inside frameworks of technique and symbolism handed down to us by ancestors who are now dead, as we shall be too before long – all this may seem too banal to be worth thinking about. On the other hand, it is these mundane facts that shape the forms and purposes of our lives (even if we live the lives of scientific objectivists), as well as our ways of making sense of them, so far as we do; and to this extent they are indispensable, or transcendental. And although the transcendental contingencies of our existence may be both accidental and scientifically irrelevant, this does not make them inconsequential. Our world – including the world of science –

would be unrecognizable, perhaps inconceivable or impossible, if they were different. The fact that the structures in which we live our lives are obvious does not mean that their significance is clear to us – for nothing is harder to understand than what is most familiar. (This paradox is perhaps the most important lesson of phenomenology and of philosophy in general.) Their familiarity makes them all the more elusive, all the more mysterious, all the more recessive to our under-standing. They may be closer to us than our own breathing, but they may be remote from us at the same time, just as we can be remote from our own inmost selves. The comforting self-evidence with which they present themselves to us may simply be the projection of our desire for homely boredom, in place of the bafflement that might be a more honest attitude to the prickly oddities of our existence.

Of course scientific thought would not get anywhere if it spent its time dithering philosophically over its ultimate presuppositions and the historical accidents that have nurtured them: taking all that for granted, you might say, is what enables science to make the kind of progress for which it is admired. But that is just where philosophy comes in: it allows us to stand aside from our everyday certainties and see them in their transcendental context. Our sense of how to sort the scientific wheat from the superstitious chaff is itself a very peculiar historical accomplishment after all. Its foundations are pretty mysteri-ous, and its implications can be quite bizarre. If it is not dismantled and reassembled from time to time, it will surely turn into another old superstition just like all the rest. With luck then, a philosophical history will allow us to catch hold of the idea of scientific objectivity before it has broken away from subjective experience, and observe it in its pristine state, at the moment when abstraction enters our lives, and sense begins to separate itself from sound.

INDEX

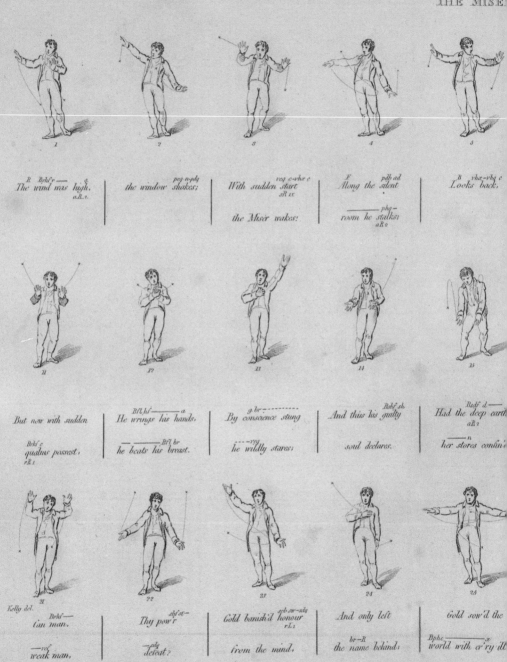

The wind was high,

the window shakes;

With sudden start

the Miser wakes:

Along the silent

room he stalks;

Looks back,

But now with sudden

qualms possest,

He wrings his hands,

he beats his breast.

By conscience stung

he wildly stares:

And this his guilty

soul declares.

Had the deep earth

her stores confine

Can man,

weak man,

Thy pow'r

defeat?

Gold banish'd honour

from the mind,

And only left

the name behind:

Gold sow'd the

world with ev'ry ill

Kelly del.